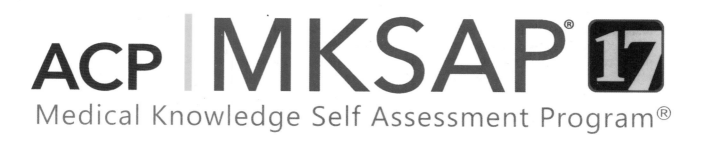

Endocrinology and Metabolism

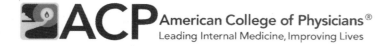

Welcome to the Endocrinology and Metabolism Section of MKSAP 17!

In these pages, you will find updated information on disorders of glucose metabolism, disorders of the pituitary gland, disorders of the adrenal glands, disorders of the thyroid gland, reproductive disorders, and calcium and bone disorders. All of these topics are uniquely focused on the needs of generalists and subspecialists *outside* of endocrinology and metabolism.

The publication of the 17th edition of Medical Knowledge Self-Assessment Program (MKSAP) represents nearly a half-century of serving as the gold-standard resource for internal medicine education. It also marks its evolution into an innovative learning system to better meet the changing educational needs and learning styles of all internists.

The core content of MKSAP has been developed as in previous editions—newly generated, essential information in 11 topic areas of internal medicine created by dozens of leading generalists and subspecialists and guided by certification and recertification requirements, emerging knowledge in the field, and user feedback. MKSAP 17 also contains 1200 all-new, psychometrically validated, and peer-reviewed multiple-choice questions (MCQs) for self-assessment and study, including 84 in Endocrinology and Metabolism. MKSAP 17 continues to include *High Value Care* (HVC) recommendations, based on the concept of balancing clinical benefit with costs and harms, with links to MCQs that illustrate these principles. In addition, HVC Key Points are highlighted in the text. Also highlighted, with blue text, are *Hospitalist*-focused content and MCQs that directly address the learning needs of internists who work in the hospital setting.

MKSAP 17 Digital provides access to additional tools allowing you to customize your learning experience, including regular text updates with practice-changing, new information and 200 new self-assessment questions; a board-style pretest to help direct your learning; and enhanced custom-quiz options. And, with MKSAP Complete, learners can access 1200 electronic flashcards for quick review of important concepts or review the updated and enhanced version of Virtual Dx, an image-based self-assessment tool.

As before, MKSAP 17 is optimized for use on your mobile devices, with iOS- and Android-based apps allowing you to sync your work between your apps and online account and submit for CME credits and MOC points online.

Please visit us at the MKSAP Resource Site (mksap.acponline.org) to find out how we can help you study, earn CME credit and MOC points, and stay up to date.

Whether you prefer to use the traditional print version or take advantage of the features available through the digital version, we hope you enjoy MKSAP 17 and that it meets and exceeds your personal learning needs.

On behalf of the many internists who have offered their time and expertise to create the content for MKSAP 17 and the editorial staff who work to bring this material to you in the best possible way, we are honored that you have chosen to use MKSAP 17 and appreciate any feedback about the program you may have. Please feel free to send us any comments to mksap_editors@acponline.org.

Sincerely,

Philip A. Masters, MD, FACP
Editor-in-Chief
Senior Physician Educator
Director, Clinical Content Development
Medical Education Division
American College of Physicians

Endocrinology and Metabolism

Committee

Cynthia A. Burns, MD, FACP, Section Editor[1]
Director, Internal Medicine Clerkship & Acting Internships
Associate Professor, Department of Internal Medicine
Section on Endocrinology & Metabolism
Wake Forest University School of Medicine
Winston-Salem, North Carolina

Howard H. Weitz, MD, MACP, Associate Editor[1]
Director, Jefferson Heart Institute
Director, Division of Cardiology
Sidney Kimmel Medical College at Thomas Jefferson
    University
Philadelphia, Pennsylvania

Jessicah Collins, MD[1]
Clinical Endocrinologist
Diabetes and Endocrinology Clinic
Augusta Health
Fishersville, Virginia

Kristen G. Hairston, MD, MPH[1]
Medical Director, Joslin Diabetes Center
Associate Professor
Department of Internal Medicine
Section on Endocrinology & Metabolism
Wake Forest University School of Medicine
Winston-Salem, North Carolina

Erika B. Johnston-MacAnanny, MD[1]
Assistant Professor
Medical Director, Center for Reproductive Medicine
Associate Faculty, Women's Health Center of Excellence
Wake Forest Center for Reproductive Medicine
Wake Forest School of Medicine
Winston-Salem, North Carolina

Wanda C. Lakey, MD, MHS[2]
Assistant Professor of Medicine
Division of Endocrinology
Duke University Medical Center
Durham VA Medical Center
Durham, North Carolina

Sarah Mayson, MD[2]
Assistant Professor
Department of Medicine
Division of Endocrinology, Metabolism and Diabetes
University of Colorado School of Medicine
Aurora, Colorado

Jennifer Sipos, MD[2]
Associate Professor of Medicine
Director, Benign Thyroid Program
Division of Endocrinology, Diabetes, and Metabolism
The Ohio State University School of Medicine
Columbus, Ohio

Editor-in-Chief

Philip A. Masters, MD, FACP[1]
Senior Physician Educator
Director, Clinical Content Development
American College of Physicians
Philadelphia, Pennsylvania

Director, Clinical Program Development

Cynthia D. Smith, MD, FACP[2]
American College of Physicians
Philadelphia, Pennsylvania

Endocrinology and Metabolism Reviewers

Amindra Singh Arora, MD[1]
Stewart F. Babbott, MD, FACP[1]
John K. Chamberlain, MD, MACP[1]
Terence Chan, MD[2]
Pieter A. Cohen, MD[2]
Benjamin P. Geisler, MD[2]
Richard Hoffman, MD, MPH[1]
Sowmya Kanikkannan, MD, FACP[1]
Mark D. Siegel, MD, FACP[2]

Endocrinology and Metabolism Reviewer Representing the American Society for Clinical Pharmacology & Therapeutics

Linda A. Hershey, MD, PhD[2]

Endocrinology and Metabolism ACP Editorial Staff

Randy Hendrickson[1], Production Administrator/Editor
Katie Idell[1], Manager, Clinical Skills and Digital Programs
Margaret Wells[1], Director, Self-Assessment and Educational
    Programs
Becky Krumm[1], Managing Editor

ACP Principal Staff

Patrick C. Alguire, MD, FACP[2]
Senior Vice President, Medical Education

Sean McKinney[1]
Vice President, Medical Education

Margaret Wells[1]
Director, Self-Assessment and Educational Programs

Becky Krumm[1]
Managing Editor

Katie Idell[1]
Manager, Clinical Skills Program and Digital Products

Valerie A. Dangovetsky[1]
Administrator

Ellen McDonald, PhD[1]
Senior Staff Editor

Megan Zborowski[1]
Senior Staff Editor

Randy Hendrickson[1]
Production Administrator/Editor

Linnea Donnarumma[1]
Staff Editor

Susan Galeone[1]
Staff Editor

Jackie Twomey[1]
Staff Editor

Julia Nawrocki[1]
Staff Editor

Kimberly Kerns[1]
Administrative Coordinator

Rosemarie Houton[1]
Administrative Representative

---

1. Has no relationships with any entity producing, marketing, reselling, or distributing health care goods or services consumed by, or used on, patients.

2. Has disclosed relationship(s) with any entity producing, marketing, reselling, or distributing health care goods or services consumed by, or used on, patients.

Disclosure of Relationships with any entity producing, marketing, reselling, or distributing health care goods or services consumed by, or used on, patients.

Patrick C. Alguire, MD, FACP
Consultantship
National Board of Medical Examiners
Royalties
UpToDate
Stock Options/Holdings
Amgen Inc, Bristol-Myers Squibb, GlaxoSmithKline, Stryker Corporation, Zimmer Orthopedics, Teva Pharmaceuticals, Medtronic, Covidien, Inc., Express Scripts

Terence Chan, MD
Honoraria
AstraZeneca (Canada)

Pieter A. Cohen, MD
Stock Options/Holdings (spouse)
Bio Reference Labs, Idexx Laboratories, Johnson & Johnson, Mettler Toledo International Inc., Stryker Corp., Biota Pharmaceuticals, Pfizer, ResMed Inc., Vertex Pharmaceuticals
Honoraria
Consumer Union, Wall Street Journal

Benjamin P. Geisler, MD
Royalties
UpToDate
Consultantship
Wing Tech Inc., Ardian Medtronic LLC, Medtronic Vascular Inc., Amgen Inc.

Linda A. Hershey, MD, PhD
Research Grants/Contracts
Baxter, Novartis, Forum Pharmaceuticals (formerly EnVivo)
Honoraria
Med Link Neurology

Wanda C. Lakey, MD, MHS
Research Grants/Contracts
Janssen, Regeneron, Amarin, Sanofi/Aventis

Sarah Mayson, MD[2]
Other (Sub-Investigator for Clinical Studies)
Novartis, Cortendo

Mark D. Siegel, MD, FACP
Consultantship
Siemens

Jennifer Sipos, MD
Consultantship
Genzyme

Cynthia D. Smith, MD, FACP
Stock Options/Holdings
Merck and Co.; spousal employment at Merck

Acknowledgments

The American College of Physicians (ACP) gratefully acknowledges the special contributions to the development and production of the 17th edition of the Medical Knowledge Self-Assessment Program® (MKSAP® 17) made by the following people:

Graphic Design: Michael Ripca (Graphics Technical Administrator) and WFGD Studio (Graphic Designers).

Production/Systems: Dan Hoffmann (Director, Web Services & Systems Development), Neil Kohl (Senior Architect),

Chris Patterson (Senior Architect), and Scott Hurd (Manager, Web Projects & CMS Services).

MKSAP 17 Digital: Under the direction of Steven Spadt, Vice President, Digital Products & Services, the digital version of MKSAP 17 was developed within the ACP's Digital Product Development Department, led by Brian Sweigard (Director). Other members of the team included Dan Barron (Senior Web Application Developer/Architect), Chris Forrest (Senior Software Developer/Design Lead), Kara Kronenwetter (Senior Web Developer), Brad Lord (Senior Web Application Developer), John McKnight (Senior Web Developer), and Nate Pershall (Senior Web Developer).

The College also wishes to acknowledge that many other persons, too numerous to mention, have contributed to the production of this program. Without their dedicated efforts, this program would not have been possible.

MKSAP Resource Site (mksap.acponline.org)

The MKSAP Resource Site (mksap.acponline.org) is a continually updated site that provides links to MKSAP 17 online answer sheets for print subscribers; the latest details on Continuing Medical Education (CME) and Maintenance of Certification (MOC) in the United States, Canada, and Australia; errata; and other new information.

ABIM Maintenance of Certification

Check the MKSAP Resource Site (mksap.acponline.org) for the latest information on how MKSAP tests can be used to apply to the American Board of Internal Medicine for Maintenance of Certification (MOC) points.

Royal College Maintenance of Certification

In Canada, MKSAP 17 is an Accredited Self-Assessment Program (Section 3) as defined by the Maintenance of Certification (MOC) Program of The Royal College of Physicians and Surgeons of Canada and approved by the Canadian Society of Internal Medicine on December 9, 2014. Approval extends from July 31, 2015 until July 31, 2018 for the Part A sections. Approval extends from December 31, 2015 to December 31, 2018 for the Part B sections.

Fellows of the Royal College may earn three credits per hour for participating in MKSAP 17 under Section 3. MKSAP 17 also meets multiple CanMEDS Roles, including that of Medical Expert, Communicator, Collaborator, Manager, Health Advocate, Scholar, and Professional.

For information on how to apply MKSAP 17 Continuing Medical Education (CME) credits to the Royal College MOC Program, visit the MKSAP Resource Site at mksap.acponline.org.

The Royal Australasian College of Physicians CPD Program

In Australia, MKSAP 17 is a Category 3 program that may be used by Fellows of The Royal Australasian College of Physicians (RACP) to meet mandatory Continuing Professional Development (CPD) points. Two CPD credits are awarded for each of the 200 *AMA PRA Category 1 Credits*™ available in MKSAP 17. More information about using MKSAP 17 for this purpose is available at the MKSAP Resource Site at mksap.acponline.org and at www.racp.edu.au. CPD credits earned through MKSAP 17 should be reported at the MyCPD site at www.racp.edu.au/mycpd.

Continuing Medical Education

The American College of Physicians (ACP) is accredited by the Accreditation Council for Continuing Medical Education (ACCME) to provide continuing medical education for physicians.

The ACP designates this enduring material, MKSAP 17, for a maximum of 200 *AMA PRA Category 1 Credits*™. Physicians should claim only the credit commensurate with the extent of their participation in the activity.

Up to 14 *AMA PRA Category 1 Credits*™ are available from December 31, 2015, to December 31, 2018, for the MKSAP 17 Endocrinology and Metabolism section.

Learning Objectives

The learning objectives of MKSAP 17 are to:
- Close gaps between actual care in your practice and preferred standards of care, based on best evidence
- Diagnose disease states that are less common and sometimes overlooked or confusing
- Improve management of comorbid conditions that can complicate patient care
- Determine when to refer patients for surgery or care by subspecialists
- Pass the ABIM Certification Examination
- Pass the ABIM Maintenance of Certification Examination

Target Audience

- General internists and primary care physicians
- Subspecialists who need to remain up-to-date in internal medicine and in areas outside of their own subspecialty area

- Residents preparing for the certification examination in internal medicine
- Physicians preparing for maintenance of certification in internal medicine (recertification)

Earn "Instantaneous" CME Credits Online

Print subscribers can enter their answers online to earn instantaneous Continuing Medical Education (CME) credits. You can submit your answers using online answer sheets that are provided at mksap.acponline.org, where a record of your MKSAP 17 credits will be available. To earn CME credits, you need to answer all of the questions in a test and earn a score of at least 50% correct (number of correct answers divided by the total number of questions). Take any of the following approaches:

1. Use the printed answer sheet at the back of this book to record your answers. Go to mksap.acponline.org, access the appropriate online answer sheet, transcribe your answers, and submit your test for instantaneous CME credits. There is no additional fee for this service.

2. Go to mksap.acponline.org, access the appropriate online answer sheet, directly enter your answers, and submit your test for instantaneous CME credits. There is no additional fee for this service.

3. Pay a $15 processing fee per answer sheet and submit the printed answer sheet at the back of this book by mail or fax, as instructed on the answer sheet. Make sure you calculate your score and fax the answer sheet to 215-351-2799 or mail the answer sheet to Member and Customer Service, American College of Physicians, 190 N. Independence Mall West, Philadelphia, PA 19106-1572, using the courtesy envelope provided in your MKSAP 17 slipcase. You will need your 10-digit order number and 8-digit ACP ID number, which are printed on your packing slip. Please allow 4 to 6 weeks for your score report to be emailed back to you. Be sure to include your email address for a response.

If you do not have a 10-digit order number and 8-digit ACP ID number or if you need help creating a user name and password to access the MKSAP 17 online answer sheets, go to mksap.acponline.org or email custserv@acponline.org.

Disclosure Policy

It is the policy of the American College of Physicians (ACP) to ensure balance, independence, objectivity, and scientific rigor in all of its educational activities. To this end, and consistent with the policies of the ACP and the Accreditation Council for Continuing Medical Education (ACCME), contributors to all ACP continuing medical education activities are required to disclose all relevant financial relationships with any entity producing, marketing, re-selling, or distributing health care goods or services consumed by, or used on, patients. Contributors are required to use generic names in the discussion of therapeutic options and are required to identify any unapproved, off-label, or investigative use of commercial products or devices. Where a trade name is used, all available trade names for the same product type are also included. If trade-name products manufactured by companies with whom contributors have relationships are discussed, contributors are asked to provide evidence-based citations in support of the discussion. The information is reviewed by the committee responsible for producing this text. If necessary, adjustments to topics or contributors' roles in content development are made to balance the discussion. Further, all readers of this text are asked to evaluate the content for evidence of commercial bias and send any relevant comments to mksap_editors@acponline.org so that future decisions about content and contributors can be made in light of this information.

Resolution of Conflicts

To resolve all conflicts of interest and influences of vested interests, the American College of Physicians (ACP) precluded members of the content-creation committee from deciding on any content issues that involved generic or trade-name products associated with proprietary entities with which these committee members had relationships. In addition, content was based on best evidence and updated clinical care guidelines, when such evidence and guidelines were available. Contributors' disclosure information can be found with the list of contributors' names and those of ACP principal staff listed in the beginning of this book.

Hospital-Based Medicine

For the convenience of subscribers who provide care in hospital settings, content that is specific to the hospital setting has been highlighted in blue. Hospital icons (H) highlight where the hospital-based content begins, continues over more than one page, and ends.

High Value Care Key Points

Key Points in the text that relate to High Value Care concepts (that is, concepts that discuss balancing clinical benefit with costs and harms) are designated by the HVC icon (HVC).

Educational Disclaimer

The editors and publisher of MKSAP 17 recognize that the development of new material offers many opportunities for error. Despite our best efforts, some errors may persist in print. Drug dosage schedules are, we believe, accurate and in accordance with current standards. Readers are advised, however, to ensure that the recommended dosages in MKSAP 17 concur with the information provided in the product information material. This is especially important in cases of new, infrequently used, or highly toxic drugs. Application of the information in MKSAP 17 remains the professional responsibility of the practitioner.

The primary purpose of MKSAP 17 is educational. Information presented, as well as publications, technologies, products, and/or services discussed, is intended to inform subscribers about the knowledge, techniques, and experiences of the contributors. A diversity of professional opinion exists, and the views of the contributors are their own and not those of the American College of Physicians (ACP). Inclusion of any material in the program does not constitute endorsement or recommendation by the ACP. The ACP does not warrant the safety, reliability, accuracy, completeness, or usefulness of and disclaims any and all liability for damages and claims that may result from the use of information, publications, technologies, products, and/or services discussed in this program.

Publisher's Information

Copyright © 2015 American College of Physicians. All rights reserved.

This publication is protected by copyright. No part of this publication may be reproduced, stored in a retrieval system, or transmitted in any form or by any means, electronic or mechanical, including photocopy, without the express consent of the American College of Physicians. MKSAP 17 is for individual use only. Only one account per subscription will be permitted for the purpose of earning Continuing Medical Education (CME) credits and Maintenance of Certification (MOC) points/credits and for other authorized uses of MKSAP 17.

Unauthorized Use of This Book Is Against the Law

Unauthorized reproduction of this publication is unlawful. The American College of Physicians (ACP) prohibits reproduction of this publication or any of its parts in any form either for individual use or for distribution.

The ACP will consider granting an individual permission to reproduce only limited portions of this publication for his or her own exclusive use. Send requests in writing to MKSAP® Permissions, American College of Physicians, 190 N. Independence Mall West, Philadelphia, PA 19106-1572, or email your request to mksap_editors@acponline.org.

MKSAP 17 ISBN: 978-1-938245-18-3
(Endocrinology and Metabolism) ISBN: 978-1-938245-25-1

Printed in the United States of America.

For order information in the United States or Canada call 800-523-1546, extension 2600. All other countries call 215-351-2600, (M-F, 9 AM – 5 PM ET). Fax inquiries to 215-351-2799 or email to custserv@acponline.org.

Errata

Errata for MKSAP 17 will be available through the MKSAP Resource Site at mksap.acponline.org as new information becomes known to the editors.

Table of Contents

Disorders of Glucose Metabolism

Diabetes Mellitus. 1
    Screening for Diabetes Mellitus. 1
    Diagnostic Criteria for Diabetes Mellitus 1
    Classification of Diabetes Mellitus. 1
    Management of Diabetes Mellitus 5
Inpatient Management of Hyperglycemia 11
    Hospitalized Patients with Diabetes Mellitus. 11
    Hospitalized Patients Without Diabetes Mellitus. . . . 12
Management of Hypoglycemia 12
    Hypoglycemia in Patients with Diabetes
    Mellitus. 12
    Hypoglycemia in Patients Without Diabetes
    Mellitus. 13
Acute Complications of Diabetes Mellitus 14
    Diabetic Ketoacidosis and Hyperglycemic
    Hyperosmolar Syndrome 14
Chronic Complications of Diabetes Mellitus 16
    Cardiovascular Morbidity. 16
    Diabetic Retinopathy 17
    Diabetic Nephropathy. 17
    Diabetic Neuropathy. 17
    Diabetic Foot Ulcers 18
    Hypoglycemic Unawareness 18

Disorders of the Pituitary Gland

Hypothalamic and Pituitary Anatomy and
Physiology 18
Pituitary Tumors. 20
    Approach to a Sellar Mass 20
    Mass Effects of Pituitary Tumors. 21
    Treatment of Clinically Nonfunctioning
    Pituitary Tumors 21
Hypopituitarism 21
    Adrenocorticotropic Hormone Deficiency
    (Secondary Cortisol Deficiency) 22
    Thyroid-Stimulating Hormone Deficiency. 23
    Gonadotropin Deficiency. 24
    Growth Hormone Deficiency. 24
    Central Diabetes Insipidus 24
    Panhypopituitarism 25
Pituitary Hormone Excess 25
    Hyperprolactinemia and Prolactinoma 25
    Acromegaly 27

Gonadotropin-Producing Adenomas 28
Thyroid-Stimulating Hormone–Secreting
Tumors. 28
Excess Antidiuretic Hormone Secretion. 28
Cushing Disease 28

Disorders of the Adrenal Glands

Adrenal Anatomy and Physiology 29
Adrenal Hormone Excess 30
    Cushing Syndrome 30
    Pheochromocytomas and Paragangliomas. 32
    Primary Hyperaldosteronism 34
    Androgen-Producing Adrenal Tumors 36
Adrenal Insufficiency 36
    Primary Adrenal Failure. 36
    Adrenal Function During Critical Illness 38
Adrenal Masses 39
    Incidentally Noted Adrenal Masses 39
    Adrenocortical Carcinoma 40

Disorders of the Thyroid Gland

Thyroid Anatomy and Physiology 40
Evaluation of Thyroid Function. 41
Functional Thyroid Disorders 42
    Thyrotoxicosis 42
    Thyroid Hormone Deficiency 45
    Drug-Induced Thyroid Dysfunction 46
Thyroid Function and Disease in Pregnancy 46
Euthyroid Sick Syndrome. 48
Thyroid Emergencies 48
    Thyroid Storm 48
    Myxedema Coma. 49
Structural Disorders of the Thyroid Gland 50
    Thyroid Nodules 50
    Goiters 51
Thyroid Cancer 52

Reproductive Disorders

Physiology of Female Reproduction 53
Amenorrhea. 54
    Clinical Features 54
    Evaluation of Amenorrhea 55
Hyperandrogenism Syndromes. 55
    Hirsutism and Polycystic Ovary Syndrome 55
    Androgen Abuse in Women. 56

Female Infertility. 56

Physiology of Male Reproduction 57

Hypogonadism 57

    Primary Hypogonadism. .57

    Secondary Hypogonadism. 57

    Androgen Deficiency in the Aging Male. 57

    Evaluation of Male Hypogonadism 58

Testosterone Replacement Therapy. 58

Anabolic Steroid Abuse in Men 60

Male Infertility. 60

Gynecomastia 60

Calcium and Bone Disorders

Calcium Homeostasis and Bone Physiology. 61

Hypercalcemia. 62

    Clinical Features of Hypercalcemia. 62

Diagnosis and Causes of Hypercalcemia 62

    Treatment of Hypercalcemia 65

Hypocalcemia 66

    Clinical Features of Hypocalcemia 66

    Diagnosis and Causes of Hypocalcemia 66

    Treatment of Hypocalcemia. 66

Metabolic Bone Disease 66

    Osteopenia and Osteoporosis 66

    Vitamin D Deficiency 69

    Paget Disease of Bone 70

Bibliography 71

Self-Assessment Test. 73

Index 137

Endocrinology and Metabolism High Value Care Recommendations

The American College of Physicians, in collaboration with multiple other organizations, is engaged in a worldwide initiative to promote the practice of High Value Care (HVC). The goals of the HVC initiative are to improve health care outcomes by providing care of proven benefit and reducing costs by avoiding unnecessary and even harmful interventions. The initiative comprises several programs that integrate the important concept of health care value (balancing clinical benefit with costs and harms) for a given intervention into a broad range of educational materials to address the needs of trainees, practicing physicians, and patients.

HVC content has been integrated into MKSAP 17 in several important ways. MKSAP 17 now includes HVC-identified key points in the text, HVC-focused multiple choice questions, and, for subscribers to MKSAP Digital, an HVC custom quiz. From the text and questions, we have generated the following list of HVC recommendations that meet the definition below of high value care and bring us closer to our goal of improving patient outcomes while conserving finite resources.

High Value Care Recommendation: A recommendation to choose diagnostic and management strategies for patients in specific clinical situations that balance clinical benefit with cost and harms with the goal of improving patient outcomes.

Below are the High Value Care Recommendations for the Endocrinology and Metabolism section of MKSAP 17.

- Lifestyle modifications are a cost-effective intervention that has been proven to decrease the risk of patients with prediabetes developing type 2 diabetes by 41% to 58%.
- The data for the role and cost-effectiveness of self-monitoring of blood glucose levels are less clear for regimens without multiple daily insulin injections and noninsulin regimens; generally this should be avoided.
- For noncritically ill patients who are eating, the use of basal and prandial subcutaneous insulin is the preferred and safest choice for achieving inpatient glycemic control; oral agents and noninsulin injectable agents do not have proven safety or efficacy data in the hospital setting.
- Isolated adult-onset growth hormone deficiency is extremely rare, and its clinical significance is debated; evaluation for growth hormone deficiency should be reserved for adults with at least one known pituitary hormone deficiency.

- Microprolactinomas in asymptomatic patients do not require treatment; however, surveillance is recommended (see Item 65).
- If the thyroid-stimulating hormone level is frankly abnormal, additional evaluation of thyroid function should be considered to determine the extent of the dysfunction; measure thyroxine (T_4) when the thyroid-stimulating hormone is elevated and measure both thyroxine (T_4) and triiodothyronine (T_3) when the thyroid-stimulating hormone is suppressed.
- There is no clinical indication for serial measurement of thyroid antibody titers to determine the need for or to guide therapy except to monitor for residual disease in patients treated for thyroid cancer
- Radioactive iodine uptake is a measure of iodine uptake by the thyroid over 24 hours; it is used to evaluate the cause of hyperthyroidism and is not indicated in patients with normal or elevated thyroid-stimulating hormone levels.
- In patients with subclinical hyperthyroidism, repeat assessment of thyroid function should be performed 6 to 12 weeks after the initial tests, as the values will normalize in up to 30% of patients.
- An elevated serum thyroid-stimulating hormone level indicates the diagnosis of primary hypothyroidism; thyroid imaging is not indicated unless there is concern for a nodule on physical examination.
- The typical pattern of euthyroid sick syndrome, nonthyroidal illness syndrome, or low triiodothyronine (T_3) syndrome is a mildly elevated thyroid-stimulating hormone level and slightly low thyroxine (T_4) and triiodothyronine (T_3) levels; this pattern should not prompt further testing in the hospital.
- After patients with euthyroid sick syndrome are discharged from the hospital, thyroid function abnormalities may persist for several weeks so follow-up thyroid function tests should not be repeated until 6 weeks after discharge.
- A serum thyroid-stimulating hormone measurement is the initial laboratory test in a patient with a thyroid nodule; if the thyroid-stimulating hormone is suppressed, then measurement of thyroxine (T_4) and triiodothyronine (T_3) should be performed, and a radionuclide scan should be considered to identify "hot" or functioning nodules, which have a very low likelihood of malignancy and typically do not require fine-needle aspiration.

- If the thyroid-stimulating hormone level is high or normal, the radionuclide scan is unnecessary as it is unlikely to reveal a hot nodule and ultrasonography is an inexpensive and highly effective method for stratification of malignancy risk for nonfunctioning thyroid nodules.
- Measurement of testosterone levels is not recommended if a patient is having regular morning erections, does not have true gynecomastia on examination, and has a normal testicular examination, as it is highly unlikely that he has testosterone deficiency.
- Mild, chronic, asymptomatic gynecomastia in the male patient does not warrant evaluation.
- 25-Hydroxyvitamin D has a relatively long half-life of several weeks, is the best indicator of whole body vitamin D status, and is the recommended test for vitamin D deficiency.
- A 25-hydroxyvitamin D level between 30 and 40 ng/mL (75-100 nmol/L) is deemed sufficient for bone health; most expert groups recommend screening all groups at least once for evidence of deficiency since U.S. incidence is 30% to 60% of the population, however, it should not be a serial, recurring screening test.
- Treatment for low bone mass in postmenopausal women involves lifestyle modification (maximizing weight-bearing exercise and avoidance of tobacco or excessive alcohol) and vitamin D and calcium supplementation; the need for pharmacologic therapy is based on the 10-year estimated fracture risk ($\geq$20% for a major osteoporotic fracture or $\geq$3% for hip fracture)(see Item 12).

Endocrinology and Metabolism

Disorders of Glucose Metabolism

Diabetes Mellitus

Diabetes mellitus is a chronic metabolic disease characterized by elevated plasma glucose levels as a consequence of insulin deficiency, impaired action of insulin secondary to insulin resistance, or a combination of both abnormalities. Prediabetes is defined as elevated plasma glucose levels below the diagnostic criteria for diabetes, but above the normal range.

Screening for Diabetes Mellitus

Patients with diabetes mellitus may exhibit classic symptoms (polyuria, polydipsia, polyphagia), or more commonly, they can be asymptomatic. Diabetes screening may detect an early asymptomatic phase. Current guidelines do not recommend routine screening for type 1 diabetes as there is no consistent evidence that early treatment during the asymptomatic stage prevents progression of the disease. Similarly, it has not been firmly established that screening improves clinical outcomes in type 2 diabetes. However, microvascular and macrovascular disease can be present at the time of diagnosis of type 2 diabetes, which is indicative of ongoing organ damage during the asymptomatic phase. Furthermore, there is evidence that the microvascular and macrovascular disease associated with type 2 diabetes may be reduced with improved glucose control early in the disease course and that treatment of prediabetes may delay the onset of type 2 diabetes. In 2008, the U.S. Preventive Services Task Force (USPSTF) recommended screening for type 2 diabetes only in asymptomatic adults with a sustained blood pressure level (treated or untreated) greater than 135/80 mm Hg. Updated USPSTF draft guidelines from 2014 have expanded screening recommendations to all adults in primary care settings with risk factors for the development of diabetes (**Table 1**). In contrast, the American Diabetes Association (ADA) recommends screening for type 2 diabetes based on BMI (≥25) with additional risk factors, including a history of gestational diabetes, or age (≥45 years).

Diagnostic Criteria for Diabetes Mellitus

Prediabetes and diabetes can be diagnosed based on the elevated results from one of the following screening tests repeated on two separate occasions: fasting plasma glucose (FPG), 2-hour postprandial glucose during an oral glucose tolerance test (OGTT), or hemoglobin A_{1c} (**Table 2**). A random plasma glucose level greater than or equal to 200 mg/dL (11.1 mmol/L) with classic hyperglycemic symptoms is diagnostic of diabetes and

does not warrant repeat measurement. The diabetes screening tests have several advantages and disadvantages to consider. FPG is cheaper and more readily available in most countries compared with hemoglobin A_{1c}, but the requirement for overnight fasting can be problematic. OGTT best reflects the pathophysiology of diabetes by identifying postprandial hyperglycemia secondary to pancreatic beta-cell deficiency; however, the test is time-intensive. Hemoglobin A_{1c} testing is more convenient with no fasting requirement, is unaffected by acute stress or illness, and provides an accurate reflection of the average plasma glucose over the previous 3 months. By contrast, hemoglobin A_{1c} testing can miss early glucose abnormalities, such as postprandial hyperglycemia. Another disadvantage is its decreased reliability in the setting of anemia, hemoglobinopathies, or kidney or liver disease. Furthermore, conditions that affect the turnover of erythrocytes, such as anemias/hemoglobinopathies and pregnancy, can affect the reliability of hemoglobin A_{1c}.

Classification of Diabetes Mellitus

Categories for classification of diabetes encompass a range of insulin abnormalities, including absolute or relative insulin deficiency, insulin resistance, or a combination of these abnormalities (**Table 3**).

Insulin Deficiency

Type 1 Diabetes Mellitus

Type 1 diabetes occurs in the setting of insulin deficiency. It accounts for 5% of diagnosed diabetes cases. The underlying mechanism is destruction of insulin-producing pancreatic beta cells, which can be autoimmune-mediated, idiopathic, or acquired.

Autoimmune-mediated type 1 diabetes mellitus can result from a combination of genetic, environmental, and autoimmune factors. There is a strong association between type 1 diabetes and specific HLA antigens. One or more precipitating events, such as viral infections, can trigger the autoimmune process of beta-cell destruction in genetically susceptible persons. Autoantibodies (one or more) can be present at the time of diagnosis, including antibodies to the following: islet cells, glutamic acid decarboxylase (GAD65), tyrosine phosphatases IA-2 and IA-2β, insulin, and zinc transporter autoantibodies. Measurements of autoantibodies to GAD65 and IA-2 are recommended for initial confirmation as both of these assays are highly automated. In addition, autoantibodies to GAD65 persist longer than those to islet cells after the development of diabetes.

Autoimmune-mediated type 1 diabetes has classically been considered a disease of children and young, thin adults,

TABLE 1. Screening Guidelines for Type 2 Diabetes Mellitus in Asymptomatic Adults

	ADA	USPSTF
Screening criteria	BMI ≥25[a] and at least one additional risk factor: Physical inactivity First-degree relative with diabetes High-risk race/ethnicity (black, Latino, Native American, Asian American, Pacific Islander) Delivery of a baby weighing >4.1 kg (9 lb) History of GDM Hypertension (≥140/90 mm Hg or on antihypertensive medication) HDL cholesterol <35 mg/dL (0.90 mmol/L) and/or triglyceride level >250 mg/dL (2.82 mmol/L) Polycystic ovary syndrome Hemoglobin A_{1c} ≥5.7%, IGT, or IFG on previous testing Other conditions associated with insulin resistance (severe obesity, acanthosis nigricans) History of CVD	2008 guidelines: Sustained BP >135/80 mm Hg treated or untreated 2014 updated draft: Screening of adults in primary care settings with at least one of the following risk factors for IFG, IGT, or type 2 diabetes mellitus: Age ≥45 years Overweight or obese First-degree relative with diabetes History of GDM History of polycystic ovary syndrome High-risk race/ethnicity (black, American Indian/Alaska Native, Asian American, Hispanic/Latino, and Native Hawaiian/Pacific Islander)
Additional screening criteria	All patients age 45 years or older	Patients age 45 years or younger with any of the other risk factors in the screening criteria
Additional screening considerations	Use of glucocorticoids or antipsychotics	—
Screening intervals	3-year intervals if results are normal. Yearly testing if prediabetes (hemoglobin A_{1c} between 5.7% and 6.5%, IGT, IFG) is diagnosed.	3-year intervals if low-risk and normal plasma glucose values. In high-risk adults or those with near abnormal test values, yearly testing may be beneficial.

[a]At-risk BMI may be lower in some ethnic groups.

ADA = American Diabetes Association; BP = blood pressure; CVD = cardiovascular disease; GDM = gestational diabetes mellitus; IFG = impaired fasting glucose; IGT = impaired glucose tolerance; USPSTF = U.S. Preventive Services Task Force.

Data from American Diabetes Association. Classification and diagnosis of diabetes. Sec. 2. *In* Standards of Medical Care in Diabetes-2015. Diabetes Care 2015;38 Suppl 1:S8-16. [PMID: 25537714]

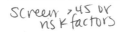

Screen >45 or risk factors

A_{1c} 5.7–6.5% = pre DMII.   *>6.5 = DM.*

TABLE 2. Diagnostic Criteria for Diabetes Mellitus[a]

Test	Normal Range	Increased Risk for Diabetes (Prediabetes)	Diabetes
Random plasma glucose	—	—	Classic hyperglycemic symptoms plus a random plasma glucose ≥200 mg/dL (11.1 mmol/L)
Fasting plasma glucose[b]	<100 mg/dL (5.6 mmol/L)	100-125 mg/dL (5.6-6.9 mmol/L)	≥126 mg/dL (7.0 mmol/L)
Plasma glucose during a 2-hour 75-g OGTT	<140 mg/dL (7.8 mmol/L)	140-199 mg/dL (7.8-11.0 mmol/L)	≥200 mg/dL (11.1 mmol/L)
Hemoglobin A_{1c}	<5.7%	5.7%-6.4%	≥6.5%

OGTT = oral glucose tolerance test.

[a]In the absence of hyperglycemic symptoms, an abnormal fasting plasma glucose, OGTT, or hemoglobin A_{1c} should be confirmed by repeat testing. The same test should be used when repeating the measurement for confirmation. If two different tests are performed and only one has abnormal results, the American Diabetes Association recommends repeating the test with the abnormal results.

[b]Fasting for at least 8 hours.

Data from American Diabetes Association. (2) Classification and diagnosis of diabetes. Diabetes Care 2015 Jan;38 Suppl:S8-S16. [PMID: 25537714]

TABLE 3. Classification of Diabetes Mellitus

Insulin Deficiency[a]

Immune-mediated

    Type 1 diabetes

    LADA

    Rare forms: "stiff man" syndrome, anti-insulin receptor antibodies

Idiopathic (seronegative)

Acquired

    Diseases of the exocrine pancreas: pancreatitis, trauma/pancreatectomy, neoplasia, cystic fibrosis, hemochromatosis, fibrocalculous, pancreatopathy

    Infections: congenital rubella

    Drug-related: Vacor (rat poison), intravenous pentamidine

Insulin Resistance

Type 2 Diabetes[b]

Ketosis prone[c]

Other or Rare Types

Genetic defects in beta-cell function (including six distinct MODY syndromes)

Genetic defects in insulin action

Endocrinopathies:

    (acromegaly, Cushing syndrome, glucagonoma, pheochromocytoma, hyperthyroidism)[d]

    (somatostatinoma, aldosteronoma)[e]

Drug-related:

    (glucocorticoids, thiazides, β-blockers, diazoxide, tacrolimus, cyclosporine, niacin, HIV protease inhibitors, atypical antipsychotics [clozapine, olanzapine])[f]

Genetic syndromes:

    Down syndrome[g]

    Wolfram syndrome (DIDMOAD)[h]

    (Klinefelter, Turner, and Prader-Willi syndromes; myotonic dystrophy)[d]

DIDMOAD = diabetes insipidus, diabetes mellitus, optic atrophy, and deafness; LADA = late autoimmune diabetes in adults; MODY = maturity-onset diabetes of the young.

[a]Beta-cell destruction usually leading to absolute insulin deficiency.

[b]Insulin resistance with progressive relative insulin deficiency.

[c]More common in nonwhite patients who present with diabetic ketoacidosis but become non-insulin dependent over time.

[d]Impaired insulin action.

[e]Impaired insulin secretion.

[f]Impaired insulin secretion, impaired insulin action or altered hepatic glucose metabolism.

[g]Insulin deficiency, immune-mediated.

[h]Insulin deficiency.

although it can occur at any age or BMI range. The initial presentation can range from modest elevations in plasma glucose levels to diabetic ketoacidosis (DKA). The time course for beta-cell destruction is also variable, although it is frequently more rapid in children compared with adults. Upon initiation of insulin therapy for type 1 diabetes, the remaining functioning pancreatic beta cells may temporarily regain the ability to produce some insulin during a "honeymoon" phase lasting several weeks to many months, although this is not an adequate or sustained effect. Insulin therapy is therefore recommended during the honeymoon phase to reduce the metabolic stress on the functioning beta cells to preserve any residual function for as long as possible. Late autoimmune diabetes in adults (LADA) presents in patients with autoantibodies to pancreatic beta-cell antigens and beta-cell destruction who did not require insulin initially but eventually progressed to an insulin requirement. Patients with autoimmune-mediated type 1 diabetes are at an increased risk to develop other autoimmune diseases, such as thyroiditis and celiac disease most commonly. Thus, screening for associated autoimmune diseases should be considered at the time of diagnosis and/or the development of signs and symptoms. Consensus on the frequency and effectiveness of repeat screening for associated autoimmune diseases is lacking.

Idiopathic type 1 diabetes can present with relative insulin deficiency and episodic DKA without evidence for autoimmunity. There is a strong genetic history of diabetes, and Asian and African ancestry appears to be a predisposing factor.

Acquired type 1 diabetes can be caused by diseases affecting the exocrine pancreas, infections, or drugs. Diffuse damage to the pancreas and beta cells or impaired insulin secretion with subsequent insulin deficiency occurs in these scenarios.

KEY POINTS

- Prediabetes and diabetes mellitus can be diagnosed based on the elevated results from one of the following screening tests repeated on two separate occasions: fasting plasma glucose, 2-hour postprandial glucose during an oral glucose tolerance test, or hemoglobin A_{1c}.

- Measurements of autoantibodies to GAD65 and IA-2 are recommended for initial confirmation of autoimmune-mediated type 1 diabetes mellitus.

Insulin Resistance

Insulin resistance is characterized by the inability of the peripheral cells to utilize insulin effectively, with a compensatory increase in the amount of insulin secreted by the pancreatic beta cells in response to hyperglycemia. The pancreas exhibits a relative insulin deficiency when it cannot produce enough insulin to overcome the hyperglycemia. Obesity predisposes to the development of insulin resistance.

Metabolic Syndrome

Metabolic syndrome is the coexistence of a group of risk factors that increases a person's probability for the development of type 2 diabetes mellitus and cardiovascular disease (CVD). In addition to impaired glucose metabolism, these risk factors include central body obesity, hypertension, and hyperlipidemia (**Table 4**). Metabolic syndrome increases the relative risk of developing CVD by twofold and diabetes by fivefold, although it is not clear whether the combination of factors associated with metabolic syndrome imparts a greater risk than that attributable to each individual risk factor present. In the presence of one

abd girth

LDL >

HDL <

Handwritten margin notes: 40 in waist   HDL e40   139/80
TG >150   HDL <50   gluc >100

TABLE 4. AHA/NHLBI Criteria for the Definition of the Metabolic Syndrome

Clinical Criteria (Must meet at least 3 of the 5 criteria)	Qualifying Measurements
Waist circumference[a]	Men 40 in (102 cm)[b]
	Women 35 in (89 cm)[c]
Fasting TG	≥150 mg/dL (1.7 mmol/L) or
	Drug therapy targeting increased TG
HDL cholesterol	Men <40 mg/dL (1.0 mmol/L)
	Women <50 mg/dL (1.3 mmol/L) or
	Drug therapy targeting decreased HDL
Blood pressure	Systolic ≥130 mm Hg or
	Diastolic ≥85 mm Hg or
	Drug therapy for hypertension
Fasting glucose	Blood glucose ≥100 mg/dL (5.6 mmol/L) or
	Drug therapy for increased glucose

AHA = American Heart Association; HDL = high-density lipoprotein cholesterol; NHLBI = National Heart, Lung, and Blood Institute; TG = triglycerides.

[a]Some individuals with minimally elevated waist circumference measurements [e.g., (men 37-39 in or 94-99 cm) or (women 31-34 in or 79-86 cm)] may still be at risk for type 2 diabetes or cardiovascular disease and will benefit from lifestyle interventions.

[b]A lower waist circumference of 35 in (89 cm) should be used for Asian American men.

[c]A lower waist circumference of 31 in (79 cm) should be used for Asian American women.

Data from Grundy SM, Cleeman JI, Daniels SR, et al. Diagnosis and management of the metabolic syndrome: An American Heart Association/National Heart, Lung, and Blood Institute Scientific Statement: Executive Summary. Circulation. 2005 Oct 25;112(17):2735-52. [PMID: 16157765]

or more risk factors for metabolic syndrome, the Endocrine Society recommends a 3-year screening interval for the metabolic syndrome components including waist circumference, fasting lipid profile, fasting plasma glucose, and blood pressure. Calculation of the 10-year CVD risk is recommended in persons with metabolic syndrome to determine the need for lifestyle modifications and therapeutic interventions to prevent or delay progression to type 2 diabetes or CVD. The Framingham Risk Score and the new Pooled Cohort Equation from the American College of Cardiology/American Heart Association are frequently used within the United States to assess CVD risk.

Type 2 Diabetes Mellitus

Type 2 diabetes mellitus accounts for most (90%-95%) diagnosed diabetes cases. It affects 10.9 million (26.9%) of adults in the United States aged 65 years or older. Asian Americans, American Indians, Alaska Natives, Hispanics, and non-Hispanic black persons are at an increased risk for developing diabetes compared with non-Hispanic white persons. The etiology of type 2 diabetes is likely multifactorial. There is often a strong family history of type 2 diabetes among first-degree relatives, although the specific genes responsible for the glucose abnormalities remain unidentified.

Insulin resistance from obesity in the setting of relative insulin deficiency contributes to the development of type 2 diabetes in the majority of patients. The degree of hyperglycemia depends on the extent of beta-cell function, which can decline over time.

Type 2 diabetes generally has an insidious onset of prolonged asymptomatic hyperglycemia. Most patients do not present with the classic symptoms of polydipsia, polyphagia, or polyuria. Patients with type 2 diabetes may present first with macrovascular or microvascular changes. Although type 2 diabetes is often considered an adult disease, the incidence is increasing along with obesity rates in children and adolescents.

Residual insulin production from the beta cells is insufficient to control glucose adequately, but it is able to suppress lipolysis for most persons with type 2 diabetes. Under extreme metabolic stress, such as an illness, some patients with type 2 diabetes cannot suppress lipolysis and present with DKA. Ketosis-prone patients with type 2 diabetes are more likely to be overweight or obese, middle-aged, male, and of black or Latino ethnicity. Insulin use during the time of metabolic stress can often restore the beta cells from the glucose toxicity with a return to diet, exercise, and oral hypoglycemic agents for glucose control. Prior to switching from insulin to oral therapy, pancreatic beta-cell function should be assessed with fasting C-peptide and glucose measurements.

Lifestyle modifications alone or combined with therapeutic interventions can prevent or delay the development of type 2 diabetes in high-risk persons. Lifestyle modifications are a cost-effective intervention. Several randomized controlled trials provide evidence that diet changes, increased daily exercise, and weight loss targets of 5% to 7% can significantly decrease the risk of developing type 2 diabetes in persons with prediabetes by 41% to 58%. Additionally, metformin has been shown to reduce the risk of diabetes in patients with prediabetes, although this effect was not as robust as lifestyle interventions. In the setting of impaired glucose tolerance, impaired fasting glucose values, or hemoglobin A_{1c} values between 5.7% and 6.4%, the ADA recommends considering metformin for prevention of type 2 diabetes.

Additional therapeutic agents, such as lipase inhibitors, α-glucosidase inhibitors, and thiazolidinediones, have been evaluated to delay or prevent type 2 diabetes; however, the effectiveness, cost, and potential side effects must be considered before implementation (**Table 5**).

KEY POINTS

- Lifestyle modifications are a cost-effective intervention that has been proven to decrease the risk of patients with prediabetes developing type 2 diabetes by 41% to 58%. **HVC**

- In high-risk persons, the American Diabetes Association recommends considering metformin for prevention of type 2 diabetes, particularly in patients who are younger than 60 years of age, have a BMI greater than 35, or have a history of gestational diabetes.

TABLE 5. Strategies to Prevent or Delay Onset of Type 2 Diabetes Mellitus

Intervention	Effectiveness
Diet and exercise	Sustained weight loss of 7%, with at least 150 minutes of moderate exercise per week, shown to delay onset of diabetes by up to 3 years
Smoking cessation	Modestly effective as long as it does not cause weight gain, but is always recommended
Bariatric surgery	Effective if used in morbidly obese persons (BMI >40)
Metformin[a]	Shown to delay onset of diabetes by up to 3 years
Lipase inhibitors (orlistat)	Shown to delay onset of diabetes by up to 3 years
α-Glucosidase inhibitors (acarbose, voglibose)	Shown to delay onset of diabetes by up to 3 years
Thiazolidinediones (troglitazone, rosiglitazone, pioglitazone)	Shown to delay onset of diabetes by up to 3 years
Insulin and insulin secretagogues (sulfonylureas, meglitinides)	Ineffective
ACE inhibitors and angiotensin receptor blockers	Ineffective
Estrogen-progestin	Modest effect only

[a]Preferred.

Gestational Diabetes Mellitus

Relative insulin deficiency during the increased insulin resistance associated with pregnancy can result in the development of gestational diabetes mellitus. Pregnant women at high risk for developing gestational diabetes include those from certain racial or ethnic groups (Hispanic/Latino Americans, blacks, and American Indians), overweight or obese women, women older than 25 years of age, and women with a strong family history of type 2 diabetes. An estimated 2% to 10% of pregnant women have gestational diabetes. Complications related to gestational diabetes include miscarriage, fetal deformities, large for gestational age infants, macrosomia, preeclampsia, complications during labor and delivery, increased perinatal complications, and mortality. Complication risk is on a continuum with increasing hyperglycemia.

Disagreement exists among consensus groups regarding the definition, screening methods, and diagnostic criteria for gestational diabetes. High-risk pregnant women should be screened for overt diabetes at the initial prenatal visit using criteria for nonpregnant women, according to the International Association of Diabetes and Pregnancy Study Group (IADPSG) and the ADA. In the absence of overt diabetes at the initial office visit, diabetes screening should occur between 24 and 28 weeks' gestation. Once a diagnosis of gestational diabetes is made, glucose monitoring should be performed at least four times daily initially, to include fasting and 1-hour or 2-hour postprandial values. Postprandial hyperglycemia in pregnancy may predict worse fetal outcomes and complications.

Lifestyle interventions and/or pharmacologic agents should be implemented when glucose goals for gestational diabetes are not met. Nutrition requirements for gestational diabetes should allow for appropriate maternal weight gain for normal fetal growth while obtaining goal glucose values. A moderate exercise program is recommended for glycemic control.

Insulin has traditionally been the mainstay of therapy for gestational diabetes when glycemic goals are not met with diet and exercise. Off-label use of metformin and glyburide in pregnancy has been studied and there appears to be equivalence in efficacy with insulin; however, long-term safety data are lacking.

Gestational diabetes resolves after pregnancy for most women; however, the risk of developing type 2 diabetes is 5% to 10% after delivery and 35% to 60% in the subsequent 10 to 20 years. The ADA recommends diabetes screening for women with a history of gestational diabetes using standard criteria at 6 to 12 weeks postpartum and every 3 years thereafter.

KEY POINTS

- Lifestyle interventions should be implemented to meet glycemic goals in women with gestational diabetes; however, when these are not met, insulin should be initiated.

- For women with a history of gestational diabetes, diabetes screening using standard criteria should occur at 6 to 12 weeks postpartum and every 3 years thereafter.

Uncommon Types of Diabetes Mellitus

Genetic defects in beta-cell function and insulin action cause some uncommon forms of diabetes (see Table 3). Maturity-onset diabetes of the young (MODY) is an autosomal dominant monogenetic defect that affects beta-cell function but not insulin action. MODY should be suspected in non-obese patients with a strong family history for diabetes when the onset of diabetes occurs before 25 years of age in the absence of autoantibodies. Genetic defects in insulin action cause insulin resistance with varying degrees of hyperglycemia, as seen with congenital lipodystrophy.

Several endocrinopathies can impair insulin action or secretion as a consequence of excess hormone production. Conditions such as Cushing syndrome and pheochromocytoma decrease the action of insulin secondary to excess cortisol and epinephrine, respectively. The hypokalemia induced by hyperaldosteronism can inhibit the secretion of insulin.

Management of Diabetes Mellitus

The most effective management of diabetes mellitus includes a multidisciplinary approach, including patient education and support, engaging patients in their care and decision making, lifestyle modifications with diet and exercise, reduced caloric intake for overweight and obese patients, and pharmacologic therapies when necessary to meet individualized glycemic goals (**Table 6**).

Patient Education

Diabetes self-management education (DSME) and diabetes self-management support (DSMS) are recommended at the time of diagnosis of prediabetes or diabetes and throughout

TABLE 6. American Diabetes Association Recommended Outpatient Glycemic Goals for Adults with Diabetes Mellitus

State of Health	Characteristics of Patients	Hemoglobin A_{1c}[a]	Preprandial Capillary Glucose[a]	Postprandial Capillary Glucose (1-2 hours after meal)[a]
Healthy	Early in disease course	<7.0% without severe recurrent hypoglycemia	70-130 mg/dL (3.9-7.2 mmol/L)	<180 mg/dL (10.0 mmol/L)
	Few comorbidities			
	Preconception	(<6.5% for select patients)[b]		
	Patient preference			
	Life expectancy >10 years			
Complex health issues	Significant comorbidities, including advanced atherosclerosis or microvascular complications	<8.0% without severe recurrent hypoglycemia		
	Longer duration of diabetes			
	Frequent hypoglycemia			
	Hypoglycemia unawareness			
	Life expectancy <10 years			
Older adults	Few comorbidities	<7.0%-7.5% without severe recurrent hypoglycemia	90-130 mg/dL (5.0-7.2 mmol/L)	
	Extended life expectancy			
	No impairment of cognition or function			
	Multiple comorbidities	<8.0% without severe recurrent hypoglycemia	90-150 mg/dL (5.0-8.3 mmol/L)	
	Hypoglycemic risk			
	Fall risk			
	Mild impairments in cognition and function			
	Poor health	<8.5% without severe recurrent hypoglycemia	100-180 mg/dL (5.6-10.0 mmol/L)	
	Chronic comorbidities with end-stage disease			
	Long-term care placement			
	Moderate-to-severe impairment in cognition and function			
	Limited life expectancy			
Pregnant women	Preexisting type 1 or type 2 diabetes	<6.0% without severe recurrent hypoglycemia	60-99 mg/dL (3.3-5.5 mmol/L)	100-129 mg/dL (5.6-7.1 mmol/L)
	Gestational diabetes		≤95 mg/dL (5.3 mmol/L)	1-hour after meal: ≤140 mg/dL (7.8 mmol/L)
				2-hours after meal: ≤120 mg/dL (6.7 mmol/L)

[a]Recommended if goal can be met without severe recurrent hypoglycemia. If severe recurrent hypoglycemia is present, there is no recommended hemoglobin A_{1c} goal, as modification of the patient's diabetes mellitus regimen to resolve severe recurrent hypoglycemia should take precedence. When severe recurrent hypoglycemia is resolved, an hemoglobin A_{1c} goal can be chosen, and treatment decisions can again be made based on that individualized hemoglobin A_{1c} goal without frequent hypoglycemia.

[b]This can be considered for patients with an early diagnosis of diabetes mellitus, no significant cardiovascular disease, or managed with lifestyle modifications or metformin.

Data from American Diabetes Association. Glycemic targets. Sec. 6. In Standards of Medical Care in Diabetes-2015. Diabetes Care. 2015;38(Suppl 1):S33-S40. [PMID: 25537705]. (Modification of Table 6.2 (p. S37).

Data from American Diabetes Association. Older adults. Sec. 10. In Standards of Medical Care in Diabetes-2015. Diabetes Care. 2015;38(Suppl 1):S67-S69. [PMID: 25537711]. (Modification of Table 10.1 (p. S68).

Data from American Diabetes Association. Management of diabetes in pregnancy. Sec. 12. In Standards of Medical Care in Diabetes-2015. Diabetes Care. 2015;38(Suppl 1): S77-S79. [PMID: 25537713].

the lifetime of the patient. DSMS is an individualized plan that provides opportunities for educational and motivational support for diabetes self-management. DSME and DSMS jointly provide an opportunity for collaboration between the patient and health care providers to assess educational needs and abilities, develop personal treatment goals, learn self-management skills, and provide ongoing psychosocial and clinical support. Improved outcomes and reduced costs have been associated with DSME and DSMS.

Self-Monitoring of Blood Glucose

Blood glucose monitoring can involve a variety of modalities, including self-monitoring of blood glucose (SMBG), hemoglobin A_{1c}, or continuous glucose monitoring (CGM).

SMBG is recommended for patients on multiple daily injection (MDI) insulin therapy or continuous subcutaneous insulin infusion (CSII) therapy. SMBG should be performed frequently during several critical time periods: preprandial, bedtime, before and after exercise, periods of symptomatic hypoglycemia or hyperglycemia, and before important activities such as operating dangerous machinery. Monitoring blood glucose levels 1 to 2 hours after food consumption (postprandial) can be useful to assess prandial insulin coverage in patients with at-goal preprandial readings but with hemoglobin A_{1c} not at goal. Overnight blood glucose monitoring can help detect hypoglycemia or dawn phenomenon. Success with SMBG requires the physician and patient to act upon the information that it provides. This can include insulin dose adjustments, changes in meal content, or changes in activity level to reach individualized glycemic goals. The data for the role and cost-effectiveness of SMBG are less clear for regimens without multiple daily insulin injections and non-insulin regimens.

It is often necessary to combine both SMBG and hemoglobin A_{1c} to determine if adequate control of glucose has been achieved. There is a strong correlation between hemoglobin A_{1c} and the average 3-month plasma glucose value. Therefore, the ADA and the American Association for Clinical Chemistry advocate reporting both the hemoglobin A_{1c} and the estimated plasma glucose levels (**Table 7**). Hemoglobin A_{1c} monitoring should be measured at the time of diagnosis and every 3 months while making changes to achieve glycemic goals. Testing intervals can be decreased to twice yearly after glycemic goals have been met.

CGM technology measures real-time glucose values from the interstitial fluid every few seconds through the temporary placement of a sensor subcutaneously for 3 to 7 days. The sensor is connected to a transmitter that sends the data through wireless radiofrequency to a display device. CGM glucose values average +/- 15% from a laboratory glucose measurement. CGM may be useful in persons with frequent hypoglycemia, hypoglycemic unawareness, or extreme fluctuations in glucose levels. CGM systems can rapidly identify hypo- or hyperglycemia that is not always detected with SMBG or hemoglobin A_{1c} measurements. Additionally, the ADA endorses the use of

TABLE 7. Comparison of Hemoglobin A_{1c} Value and Estimated Plasma Glucose Level

Hemoglobin A_{1c} (%)	Estimated Average Plasma Glucose Level
	mg/dL(mmol/L)
6	126 (7.0)
7	154 (8.6)
8	183 (10.2)
9	212 (11.8)
10	240 (13.4)
11	269 (14.9)
12	298 (16.5)

Adapted with permission of American Diabetes Association, from Translating the A1C assay into estimated average glucose values. Nathan DM, Kuenen J, Borg R, Zheng H, Shoenfeld D, Heine RJ; A1C-derived average glucose study group. [erratum in Diabetes Care. 2009;32(1):207]. Diabetes Care. 2008;31(8):1476. [PMID: 18540046]

CGM combined with intensive insulin therapy in adults (≥25 years of age) with type 1 diabetes as a successful modality to lower hemoglobin A_{1c} levels. The greatest improvements in glycemic control are associated with longer periods of CGM use. In patients using a CGM system, it is important to note that it does not replace SMBG. Calibration with SMBG is required at least twice daily with CGM systems. All CGM glucose values that warrant an immediate intervention should be confirmed with SMBG prior to action due to a lag time ranging from 5 to 21 minutes for several CGM brands between capillary blood glucose and interstitial glucose. Rapid glucose fluctuations further increase the lag time.

KEY POINTS

- Blood glucose monitoring, including self-monitoring of blood glucose levels, hemoglobin A_{1c} levels, or continuous glucose monitoring, is recommended for patients with diabetes mellitus requiring multiple daily insulin injections or continuous intravenous insulin injection therapy.
- The data for the role and cost-effectiveness of self-monitoring of blood glucose levels are less clear for regimens without multiple daily insulin injections and noninsulin regimens; generally this should be avoided.

HVC

Nonpharmacologic Approaches

Nonpharmacologic approaches to diabetes management should be implemented throughout the lifespan of the patient. These approaches can be used alone or as adjunct therapy in type 2 diabetes to improve the success rate of pharmacologic agents. Medical nutrition therapy and exercise can be used in conjunction with insulin therapy for patients with type 1 diabetes.

Medical nutrition therapy is an essential component of any successful management plan for patients with prediabetes or diabetes. Modest weight loss (2.0-8.0 kg [4.4-17.6 lb] or 7%)

through caloric reduction can benefit some overweight or obese adults with type 2 diabetes.

Consistent exercise provides beneficial effects on glucose control, weight, and cardiovascular status. For persons with diabetes in whom no contraindications exist, aerobic exercise should consist of at least 150 minutes/week at a moderate intensity level, 75 minutes/week at a vigorous activity level, or a combination of these two. Resistance training should be incorporated into the exercise routine at least 2 days per week. Hypoglycemia and extreme hyperglycemia can worsen if present at the time of exercise and should be corrected before proceeding with increased physical activity.

Bariatric surgical procedures (restrictive and bypass) can be considered in obese patients with type 2 diabetes. Weight loss and diabetes remission rates are significant with these procedures, but the long-term benefits require additional studies. See MKSAP 17 Gastroenterology and Hepatology and MKSAP 17 General Internal Medicine for more information.

Depression, anxiety, and diabetes-related stress are common among patients with diabetes and may impair their ability to achieve success with a diabetes management plan. Screening should occur continuously during the course of diabetes treatment.

Pharmacologic Therapy

An individualized treatment goal will help guide the selection of the optimal treatment regimen. For many persons with diabetes, a reasonable goal for hemoglobin A_{1c} is less than 7.0% (or less than 6.5%, if this can be achieved without significant hypoglycemia). If severe recurrent hypoglycemia is present, there is no recommended hemoglobin A_{1c} goal, as modification of the patient's diabetes regimen to resolve severe recurrent hypoglycemia should take precedence. The increased risks of hypoglycemia outweigh the risks of diabetes complications in older patients with longer disease duration, which necessitates consideration of a less-stringent glycemic goal. The recommended goals from the ADA for blood glucose and hemoglobin A_{1c} levels are located in Table 6.

Therapy for Type 1 Diabetes Mellitus

Lifelong insulin therapy is the first-line treatment for type 1 diabetes. Physiologic insulin therapy, also known as intensive insulin therapy, is the ideal insulin regimen as it attempts to mimic the actions of normal pancreatic beta cells. Intensive insulin therapy includes multiple daily injections (MDI) (≥3 per day) with an intermediate or long-acting insulin for basal coverage and multiple preprandial injections throughout the day with analogue or regular insulin. Intensive insulin therapy can also include continuous subcutaneous insulin infusion (CSII) and meal-time boluses with an insulin pump. Data support targeting normal glycemic levels with a goal hemoglobin A_{1c} of less than 7% for most persons with type 1 diabetes to reduce long-term complications. Long-term physiologic insulin therapy reduces early microvascular disease by 34% to 76% and reduces cardiovascular events by

42% to 57%. Intensive insulin therapy has risks, including significant increases in hypoglycemia and weight gain. Therapy should therefore be individually tailored for each patient's preferences, lifestyle, education level, financial resources, and comorbidities.

Available insulin preparations and their activity profiles are indicated in **Table 8**. Most persons with type 1 diabetes are sensitive to the effects of exogenous insulin therapy, with initial total daily doses of insulin typically ranging from 0.3 to 1 U/kg/d. A basal insulin dose should account for half of the total daily dose of insulin, while the remaining insulin should be divided to cover the number of meals consumed during the day. Basal insulin coverage can be provided with one to two daily injections of insulin detemir, glargine, or neutral protamine Hagedorn (NPH) insulin. CSII can also provide basal coverage with analogue insulin. For prandial coverage, analogue or regular insulin is injected prior to meal consumption or analogue insulin is bolused with CSII prior to meals. Insulin dosing immediately after a meal is appropriate in certain situations, particularly when food intake is unpredictable. Postprandial insulin dosing allows for a reduction in the insulin dose that is commensurate with the amount of food ingested to avoid hypoglycemia that could have resulted from the full insulin dose. For example, the postprandial insulin dose is reduced by 50% if only half of the meal is consumed.

TABLE 8. Pharmacokinetic Properties of Insulin Products[a]

Insulin Type	Onset	Peak	Duration
Rapid-acting or analogue (lispro, aspart, glulisine)	5-15 min	45-90 min	2-4 h
Short-acting (regular)	0.5-1 h	2-4 h	4-8 h
NPH insulin	1-3 h	4-10 h	10-18 h
Detemir	1-2 h	None[b]	12-24 h[c]
Glargine	2-3 h	None[b]	20-24+ h
Pre-mixed insulins			
70% NPH/30% regular	0.5-1 h	2-10 h	10-18 h
50% NPH/50% regular	0.5-1 h	2-10 h[d]	10-18 h
75% NPL/25% lispro	10-20 min	1-6 h	10-18 h
50% NPL/50% lispro	10-20 min	1-6 h[d]	10-18 h
70% NPA/30% aspart	10-20 min	1-6 h	10-18 h

NPA = neutral protamine aspart; NPH = neutral protamine Hagedorn; NPL = neutral protamine lispro.

[a]The time course of each insulin varies significantly between persons and within the same person on different days. Therefore, the time periods listed should be considered general guidelines only.

[b]Both insulin detemir and insulin glargine can produce a peak effect in some persons, especially at higher doses.

[c]The duration of action for insulin detemir varies depending on the dose given.

[d]Premixed insulins containing a larger proportion of rapid- or short-acting insulin tend to have larger peaks occurring at an earlier time than mixtures containing smaller proportions of rapid and short-acting insulin.

Regular insulin requires a longer time interval between prandial injection and food consumption compared with analogue insulin due to its longer onset of action. Classic carbohydrate counting with prandial analogue insulin allows flexibility and variety in the types and sizes of meals consumed by adjusting the dose based on the number of carbohydrates ingested. Typically, 1 U of analogue insulin is used to cover every 10 to 20 g of carbohydrate in the meal. Modified carbohydrate counting for patients who are unwilling or cannot count carbohydrates includes fixed prandial doses of regular or analogue insulin that can be adjusted by 50% based upon the size of the meal: regular (100% dose), small (50% dose), or large (150% dose). In the setting of pre-meal hyperglycemia, the prandial dose of insulin determined by the classic or modified carbohydrate counting methods can be combined with a supplemental insulin dose to correct the hyperglycemia. There are a variety of methods to determine the supplemental insulin dose needed for correction; however, an additional 1 U of analogue or regular insulin for every 50 mg/dL (2.8 mmol/L) above the target blood glucose at the pre-meal measurement is a reasonable starting point. For example, an additional 2 U of regular or analogue insulin would be administered for a patient with a blood glucose level of 210 mg/dL (11.7 mmol/L) if the target blood glucose is 150 mg/dL (8.3 mmol/L) or less. When administering any prandial or supplemental insulin doses, the duration of action of previous analogue or regular insulin injections must be considered, as the risk of insulin-stacking and subsequent hypoglycemia increases if the dosing is too frequent. Allowing at least 3 to 4 hours between injections can decrease this risk. Premixed insulins containing a fixed percentage of a long-acting and regular or analogue insulin are given twice daily, particularly in patients who are unable to comply with more frequent daily injections, although greater glycemic variability and hypoglycemia are concerns when utilizing a nonphysiologic regimen.

CSII should be considered for select patients with type 1 diabetes if adequate glycemic control is not achieved with adherence to MDI therapy. CSII may be beneficial in several scenarios, including significant early morning hyperglycemia ("dawn phenomenon"), labile plasma glucose values and frequent DKA, frequent severe hypoglycemia or hypoglycemic unawareness, preconception and pregnancy, or active lifestyles/patient preference. If a patient is not adherent with insulin injections and blood glucose monitoring, adherence is unlikely to increase because a pump is prescribed; therefore, pump therapy is not recommended in the nonadherent patient.

Cost of the insulin regimen chosen should be weighed against potential benefits. MDI regimens require more insulin supplies and glucose monitoring. Insulin analogues demonstrate fewer hypoglycemic events, but cost more than regular human insulin. Insulin pens increase both convenience and cost when compared with insulin in vials. Insulin pump supplies are expensive compared with other insulin therapies; however, data from several analyses indicate that overall CSII is a cost-effective treatment modality.

KEY POINTS

- Lifelong insulin therapy is the first-line treatment for type 1 diabetes; physiologic insulin therapy reduces early microvascular disease by 34% to 76% in patients with type 1 diabetes mellitus compared with nonphysiologic regimens.

- Continuous subcutaneous insulin infusion is a cost-effective treatment modality and should be considered for select patients with type 1 diabetes mellitus if adequate glycemic control is not achieved with adherence to multiple daily injection therapy.

Therapy for Type 2 Diabetes Mellitus

Lifestyle modifications must often be combined with oral pharmacologic agents for optimal glycemic control, particularly as type 2 diabetes progresses with continued loss of pancreatic beta-cell function and insulin production. Multiple oral agents may be required or used in conjunction with noninsulin injectable agents or insulin as glycemic control worsens. There are many options for oral agents, with major differences in cost, timing of administration, mechanism of action, and side-effect profiles (**Table 9**).

Metformin is the recommended first-line therapy to be initiated either in conjunction with lifestyle modifications at the time of diagnosis or within 6 weeks of failing to obtain glycemic control with lifestyle changes alone. Metformin has a lower incidence of hypoglycemia and weight gain compared with some of the other oral agents and insulin. Gastrointestinal side effects (such as abdominal cramping or diarrhea) are common with metformin; initial low doses with gradual increases and administration of the tablet following a substantial meal can improve tolerance to the medication. Due to the potential risk of lactic acidosis, contraindications to metformin therapy include serum creatinine greater than 1.5 mg/dL (133 µmol/L) in men and 1.4 mg/dL (124 µmol/L) in women, symptomatic heart failure or liver disease, and illness with hemodynamic instability. Metformin must be withheld for 48 hours in the setting of intravenous contrast dye. In a nonhospitalized patient, metformin should be withheld with any illness that may cause dehydration.

If lifestyle modifications and maximally tolerated doses of metformin fail to adequately control glucose, additional agents should be added every 3 months until glycemic goals have been met. Without strong comparative-effectiveness data to identify the best class of second-line drugs to be implemented, several factors must be considered. Patient preferences and financial resources are key components to developing an individualized treatment plan. Another important determining factor in selection of the second-line drug class is the patient's weight. Weight-neutral drug classes include α-glucosidase inhibitors and dipeptidyl peptidase-4 (DPP-4) inhibitors. If weight loss is a desired effect, glucagon-like peptide 1 (GLP-1) mimetics, pramlintide, and sodium-glucose transporter-2 (SGLT2) inhibitors are

TABLE 9. Pharmacologic Agents Used to Lower Blood Glucose Levels in Type 2 Diabetes Mellitus

Class	Mechanism of Action	Effect on Weight	Risks and Concerns	Long-Term Studies on Definitive Outcomes
Insulin[a]	Decreases hepatic glucose production, increases peripheral glucose uptake	Increase	Hypoglycemia; insulin allergy (rare)	Decrease in both microvascular and macrovascular events
Sulfonylureas (tolbutamide, chlorpropamide, glipizide, glyburide, gliclazide, glimepiride)[b]	Stimulate insulin secretion	Increase	Hypoglycemia (especially in drugs with long half-lives or in older populations); weight gain	Decrease in microvascular events but possible increase in macrovascular events with tolbutamide, chloropropamide, glyburide, and glipizide; not seen with gliclazide or glimepiride
Biguanides (metformin)[b]	Decrease hepatic glucose production, increase insulin-mediated uptake of glucose in muscles	Neutral	Diarrhea and abdominal discomfort; lactic acidosis (rare); contraindicated in presence of progressive liver, kidney or cardiac failure	Decrease in both microvascular and macrovascular events
α-Glucosidase inhibitors (acarbose, miglitol, voglibose)[b]	Inhibit polysaccharide absorption	Neutral	Flatulence; abdominal discomfort	May reduce CVD events
Thiazolidinediones (rosiglitazone, pioglitazone)[b]	Increase peripheral uptake of glucose, decrease hepatic glucose production	Increase	Fluid retention; heart failure; macular edema; osteoporosis (possible increased risk of bladder cancer with pioglitazone)	Unclear whether pioglitazone causes net harm or good
Meglitinides (repaglinide, nateglinide)[b]	Stimulate insulin release	Increase	Hypoglycemia	None
Amylinomimetics (pramlintide)[a]	Slow gastric emptying, suppress glucagon secretion, increase satiety	Decrease	Nausea; vomiting; increased hypoglycemic risk with insulin	None
GLP-1 mimetics (exenatide and liraglutide)[a]	Slow gastric emptying, suppress glucagon secretion, increase satiety	Decrease	Hypoglycemia when used in combination with sulfonylureas; nausea and vomiting; possible increased risk of pancreatitis and chronic kidney disease	None
DPP-4 inhibitors (sitagliptin, saxagliptin, vildagliptin, linagliptin, alogliptin)[b]	Slow gastric emptying, suppress glucagon secretion	Neutral	Hypoglycemia when used in combination with sulfonylureas; nausea; increased risk of infections; possible increased risk of pancreatitis	No increase in ischemic cardiovascular events; increased rate of hospitalization for heart failure with saxagliptin
SGLT2 inhibitors (dapagliflozin and canagliflozin)[b]	Increases kidney excretion of glucose	Decrease	Hypoglycemia with insulin secretagogues and insulin; hypotension; kidney impairment; hypersensitivity reactions; increased candidal genital infections and urinary tract infections	None

CVD = cardiovascular disease; DPP-4 = dipeptidyl peptidase-4; GLP-1 = glucagon-like peptide-1; SGLT2 = sodium-glucose co-transporter 2.

[a]Injection.

[b]Oral.

candidates to consider. Weight gain is likely with the use of insulin, sulfonylureas, thiazolidinediones, and meglitinides. The risk of hypoglycemia must be considered with the selection of any therapeutic agent, particularly when it is combined with insulin secretagogues or insulin. Gastrointestinal side effects from GLP-1 mimetics and pramlintide may decrease tolerability for some patients and should not be used in patients with gastroparesis. Patients with frequent candidal genital infections would not be ideal candidates for SGLT2 inhibitor therapy.

Insulin therapy should be strongly considered in the setting of symptomatic hyperglycemia or markedly elevated hemoglobin A_{1c} (>8.5% to 9%) at the time of diagnosis or when lifestyle modifications and/or noninsulin therapies fail to achieve glycemic goals. The American Association of Clinical Endocrinologists (AACE) recommends weight-based initiation of basal insulin at initial doses of 0.1 to 0.3 U/kg. The dose should be increased several units every 2 to 3 days to reach fasting plasma glucose goals, based on the patient's SMBG readings. Reductions of insulin doses by 10% to 40% should be made in the setting of hypoglycemia with insulin titrations. If glycemic goals are not met with basal insulin, then prandial insulin should be added to the regimen with frequent titration of doses for optimal glucose control. When premeal glucose values are not at a patient-specific goal, the preceding prandial insulin dose should be increased or decreased by 10% to 20% in the setting of hyper- or hypoglycemia, respectively. (Also see section on Therapy for Type 1 Diabetes Mellitus.)

KEY POINTS

- For patients with type 2 diabetes mellitus, metformin is recommended first-line therapy and should be initiated in conjunction with lifestyle modifications; it has a lower incidence of hypoglycemia and weight gain compared with some of the other oral agents and insulin.

- In older patients with type 2 diabetes mellitus of longer disease duration, treatment of severe recurrent hypoglycemia should take precedence over controlling hemoglobin A_{1c} values; the increased risks of hypoglycemia outweigh the risks of diabetes complications.

Inpatient Management of Hyperglycemia

Inpatient hyperglycemia, defined as consistently elevated plasma glucose values above 140 mg/dL (7.8 mmol/L), is associated with poor outcomes. Attempts to decrease morbidity and mortality with tight glycemic control (80-110 mg/dL [4.4–6.1 mmol/L]) have not consistently demonstrated improvements in adverse outcomes and, in some settings, have shown increased rates of severe hypoglycemic events and mortality. As a result, revised inpatient glycemic targets are less stringent than outpatient glucose targets to avoid both hypoglycemia

and severe hyperglycemia that can lead to volume depletion and electrolyte abnormalities.

Hospitalized Patients with Diabetes Mellitus

Critically ill patients with type 1 diabetes mellitus will require insulin therapy upon admission to the hospital. For critically ill patients with type 2 diabetes, intravenous insulin infusion therapy should be initiated when plasma glucose levels exceed 180 to 200 mg/dL (10-11.1 mmol/L). Glucose goals on intravenous insulin are 140 to 200 mg/dL (7.8-11.1 mmol/L) with frequent bedside point-of-care (POC) monitoring every 1 to 2 hours for insulin adjustments.

In noncritically ill patients, the ADA and AACE advocate a premeal glucose goal of less than 140 mg/dL (7.8 mmol/L) and random plasma glucose values less than 180 mg/dL (10 mmol/L). Therapy adjustments should be considered when plasma glucose levels are less than 100 mg/dL (5.6 mmol/L) and are necessary when glucose values fall below 70 mg/dL (3.9 mmol/L) to avoid continued hypoglycemia. In contrast, the American College of Physicians (ACP) recommends avoiding glucose levels less than 140 mg/dL (7.8 mmol/L) owing to the increased risk of hypoglycemia with tighter glycemic control.

Insulin is the preferred therapy and likely the safest choice for achieving inpatient glycemic control. Use of sliding scale insulin alone is not recommended, as it is not physiologic and frequently causes large glucose fluctuations owing to the inherent reactive nature of its dosing, coupled with the near universal lag time between measurement of glucose and injection of insulin that occurs in most hospitals. The recommended insulin regimen should incorporate both basal and prandial coverage. In the setting of preprandial hyperglycemia, prandial coverage can be supplemented with additional insulin (correction factor insulin). Prandial coverage should account for the carbohydrates consumed at each meal and be adjusted accordingly. POC glucose monitoring should coincide with insulin administration before meals and at bedtime, with overnight measurements to monitor for hypoglycemia only if fasting readings are elevated or the patient is symptomatic. This glucose monitoring regimen will simulate the patient's home routine after discharge. POC monitoring should occur every 6 hours when a patient is on insulin therapy and receives nothing by mouth.

Outpatient CSII therapy can be continued if the patient is physically and mentally able to safely administer this therapy under proper supervision from health care providers with CSII expertise. POC glucose monitoring, basal rates of insulin, and patient-initiated bolus amounts of insulin should be documented in the medical record.

Oral agents and noninsulin injectable agents do not have safety or efficacy data in the hospital setting. The safest recommendation is to discontinue these agents upon admission to the hospital, although continuation can be considered in a stable patient with glycemic control at goal and no anticipated changes in nutrition or hemodynamic status. These agents can be particularly dangerous in fasting states or when organ perfusion or

CONT.

function is compromised. Resumption of these medications may be considered once a patient is stable with regular activities and nutrition or at the time of hospital discharge. H

KEY POINTS

- For critically ill patients with type 2 diabetes mellitus, intravenous insulin infusion therapy should be initiated when plasma glucose levels exceed 180 to 200 mg/dL (10-11.1 mmol/L); glucose goals on intravenous insulin are 140 to 200 mg/dL (7.8-11.1 mmol/L) with frequent bedside point-of-care monitoring every 1 to 2 hours.

HVC
- For noncritically ill patients, basal and prandial subcutaneous insulin is the preferred and safest choice for achieving inpatient glycemic; oral agents and noninsulin injectable agents do not have proven safety or efficacy data in the hospital setting.

Hospitalized Patients Without Diabetes Mellitus

Hyperglycemia as a result of acute stress related to illness, concomitant medications, or enteral/parenteral nutrition can occur in patients without a previous history of glucose abnormalities. The glycemic goals and glucose-management strategies in this population should follow those for hospitalized patients with diabetes. Hyperglycemia in hospitalized patients may also indicate the presence of previously undiagnosed diabetes. Measurement of hemoglobin A_{1c} in hyperglycemic non-hospitalized patients, if feasible, can provide insight into the length of the hyperglycemia. A hemoglobin A_{1c} level greater than 6.5% suggests long-standing hyperglycemia. Follow-up diabetes screening and care should be implemented after discharge from the hospital.

Management of Hypoglycemia

Hypoglycemia in Patients with Diabetes Mellitus

Hypoglycemia is a common complication of intensive therapeutic regimens in patients with diabetes mellitus, often limiting the ability to safely reach glycemic goals for many patients. Avoidance of hypoglycemia prior to focusing on a patient's hemoglobin A_{1c} goal is of utmost importance because of the significant morbidity and mortality associated with low plasma glucose levels.

Hypoglycemia is defined as a plasma glucose level less than 70 mg/dL (3.9 mmol/L). Insulin secretion ceases when the glucose level falls below 80 mg/dL (4.4 mmol/L). Hyperadrenergic symptoms begin to alert the patient to hypoglycemia through an increase in heart rate, sweating, tremors, hunger, and anxiety when glucose levels decline. Typically, the body responds to hypoglycemia by secreting counterregulatory hormones, such as glucagon, epinephrine, norepinephrine, cortisol, and growth hormone, in succession based on the escalating degree of hypoglycemia. If the counterregulatory measures fail or the hypoglycemia is not corrected, cognitive function begins to decline and can be rapidly followed by loss of consciousness, seizures, and death. Relative hypoglycemia occurs when a patient has symptoms of hypoglycemia but the plasma glucose level is greater than 70 mg/dL (3.9 mmol/L). This can occur with rapid decreases in glucose or with correction of glucose to near-normal glycemic levels in a patient with a history of prolonged hyperglycemia (plasma glucose >200 mg/dL [11.1 mmol/L]). Relative hypoglycemia can be diminished if glucose levels are maintained closer to normal ranges and if treatment to goal glucose level is achieved over a longer period of time in patients with a history of prolonged uncontrolled diabetes.

The etiology of hypoglycemia can be quite variable. Exercise can lead to hypoglycemia if appropriate measures are not taken to avoid it. Prior to exercise, consumption of a snack with 15 to 30 g of carbohydrates can help reduce the risk of hypoglycemia, or a patient can reduce the dose of prandial insulin given at the meal prior to the planned exercise, if on an MDI regimen. A snack with complex carbohydrates is often required after prolonged exercise to replenish glycogen stores since glucose utilization can be prolonged in muscles and the liver. In overweight/obese patients, decreasing the insulin dose instead of ingesting snacks before exercise can avoid additional weight gain. Poor timing or skipping of meals or consumption of smaller amounts of food without an adjustment to insulin doses or oral hypoglycemic agents can cause hypoglycemia. Use of a nonphysiologic sliding scale insulin regimen or use of an aggressive supplemental insulin correction factor regimen is often the etiology of hypoglycemic events. A reduction in kidney function, particularly in elderly patients, can decrease clearance of insulin or insulin secretagogues and lead to prolonged hypoglycemia. Alcohol consumption can cause delayed hypoglycemia.

Treatment of hypoglycemia is twofold: immediate correction of hypoglycemia and prevention of future events. If a patient is conscious, 15 to 20 g of a carbohydrate with glucose should be consumed. Glucose tablets or glucose gel are ideal treatment regimens. The blood glucose level should be checked again after 15 minutes, and consumption of 15 to 20 g of glucose should occur again if the hypoglycemia does not improve to greater than 70 mg/dL (3.9 mmol/L). Since the effects of the insulin or oral hypoglycemic agents are likely still present, a meal or snack should be consumed after the glucose has been corrected to avoid continued hypoglycemia. Every patient with diabetes on medications associated with hypoglycemia should receive a prescription for a glucagon kit, which should be used when oral consumption of glucose is not possible or safe.

Relaxing the glycemic targets and hemoglobin A_{1c} goals and reducing doses of therapeutic agents will decrease the risk of future hypoglycemia. A review of a patient's diabetes self-management skills can also help identify recurring risk factors for hypoglycemia. H

KEY POINTS

- Hypoglycemia is defined as a plasma glucose level less than 70 mg/dL (3.9 mmol/L) and is associated with significant morbidity and mortality.
- Relaxing the glycemic targets and hemoglobin A_{1c} goals and reducing doses of therapeutic agents will decrease the risk of future hypoglycemia.

Hypoglycemia in Patients Without Diabetes Mellitus

Hypoglycemia in patients without diabetes is rare, thus evaluation for pathologic hypoglycemia should only occur when Whipple triad is present: symptomatic hypoglycemia, documented hypoglycemia at 55 mg/dL (3.1 mmol/L) or lower, and prompt symptomatic relief with correction of hypoglycemia. Hypoglycemia should not be confirmed with POC glucose monitors, but instead with a more accurate established laboratory method. Hypoglycemia in patients without diabetes is usually related to drugs, illness, hormonal deficiency, non-islet cell tumor, endogenous hyperinsulinism/noninsulinoma, pancreatogenous hypoglycemia, depletion of hepatic glycogen stores, or alcohol ingestion. Diagnostic studies should be obtained during a spontaneous hypoglycemic episode or during an attempt to recreate a scenario known to cause hypoglycemia, such as prolonged fasting or after a mixed meal, which consists of the type of food that induces the hypoglycemia, typically a simple carbohydrate-rich meal, such as orange juice, pancakes, and syrup. Hypoglycemia has classically been categorized as occurring in the fasting versus postprandial state, although the etiologies of each of these classifications of hypoglycemia are not mutually exclusive. The differential diagnoses based on the laboratory test results are found in **Table 10**. Imaging studies should not occur unless biochemical evidence of endogenous hyperinsulinism is confirmed and is related to a tumor or pancreatic abnormality.

Fasting Hypoglycemia

Suspected hypoglycemia that is either spontaneous or begins after a fast should be evaluated by the following simultaneous laboratory measurements: glucose, insulin, C-peptide, proinsulin, β-hydroxybutyrate, and insulin secretagogue screen. C-peptide and proinsulin are measures of the endogenous production of insulin. β-Hydroxybutyrate is suppressed by endogenous and exogenous insulin, but would be unsuppressed in a normal physiologic state of hypoglycemia or in a non–insulin-mediated condition. If hypoglycemia is not present at the time of evaluation, a 72-hour fast is indicated, which is typically performed in consultation with an endocrinologist. This test involves measurement of the above-mentioned laboratory values every 6 hours until the plasma glucose level reaches 60 mg/dL (3.3 mmol/L) and subsequently every 1 to 2 hours until specific plasma glucose, symptom, or time criteria are met. This test also involves measuring the response to glucagon administration. Evaluation for anti-insulin antibodies can detect the rare condition of insulin autoimmune hypoglycemia as the underlying etiology for the hypoglycemia.

Postprandial Hypoglycemia

Postprandial hypoglycemia without a history of a prior bariatric procedure is rare. It typically occurs within 5 hours of food consumption. A mixed meal tolerance test is usually performed in consultation with an endocrinologist and measures the glucose level as symptoms occur. Glucose, insulin, proinsulin, and C-peptide levels are measured prior to the meal and repeated at 30-minute intervals or at the time of symptomatic hypoglycemia (blood glucose level <60 mg/dL [3.3 mmol/L]) within the 5 hours after meal consumption. If symptomatic hypoglycemia occurs, insulin antibodies are measured and an oral hypoglycemic agent screening test is obtained. Treatment, with or without the detection of pathologic hypoglycemia on the mixed meal test, often involves small, frequent complex

TABLE 10. Differential Diagnosis of Spontaneous Fasting Hypoglycemia[a] in a Patient Without Diabetes

Diagnosis	Serum Insulin	Plasma C-Peptide	Plasma Proinsulin	Serum β-hydroxybutyrate	Serum Insulin Antibodies	Urine or Blood Metabolites of Sulfonylureas or Meglitinides
Insulinoma	↑	↑	↑	↓	Negative	Negative
Surreptitious use of sulfonylureas of meglitinides	↑	↑	↑	↓	Negative	Positive
Surreptitious use of insulin	↑	↓	↓	↓	Negative	Negative
Insulin autoimmune hypoglycemia	↑	↑	↑	↓	Positive	Negative

[a]Symptomatic hypoglycemia, fasting plasma glucose 55 mg/dL (3.1 mmol/L) or lower, and prompt symptomatic relief with correction of hypoglycemia (Whipple triad).

Data from Cryer PE, Axelrod L, Grossman AB, et al. Evaluation and management of adult hypoglycemic disorders: an Endocrine Society Clinical Practice Guideline. J Clin Endocrinol Metab. 2009 Mar;94(3):709-28. [PMID: 19088155]

Bromocriptine (dopa)
to suppress prolactin

meals composed of protein, fat, and carbohydrate to avoid the sensation of hypoglycemia.

Acute Complications of Diabetes Mellitus

Diabetic Ketoacidosis and Hyperglycemic Hyperosmolar Syndrome

Diabetic ketoacidosis (DKA) and hyperglycemic hyperosmolar syndrome (HHS) are acute complications of uncontrolled hyperglycemia with life-threatening consequences if not recognized and treated early. DKA typically occurs in the setting of hyperglycemia with relative or absolute insulin deficiency and an increase in counterregulatory hormones. Sufficient amounts of insulin are not present to suppress lipolysis and oxidation of free fatty acids, which results in ketone body production and subsequent metabolic acidosis. DKA occurs more frequently with type 1 diabetes, although 10% to 30% of cases occur in patients with type 2 diabetes. HHS occurs in the setting of partial insulin deficiency that is more typical of type 2 diabetes. There is sufficient insulin in patients with HHS to suppress lipolysis and production of ketone bodies, but inadequate amounts to prevent the hyperglycemia, dehydration, and hyperosmolality characteristic of HHS.

Several risk factors can precipitate the development of extreme hyperglycemia: infection, intentional or inadvertent insulin therapy nonadherence, myocardial infarction, stress, trauma, and confounding medications, such as glucocorticoids or atypical antipsychotic agents. In addition, DKA may be the initial clinical presentation in some patients with previously undiagnosed type 1 or type 2 diabetes. An illness or event that leads to dehydration will often precipitate the hyperglycemia associated with HHS.

Symptoms of extreme hyperglycemia in DKA and HHS include polyuria, polydipsia, unintentional weight loss, vomiting, weakness, and mentation changes. Dehydration and metabolic abnormalities worsen as hyperglycemia progresses, which can lead to respiratory failure, lethargy, obtundation, coma, and death. DKA can occur within several hours of the inciting event. The development of HHS is less acute than DKA and may take days to weeks to develop. HHS typically presents with more extreme hyperglycemia and mental status changes compared with DKA.

The initial evaluation of severe hyperglycemia includes serologic studies (plasma glucose, serum ketones, blood urea nitrogen, creatinine, electrolytes, calculated anion gap, arterial blood gases, osmolality, complete blood count with differential, blood cultures), urine studies (ketones, urinalysis, urine culture), chest radiograph, and an electrocardiogram.

Urine and serum ketones are elevated in DKA; however, a negative measurement initially does not exclude DKA. β-Hydroxybutyrate is the major ketone body in DKA, but ketone laboratory measurements often use the nitroprusside reaction, which only estimates acetoacetate and acetone levels that may not be elevated initially. Although hyperglycemia is the typical finding at presentation with DKA, patients can present with a range of plasma glucose values, including those in the normal range (**Figure 1**). The anion gap is elevated. Stress-related mild leukocytosis is often present. Higher levels of leukocytosis may indicate an infectious process as the etiology of the hyperglycemia. Serum sodium levels can be low due to osmotic shifts of water from the intracellular to extracellular spaces. Normal or elevated serum sodium levels are indicative of severe volume depletion. Serum potassium levels may be elevated due to shifts from the intracellular to extracellular spaces due to ketoacidosis and the absence of sufficient insulin. Normal or low potassium levels on presentation indicate low potassium stores in the body with need for correction prior to initiation of insulin therapy to avoid cardiac arrhythmias. Serum amylase and lipase levels also can be elevated in the absence of pancreatitis.

HHS typically presents with normal or small amounts of urine or serum ketones. Plasma glucose values in HHS are typically greater than in DKA and can exceed 1200 mg/dL (66.6 mmol/L). The serum osmolality is elevated greater than 320 mOsm/kg H_2O. The serum bicarbonate level is greater than 18 mEq/L (18 mmol/L), and the pH remains greater than 7.3.

Treatment of DKA and HHS requires correction of hyperglycemia with intravenous insulin infusions, frequent monitoring and replacement of electrolytes, correction of hypovolemia with intravenous fluids, and possible correction of acidosis (**Table 11**). The ICU is the best place for management of severe hyperglycemia because of the frequent monitoring required with intravenous insulin therapy, the need for monitoring for potential electrolyte-induced arrhythmias, and the potential for rapid decompensation. Plasma glucose levels should be monitored initially every hour while on insulin infusion therapy. Electrolytes should be monitored every 2 to 4 hours, depending on the initial electrolyte deficits and level of acidosis. ⊞

KEY POINTS

- The development of hyperglycemic hyperosmolar syndrome is less acute than that of diabetic ketoacidosis and may take days to weeks to develop; however, hyperglycemic hyperosmolar syndrome typically presents with more extreme hyperglycemia and mental status changes compared with diabetic ketoacidosis.

- Treatment of diabetic ketoacidosis and hyperglycemic hyperosmolar syndrome requires correction of hyperglycemia with intravenous insulin infusions, frequent monitoring and replacement of electrolytes, correction of hypovolemia with intravenous fluids, and possible correction of acidosis.

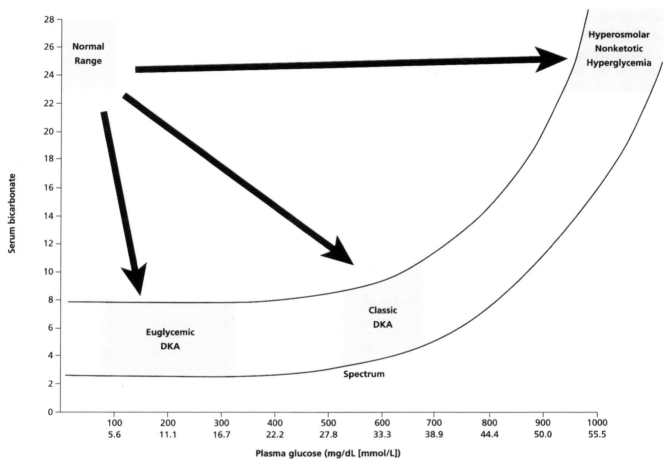

FIGURE 1. Spectrum of metabolic decompensation that occurs in diabetic ketoacidosis. DKA = diabetic ketoacidosis.

TABLE 11. Management of Hyperglycemic Crisis (DKA and HHS)			
Fluids	**Insulin (Regular)**	**Potassium**	**Correction of Acidosis**
Assess for volume status, then give 0.9% saline at 1 L/h initially in all patients, and continue if patient is severely hypovolemic. Switch to 0.45% normal saline at 250-500 mL/h if corrected serum sodium level becomes normal or high. When the plasma glucose level reaches 200 mg/dL (11.1 mmol/L) in patients with DKA or 300 mg/dL (16.7 mmol/L) in HHS, switch to 5% dextrose with 0.45% normal saline at 150-250 mL/h.	Give regular insulin 0.1 U/kg, as an intravenous bolus followed by 0.1 U/kg/h as an intravenous infusion; if the plasma glucose level does not decrease by 10% in the first hour, give an additional bolus of 0.14 U/kg and resume previous infusion rate; when the plasma glucose level reaches 200 mg/dL (11.1 mmol/L) in DKA and 300 mg/dL (16.7 mmol/L) in HHS, reduce to 0.02-0.05 U/kg/h, and maintain the plasma glucose level between 150-200 mg/dL (8.3-11.1 mmol/L) until anion gap acidosis is resolved in DKA.	Assess for adequate kidney function, with adequate urine output (approximately 50 mL/h). If serum potassium is <3.3 mEq/L (3.3 mmol/L), do not start insulin but instead give intravenous potassium chloride, 20-30 mEq/h, through a central line catheter until the serum potassium level is >3.3 mEq/L (3.3 mmol/L); then add 20-30 mEq of potassium chloride to each liter of intravenous fluids to keep the serum potassium level in the 4.0-5.0 mEq/L (4.0-5.0 mmol/L) range. If the serum potassium level is >5.2 mEq/L (5.2 mmol/L), do not give potassium chloride but instead start insulin and intravenous fluids and check the serum potassium level every 2 hours.	If pH is <6.9, give sodium bicarbonate, 100 mmol in 400 mL of water, and potassium chloride, 20 mEq, infused over 2 hours. If pH is 6.9 or greater, do not give sodium bicarbonate.

DKA = diabetic ketoacidosis; HHS = hyperglycemic hyperosmolar syndrome.

Chronic Complications of Diabetes Mellitus

Cardiovascular Morbidity

Cardiovascular disease (CVD) is a major contributor to morbidity and mortality among patients with diabetes mellitus. Diabetes alone is an independent risk factor for CVD and is considered a CVD equivalent. Concomitant risk factors in patients with diabetes, such as hypertension, obesity, and dyslipidemia, also contribute to the development of CVD and should be identified early through screening (**Table 12**).

The 8th Joint National Committee (JNC-8) recently revised its recommended blood pressure goals for patients with diabetes to 140/90 mm Hg or less, citing a lack of data to support lower targets. In contrast, the American Diabetes Association (ADA) recommends a blood pressure goal of less than 140/80 mm Hg. The ADA advocates for a lower systolic blood pressure (<130 mm Hg) in select patients (young, long life expectancy, increased risk of stroke), if this can be accomplished safely. Although JNC-8 does not specify use of an ACE inhibitor or an angiotensin receptor blocker (ARB) as initial therapy for patients with diabetes and hypertension in the absence of chronic kidney disease, the ADA recommends preferential use of these agents in treating hypertension in these patients.

The most recent American College of Cardiology/American Heart Association guidelines base treatment recommendations for patients with diabetes on age, the presence of atherosclerotic cardiovascular disease (ASCVD), or estimated 10-year ASCVD risk using the Pooled Cohort Equations; a specific goal LDL cholesterol level is no longer used in these guidelines. Treat patients with diabetes and known cardiovascular or other vascular disease with high-intensity statin therapy. In the absence of known cardiovascular or vascular disease, provide high intensity statin therapy to patients with diabetes if the LDL cholesterol level is greater than 190 mg/dL (4.9 mmol/L) or the 10-year ASCVD risk is equal to or greater than 7.5%. Provide moderate-intensity statin therapy for patients with diabetes and a 10-year ASCVD risk less than 7.5%. Consider withholding statin therapy in patients with diabetes younger than 40 years without additional cardiovascular risk factors. In contrast, ADA guidelines continue to recommend an LDL cholesterol goal in patients with diabetes of less than 100 mg/dL (2.6 mmol/L), with the option of LDL cholesterol less than 70 mg/dL (1.8 mmol/L) in patients with clinical ASCVD. Therefore, it is recommended that statin therapy be added to lifestyle modifications in patients with diabetes who have clinical ASCVD, are older than 40 years of age with CVD risk factors, or are younger than 40 years of age with LDL cholesterol not at goal.

TABLE 12. Screening Recommendations for Chronic Complications of Diabetes Mellitus

Chronic Complication	Clinical Situation	When to Start Screening	Screening Frequency	Preferred Screening Test
Retinopathy	Type 1 diabetes	At 5 years after diagnosis	Annually[a]	Dilated and comprehensive eye examination
	Type 2 diabetes	At diagnosis	Annually[a]	Dilated and comprehensive eye examination
	In pregnant women with either type of diabetes	First trimester	Every trimester and then closely for 1 year postpartum	Dilated and comprehensive eye examination
	In women with either type of diabetes planning to conceive	During preconception planning	Same as recommendations for pregnant women once conception occurs	Dilated and comprehensive eye examination
Nephropathy	Type 1 diabetes	At 5 years after diagnosis	Annually[b]	Albumin-creatinine ratio on random spot urine
	Type 2 diabetes	At diagnosis	Annually[b]	Albumin-creatinine ratio on random spot urine
Neuropathy (distal symmetric polyneuropathy)	Type 1 diabetes	At 5 years after diagnosis	Annually	10-g monofilament, 128-Hz tuning fork, ankle reflexes
	Type 2 diabetes	At diagnosis	Annually	10-g monofilament, 128-Hz tuning fork, ankle reflexes
Cardiovascular disease	Hypertension	At diagnosis	Every visit	Blood pressure measurement
	Dyslipidemia	At diagnosis	Annually[c]	Fasting lipid profile

[a]It is reasonable to screen every 2 years if no diabetic retinopathy is present and to screen more often than annually if diabetic retinopathy is advanced or progressing rapidly.

[b]The American Diabetes Association guidelines state that it is reasonable to assess progression of disease and response to therapeutic interventions with continued monitoring of urine albumin excretion.

[c]It is reasonable to screen every 2 years if lipid parameters are at goal.

KEY POINTS

- High-intensity statin therapy is indicated for patients with diabetes and known cardiovascular or vascular disease; LDH cholesterol greater than 190 mg/dL (4.9 mmol/L), or atherosclerotic cardiovascular disease 10-year risk of equal to or greater than 7.5%.

- Moderate intensity statin therapy is indicated for patients with diabetes 40 years of age and older and an atherosclerotic cardiovascular disease 10-year risk less than 7.5%.

Diabetic Retinopathy

Among adults aged 20 to 74 years, diabetic retinopathy is the leading preventable cause of blindness. Changes associated with nonproliferative retinopathy include retinal thickening from macular edema, infarcts (resulting in "cotton wool" spots or soft exudates), hard exudates, and hemorrhages. With proliferative retinopathy, neovascularization occurs secondary to chronic retinal ischemia. These new vessels may rupture, causing intraocular hemorrhage and subsequent fibrosis and retinal detachment.

Risk factors for diabetic retinopathy include long-term diabetes, poorly controlled diabetes, hypertension, and nephropathy. Retinopathy can be accelerated in pregnant women with type 1 diabetes. Rapid improvements in glycemic levels for pregnant women and nonpregnant patients can temporarily worsen preexisting retinopathy.

Screening guidelines vary depending on the type of diabetes, time of diagnosis, and pregnancy status (see Table 12).

Optimal blood glucose and blood pressure control can prevent or delay the progression of diabetic retinopathy. Laser photocoagulation is used to treat retinopathy as severity progresses. Focal laser photocoagulation of the retina can restore some vision and reduce the risk of further vision loss with macular edema. Panretinal laser photocoagulation reduces continued vision loss in proliferative diabetic retinopathy and severe nonproliferative diabetic retinopathy. Laser photocoagulation can also reduce the risk of retinopathy progression associated with pregnancy. Intravitreal injections of antiangiogenic agents, such as vascular endothelial growth factor inhibitors, may also be included in the management of proliferative retinopathy and macular edema.

KEY POINT

- Optimal blood glucose and blood pressure control can prevent or delay the progression of diabetic retinopathy; however, laser photocoagulation is used to treat diabetic retinopathy as the severity progresses.

Diabetic Nephropathy

Diabetic nephropathy not only increases the risk of progression to end-stage kidney disease, but is also a risk factor for CVD.

Measurement of increased protein excretion can be performed by two methods: albumin-creatinine ratio on a ran-

dom spot urine collection or a 24-hour urine collection. Persistently elevated levels of urine albumin excretion are defined as greater than or equal to 30 mg/g in a spot urine measurement or 30 to 299 mg/24 h and greater than or equal to 300 mg/24 h. Urine albumin levels should be elevated on multiple samples over 3 to 6 months to diagnose albuminuria, as false-positive elevations can occur in the setting of illness, menstruation, recent exercise, extreme hyperglycemia or hypertension, and heart failure. Screening timelines for urine albumin excretion are found in Table 12. Annual measurements of serum creatinine and an estimated glomerular filtration rate (GFR) can be utilized in conjunction with the urine albumin measurement to determine the stage of chronic kidney disease. When the estimated GFR is less than 30 mL/min/1.73 m^2, a referral to a nephrologist is recommended.

Diabetic nephropathy can be prevented or delayed with optimal plasma glucose and blood pressure control. In nonpregnant normotensive patients with persistently elevated urine albumin excretion, an ACE inhibitor or angiotensin receptor blocker (ARB) is recommended to decrease progression of nephropathy. In nonpregnant hypertensive patients with persistently elevated urine albumin excretion and hypertension, the ACE inhibitor or ARB should be titrated to achieve a blood pressure goal of less than 130/80 mm Hg. Measurement of urine albumin annually after initiation of therapy with an ACE inhibitor or ARB is reasonable to assess disease progression and therapeutic response as evidenced by stabilization or reduction of urine albumin excretion. Data are conflicting regarding the ability of low-protein diets to slow the progression of kidney disease, but these diets may be considered if nephropathy progresses while using an ACE inhibitor or ARB or after achieving target plasma glucose and blood pressure goals. ACE inhibitor/ARB combination treatment is not recommended.

KEY POINTS

- Elevated urinary albumin excretion is defined as greater than or equal to 30 mg/g in a spot urine measurement; annual measurements of serum creatinine and an estimated glomerular filtration rate can be utilized in conjunction with the urine albumin measurement to determine the presence of diabetic nephropathy and, if present, the stage of chronic kidney disease.

- In nonpregnant normotensive patients with persistently increased urine albumin excretion, an ACE inhibitor or angiotensin receptor blocker is recommended to decrease progression of diabetic nephropathy.

Diabetic Neuropathy

There are several categories of diabetic neuropathy, which may present separately or in combination. Symptoms of diabetic neuropathy depend on the nerve(s) or nerve root that is affected and may present as focal or diffuse disease. Achieving optimal glycemic control early in the course of diabetes can prevent the development of neuropathy, and sustained optimal glucose levels can delay the progression of neuropathy.

Distal symmetric polyneuropathy (DPN) is the most common form of diabetic neuropathy. It is characterized by a "stocking-glove" distribution that ascends proximally. DPN frequently presents as a sensation of numbness, tingling, burning, heaviness, pain, or sensitivity to light touch. The pain may worsen at night and with walking. Muscle weakness may occur in severe cases. DPN is a risk factor for muscle and joint deformities, such as Charcot foot, and foot ulcers. DPN evaluation includes assessment of ankle reflexes, vibration sensation with a 128-Hz tuning fork, and touch with a 10-g monofilament and pinprick. Screening intervals are found in Table 12. Management of DPN symptoms may require one or more classes of drugs, including antidepressants (amitriptyline, venlafaxine, duloxetine, paroxetine), anticonvulsants (pregabalin, gabapentin, valproate), or capsaicin cream.

Autonomic neuropathy can affect a single organ or multiple organs. Symptoms may include gastroparesis, diarrhea, constipation, neurogenic bladder, abnormal hidrosis, and erectile dysfunction. Cardiac symptoms include resting sinus tachycardia, orthostatic or postprandial hypotension, exercise intolerance, and silent myocardial infarction. Cardiovascular autonomic neuropathy is an independent risk factor for mortality, which underscores the need to reduce other cardiovascular risk factors in these patients.

Diabetic amyotrophy occurs in older patients or those with type 2 diabetes, and may be due to infarcts in the major nerve trunks of the leg. It can present acutely with severe pain and asymmetric proximal weakness or pain in the leg, weight loss, and autonomic neuropathy. Partial remission may occur over many months. Without any approved treatments for diabetic amyotrophy, management consists of symptomatic therapy for neuropathic pain and ambulatory aids, if necessary.

Mononeuropathies can occur acutely with a cranial or peripheral distribution. There are no specific treatments for these mononeuropathies, as the symptoms usual resolve within a few months. Nerve compression syndromes, such as carpal tunnel syndrome or peroneal palsy, occur frequently in patients with diabetes. See MKSAP 17 Neurology for more information regarding diabetic neuropathy. Referral to a neurologist for electrodiagnostic testing or evaluation for nondiabetic-related etiologies should occur with severe, rapidly progressive, or atypical neuropathies.

Diabetic Foot Ulcers

Diabetic foot ulcers increase the risk for amputation and subsequent morbidity and disability. The etiology is often multifactorial. Loss of peripheral sensation can result in significant injuries that may be undetected by the patient. Peripheral arterial disease predisposes to the development of lower extremity ischemic ulcers and impairs healing. Altered leukocyte function from hyperglycemia can impede wound healing of injuries.

Clinicians should evaluate the feet at least annually to assess for pedal pulses, sensation, ulcers, skin or nail infec-

tions, pain, ankle reflexes, and foot deformities. Patients should inspect their feet daily for early detection of any abnormality and wear appropriate footwear. Although patients with diabetes have different footwear needs, the selection of shoes should take into account several important factors: intended use, plantar protection, shape and fit on the foot, and stability issues (see MKSAP 17 Infectious Disease).

Hypoglycemic Unawareness

Frequent severe hypoglycemia can diminish the ability to detect life-threatening hypoglycemia. This unawareness is caused by failure of the release of counterregulatory hormones to trigger an autonomic response to decreased glucose levels. Continual avoidance of hypoglycemia for several weeks or longer may help restore the body's ability to detect hypoglycemia. Plasma glucose levels should be kept greater than 150 mg/dL (8.3 mmol/L) during the time period when restoration of hypoglycemic symptoms is the goal to avoid unintended and unexpected hypoglycemia. Continuous glucose monitoring systems can be useful for hypoglycemia management by alerting the patient to rapid decreases in glucose levels to allow prompt correction and avoidance of hypoglycemia (see Self-Monitoring of Blood Glucose).

KEY POINT

- Distal symmetric polyneuropathy (DPN) is the most common form of diabetic neuropathy, and it presents as a sensation of numbness or burning pain in a stocking-glove distribution; management may require one or more classes of drugs, including antidepressants (amitriptyline, venlafaxine, duloxetine, paroxetine), anticonvulsants (pregabalin, gabapentin, valproate), or capsaicin cream

Disorders of the Pituitary Gland

Hypothalamic and Pituitary Anatomy and Physiology

The anterior pituitary is made up of glandular tissue that receives its blood supply from the hypothalamus through the hypothalamic-pituitary portal plexus, whereas the posterior pituitary consists of direct extension of neurons from the hypothalamus. Both the portal blood system and the hypothalamic neurons transverse from the hypothalamus to the pituitary by way of the pituitary stalk. The hypothalamus regulates anterior pituitary gland function by synthesizing specific stimulating and inhibiting hormones, which are released in the portal blood. Posterior pituitary hormones are synthesized in the hypothalamus and travel through hypothalamic neurons to be secreted by the posterior pituitary gland. The anterior and posterior lobes are joined by the Rathke pouch. **Table 13** lists the pituitary hormones and initial testing for suspected pituitary hormone excess or deficiency.

TABLE 13. Initial Testing for Pituitary Hormone Deficiency and Excess

Pituitary Hormone Excess		
Pituitary Hormone	**Peripheral Hormone**	**Initial Test(s)**
ACTH	Cortisol	24 hour urine free cortisol (×2) OR nocturnal salivary cortisol (×2) OR overnight low dose dexamethasone test
ADH	ADH	Simultaneous serum, urine sodium, and urine osmolality
GH	IGF-1	IGF-1
TSH	Thyroxine, triiodothyronine	TSH, free (or total) thyroxine

Pituitary Hormone Deficiency			
Pituitary Hormone	**Peripheral Hormone**	**Initial Test(s)**	**Confirmatory Test**[a]
ACTH	Cortisol	Simultaneous ACTH, cortisol	ACTH stimulation test
ADH	ADH	Simultaneous serum sodium, urine and serum osmolality	Water deprivation test
LH and FSH[b]	Sex hormones	Simultaneous LH, FSH, testosterone (male), estriol (female)	
TSH	Thyroxine, triiodothyronine	Simultaneous TSH, free (or total) thyroxine	

ACTH = adrenocorticotropic hormone; ADH = antidiuretic hormone; FSH = follicle–stimulating hormone; GH = growth hormone; IGF-1 = insulin-like growth factor 1; LH = luteinizing hormone; TSH = thyroid-stimulating hormone.

[a]See Table 15 for additional information on confirmatory testing for pituitary dysfunction.

[b]Routine testing for deficiency is not recommended without specific signs of deficiency such as amenorrhea, gynecomastia, or impotence.

The anterior pituitary gland secretes and releases six hormones: adrenocorticotropic hormone (ACTH), thyroid-stimulating hormone (TSH), the gonadotropins–luteinizing hormone (LH) and follicle-stimulating hormone (FSH), growth hormone (GH), and prolactin. ACTH is released in response to corticotrophin-releasing hormone (CRH) and acts on the adrenal glands to promote the synthesis and secretion of cortisol. TSH is released in response to thyrotropin-releasing hormone (TRH) and acts on the thyroid to stimulate thyroid hormone production. LH and FSH are differentially released from the pituitary gland in response to pulses of gonadotropin-releasing hormone (GnRH). LH and FSH regulate normal male and female reproductive function. GH production is regulated by somatostatin. Prolactin controls lactation and is inhibited by dopamine. *prolactin ← dopa*

The posterior pituitary gland secretes oxytocin, which is necessary for parturition, and antidiuretic hormone (ADH, also called vasopressin), which regulates water balance.

The pituitary gland is posterior and superior to the sphenoid sinus, which provides surgical access to the gland, and is adjacent to the optic chiasm, the carotid arteries, and the cavernous sinuses (**Figure 2**).

post pit = oxytocin + ADH

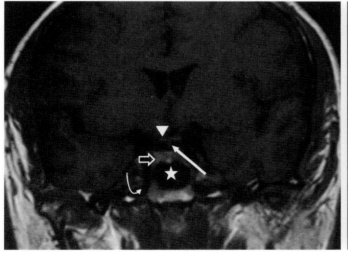 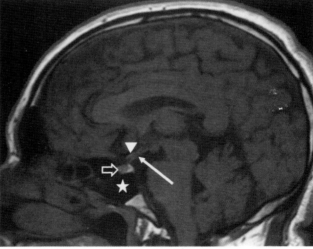

FIGURE 2. A coronal MRI (*left*) and sagittal MRI (*right*) showing the pituitary gland (*open arrow*), pituitary stalk (*thin arrow*), optic chiasm (*arrowhead*), sphenoid sinus (*star*), and carotid artery (*curved arrow*).

The pituitary gland is best imaged using MRI with gadolinium. Because the normal pituitary is relatively small, a dedicated pituitary protocol that obtains thin MRI slices through the sella is used.

Pituitary Tumors

Pituitary adenomas, which are benign, are the most common tumor of the pituitary gland. A tumor less than 1 cm is defined as a microadenoma, and a tumor 1 cm or larger is termed a macroadenoma (**Figure 3**). Pituitary adenomas are common. Autopsy studies document that 10% of the general population had undiagnosed pituitary adenomas. Frequently, pituitary adenomas are incidental findings on imaging studies completed for other reasons. When patients undergo brain MRI, 10% to 38% are found to have incidental pituitary microadenomas and 0.2% have incidental pituitary macroadenomas. Certain genetic mutations increase the chance of developing a pituitary tumor.

Approach to a Sellar Mass

When a sellar mass is noted, pituitary adenomas are most likely; however, they need to be distinguished from other pituitary lesions and nonpathologic pituitary enlargement.

The pituitary gland is enlarged diffusely in untreated primary hypothyroidism and during pregnancy. When possible, imaging of the pituitary gland should be avoided or delayed in pregnancy and in untreated primary hypothyroidism because gland enlargement on imaging may prompt an expensive and unnecessary evaluation for pituitary hormone abnormality and tumor.

Pituitary tumors are almost always nonmalignant. Two exceptions are metastatic disease and the very rare pituitary carcinoma. Additional kinds of noncancerous pituitary lesions include craniopharyngiomas, meningiomas, and Rathke cleft cysts. Inflammatory and infiltrative disorders, including lymphocytic hypophysitis, sarcoidosis, hemochromatosis, amyloidosis, Langerhans cell histiocytosis, lymphoma, and tuberculosis, can affect the pituitary gland.

Lymphocytic hypophysitis is an inflammatory pituitary lymphocytic infiltration that most commonly occurs in pregnant and postpartum women. It may cause transient or permanent pituitary insufficiency. Lymphocytic hypophysitis is treated with glucocorticoids.

A sellar mass can compress normal surrounding tissue and impair normal neurologic and pituitary function. Pituitary adenomas may also be functional and secrete excess hormone.

Incidentally Noted Pituitary Masses

When a pituitary tumor is incidentally noted, investigation must determine (1) whether it is causing a mass effect, (2) whether it is secreting excess hormones, and (3) whether it has a propensity to grow and cause problems in the future. After a thorough history and physical examination, biochemical testing can be undertaken in a targeted fashion based on the patient's clinical signs and symptoms. Initial tests could include measurement of 8 AM cortisol, TSH, free (or total) thyroxine (T_4), prolactin, and insulin-like growth factor 1 (IGF-1).

If the tumor is not causing mass effect and there is no evidence of hormone excess, a pituitary MRI should be repeated in 6 months for a macroadenoma and 12 months for

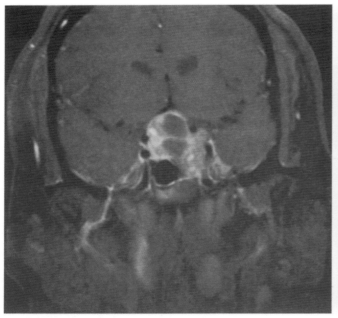
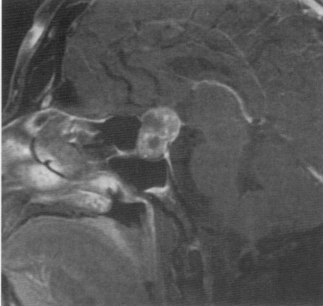

FIGURE 3. A coronal MRI (*left*) and sagittal MRI (*right*) showing a large pituitary macroadenoma. The normal pituitary gland and the optic chiasm cannot be seen because of compression from the tumor. The tumor is invasive into the left cavernous sinus. Likely, the tumor appears heterogeneous because of internal necrosis.

a microadenoma to assess for growth. If no growth occurs, MRIs should be repeated every 1 to 2 years for the next 3 years and then intermittently thereafter. In a patient at risk for cancer or with a history of cancer, metastatic disease must be excluded.

Empty Sella

Empty sella is diagnosed when the normal pituitary gland is not visualized or is excessively small on MRI; it is a radiologic finding and not a distinct clinical condition. The pituitary sella is said to be "empty" because normal tissue is not seen. The finding may be primarily due to increased cerebrospinal fluid entering and enlarging the sella, or it may be secondary to a tumor, previous pituitary surgery, radiation, or infarction. Empty sella can also occur as a congenital abnormality when the sella is normal size, but the pituitary is small. When empty sella is found incidentally on imaging, an evaluation should be completed to determine if there is a known cause for secondary empty sella and if the patient has signs or symptoms of pituitary hormone deficiency. A patient without signs or symptoms should be screened for cortisol deficiency and hypothyroidism with 8 AM cortisol, TSH, and free (or total) T_4. A patient with signs of pituitary hormone deficiency should receive a more complete biochemical evaluation of the pituitary axes, based on the signs and symptoms found.

Repeat imaging is not necessary unless indicated as surveillance for the underlying pathology that resulted in the empty sella.

KEY POINTS

- Incidentally noted pituitary tumors are common, and biochemical testing is informed by findings on history and physical examination.
- Initial tests for pituitary incidentally noted masses include measurement of 8 AM cortisol, thyroid-stimulating hormone, free (or total) thyroxine (T_4), prolactin, and insulin-like growth factor 1.
- Empty sella is diagnosed when the normal pituitary gland is not visualized or is excessively small on MRI; it is a radiologic finding and not a distinct clinical condition.

Mass Effects of Pituitary Tumors

Pituitary tumors may cause headaches in some but not all patients; the size of the tumor does not always correlate with the presence and severity of headache.

Pituitary masses can compress the normal pituitary gland, causing hormone deficiencies. A large pituitary mass may cause panhypopituitarism in which there is impaired secretion of all pituitary hormones.

Because the optic chiasm is located superior to the pituitary gland, a large pituitary mass may compress the optic chiasm resulting in vision changes. Depending on the size of the tumor and severity of optic nerve damage, a pituitary tumor may cause minimal peripheral vision loss, bitemporal hemianopsia, or complete blindness. Visual field testing is a sensitive measure of optic nerve damage and should be evaluated by an ophthalmologist in patients who report a change in vision, who have a pituitary tumor that abuts or compresses the chiasm on MRI, or who have any evidence of gross peripheral vision loss on physical examination. Change in vision due to optic chiasm compression is an indication for treating a pituitary tumor.

Pituitary tumors can also invade surrounding brain tissue leading to seizures and neurologic manifestations. Pituitary tumors can invade the cavernous sinus, causing damage to cranial nerves III, IV, and VI that pass through the sinus causing diplopia and extraocular muscle palsies/paralysis.

KEY POINT

- Pituitary masses can compress the normal pituitary gland, causing hormone deficiencies; a large pituitary mass may cause panhypopituitarism in which there is impaired secretion of all pituitary hormones.

Treatment of Clinically Nonfunctioning Pituitary Tumors

Nonfunctioning pituitary tumors that are growing or causing mass effect are treated with neurosurgery. The most common surgical approach is transsphenoidal through the nares or the mouth. A very large or invasive tumor may require craniotomy for decompression. Indications for surgery include mass effect, particularly a visual field defect; tumor that abuts the optic chiasm; tumor growth; or an invasive tumor (invading the brain or cavernous sinus). Surgery should also be considered in a patient with a tumor close to the optic chiasm who plans to become pregnant (due to the physiologic enlargement of the pituitary associated with pregnancy).

Functional pituitary tumors will be discussed later in this chapter, based on the hormone in excess (see Pituitary Hormone Excess).

KEY POINT

- Nonfunctioning pituitary tumors that are growing or causing mass effect are treated with neurosurgery.

Hypopituitarism

Hypopituitarism is caused by one or more pituitary hormone deficiencies, usually resulting from damage to the normal pituitary gland by a tumor. Hypopituitarism can also occur as a complication from surgery if the normal gland or the pituitary stalk is damaged during tumor resection or radiation therapy. Additional causes of hypopituitarism are listed in **Table 14**.

Pituitary apoplexy is acute hemorrhage into the pituitary gland often at the site of a preexisting pituitary adenoma (typically a macroadenoma). Pituitary apoplexy can cause acute pituitary hormone deficiency or mass effect from rapid

TABLE 14.	Causes of Hypopituitarism
Pituitary adenoma	
Pituitary surgery	
Pituitary radiation	
Pituitary apoplexy	
Pituitary infarction	
Craniopharyngioma	
Metastatic tumor	
Meningioma	
Lymphocytic hypophysitis	
Sarcoidosis	
Langerhans cell histiocytosis	
Lymphoma	
Hemochromatosis	
Congenital deficiencies	
Hypothalamic disease	

expansion of the sellar contents due to bleeding. It is an endocrine and neurosurgical emergency. Acute ACTH deficiency is common and can be life-threatening. If suspected, stress-dose glucocorticoid replacement should be initiated emergently. Patients with vision changes or loss associated with apoplexy require urgent surgical decompression. **H**

Hypopituitarism can occur due to postpartum pituitary infarction (Sheehan syndrome) because of excessive postpartum hemorrhage causing hypotension and hypoperfusion. Patients who may have Sheehan syndrome should be emergently tested and treated for secondary cortisol deficiency. A patient with Sheehan syndrome will not lactate because of prolactin deficiency; no treatment is available to induce lactation. Other hormone deficiencies can be evaluated 6 weeks after delivery.

GH and gonadotropin deficiencies often occur early when the pituitary gland is damaged by tumor, radiation, surgery, or hemorrhage because the cell lines that synthesize GH (somatotrophs) and LH and FSH (gonadotrophs) are most sensitive to injury. Secondary hypothyroidism (TSH deficiency) and secondary cortisol deficiency (ACTH deficiency) often occur later in the disease process. Pituitary adenomas can cause elevation in prolactin due to stalk compression, leading to a decrease in dopaminergic inhibition of prolactin secretion.

KEY POINTS

- Pituitary tumors and surgery for pituitary tumors are the most common causes of hypopituitarism.
- Stress-dose glucocorticoid replacement should be initiated emergently in patients with pituitary apoplexy or infarction, as well as emergent neurosurgical intervention; patients with vision loss associated with apoplexy require urgent surgical decompression.

Adrenocorticotropic Hormone Deficiency (Secondary Cortisol Deficiency)

Although secondary cortisol deficiency may result from damage to the pituitary gland or pituitary stalk that impairs ACTH production, it is most commonly iatrogenic due to exogenous glucocorticoid use that suppresses pituitary ACTH secretion. Patients with secondary cortisol deficiency have only glucocorticoid deficiency. The remainder of the adrenal gland functions normally and the renin-angiotensin system is intact, so these patients do not have mineralocorticoid deficiency (see Disorders of the Adrenal Glands for a discussion of primary adrenal failure). Although patients with secondary cortisol deficiency do require stress-dose glucocorticoids, they are at less risk for hypotension, hyponatremia, and adrenal crisis than those with primary cortisol deficiency (failure of the adrenal glands) because the production of mineralocorticoid is retained. Also, unlike patients with primary cortisol deficiency, patients with secondary cortisol deficiency do not develop hyperpigmentation or bronzing of the skin because ACTH and its prohormone responsible for these changes, pro-opiomelanocortin (POMC), are not hypersecreted.

Oral, injectable (including joint injections), and even topical glucocorticoids are able to suppress ACTH secretion. Glucocorticoids prescribed at doses above physiologic replacement for longer than 3 weeks should be tapered when discontinued to allow recovery of the pituitary-adrenal axis; if therapy has lasted less than 3 weeks, no taper is required for pituitary-adrenal axis recovery.

When tapering glucocorticoids, the patient can be transitioned to a hydrocortisone dose that is 10% to 20% lower than the equivalent, current glucocorticoid dose. The dose can then be decreased by 2.5 to 5 mg of hydrocortisone every 1 to 2 weeks. When tapering with prednisone, taper large doses by 25% to 50% weekly until the patient is on a dose of 5 mg daily and then taper by 1 mg every 1 to 2 weeks. It is difficult to taper dexamethasone due to the limited mg tablets available. The taper can be slower if symptoms such as lightheadedness persist.

After prolonged glucocorticoid use, recovery of the pituitary-adrenal axis should be tested prior to discontinuing glucocorticoid replacement. Specifically, morning serum cortisol should normalize to greater than 11 µg/dL (303.6 nmol/L) when glucocorticoids are withheld for 36 to 48 hours following the taper. Even after endogenous ACTH production has returned, patients may require more time to mount an adequate ACTH response to stress. After discontinuing the glucocorticoid taper, the patient can undergo an ACTH stimulation test (**Table 15**) to document adequate glucocorticoid response to stress. The diagnosis relies on demonstrating a low basal serum cortisol level that does not increase appropriately after stimulation with the ACTH analogue cosyntropin. This is done by measuring early morning (8 AM) serum cortisol. A serum cortisol level less than 3 µg/dL (82.8 nmol/L) is consistent with cortisol deficiency. A normal response is a peak serum cortisol

Handwritten annotations: am cort <3 / + cosyntropin >20 —

TABLE 15. Dynamic Testing for Pituitary Dysfunction

Indication	Test	Technique	Interpretation
ACTH (cortisol) deficiency	ACTH stimulation test	Measure baseline serum cortisol level. Administer 250 µg of synthetic ACTH. Measure cortisol levels at 30 and 60 minutes.	Serum cortisol level >18 µg/dL (496.8 nmol/L) indicates a normal response.
ADH deficiency (DI)	Water deprivation test, followed by desmopressin challenge if indicated	Patient empties bladder, and baseline weight is measured. Measure urine volume and osmolality hourly. Measure serum sodium, osmolality, and weight every 2 hours. The test is stopped when one of the following occurs: - Urine osmolality exceeds 600 mOsm/kg H_2O - Patient has lost 5% of body weight - Urine osmolality is stable for 2-3 h while serum osmolality rises - Plasma osmolality >295 mOsm/kg H_2O - Serum sodium >145 mEq/L (145 mmol/L) Desmopressin challenge if final urine osmolality <600 mOsm/kg H_2O, serum osmolality >295 mOsm/kg H_2O, or serum sodium >145 mEq/L (145 mmol/L): Give desmopressin 1 µg subcutaneously. Measure urine osmolality every 30 minutes for 2 hours.	*Water deprivation test interpretation:* Urine osmolality >600 mOsm/kg H_2O is a normal response to water deprivation, indicating ADH production and peripheral effect are intact. Urine osmolality <600 mOsm/kg H_2O, serum osmolality >295 mOsm/kg H_2O and/or serum sodium >145 mEq/L (145 mmol/L) are diagnostic of DI. *Desmopressin challenge interpretation:* >100% increase in urine osmolality is diagnostic of complete central DI. 0% increase in urine osmolality is diagnostic of complete nephrogenic DI. >50% increase in urine osmolality is diagnostic of partial central DI. <50% increase in urine osmolality is diagnostic of partial nephrogenic DI.
Growth hormone excess (acromegaly)	Glucose tolerance test	75 g oral glucose tolerance test. Measure glucose and GH at 0, 30, 60, 90, 120, and 150 minutes.	GH <0.2 ng/mL (0.2 µg/L) is a normal response. GH ≥1.0 ng/mL (1.0 µg/L) (or ≥0.3 ng/mL [0.3 µg/L] on an ultrasensitive assay) is diagnostic of acromegaly.

ACTH = adrenocorticotropic hormone; ADH = antidiuretic hormone; DI = diabetes insipidus; GH = growth hormone.

Handwritten annotations: UNa very low – dumping water. ; no response ; → give ADH + it corrects (central DI)

greater than 20 µg/dL (552 nmol/L). When the test result is normal, patients no longer require daily cortisol replacement, but should follow "sick day rules" (increasing cortisol replacement dose during illness) for up to a year after cessation of daily cortisol replacement.

Symptoms of secondary cortisol deficiency include weight loss, nausea, vomiting, lightheadedness, hypoglycemia, hypotension, and hyponatremia. Secondary cortisol deficiency is also diagnosed using an ACTH stimulation test. Secondary cortisol deficiency can be life threatening and must be treated with glucocorticoid replacement, often with hydrocortisone, although prednisone or dexamethasone may also be used. Hydrocortisone (15-30 mg/d) should be administered in 2 to 3 divided doses, or hydrocortisone should be dosed 10 to 20 mg in the morning and 5 to 10 mg in the early afternoon.

Patients require stress doses of glucocorticoids when acutely ill, hospitalized, or undergoing the stress of surgery. For moderate physiologic stress (minor or moderate surgery with general anesthesia), hydrocortisone should used (45-75 mg/d orally or intravenously in 3-4 divided doses for 2-3 days). Prednisone (10-20 mg or dexamethasone 2-3 mg/d in 1-2 divided doses) may be used alternatively. For major

physiologic stress (major surgery, trauma, critical illness, or childbirth), hydrocortisone (150-200 mg/d intravenously in 3-4 divided doses; 100 mg/d the next day; taper to baseline in 3-5 days) may be used. An alternative would be dexamethasone (6-8 mg/d intravenously in 2-3 divided doses). If the patient has pituitary apoplexy and urgent/emergent neurosurgery is planned with no time for ACTH-stimulation testing, the patient should empirically be treated with glucocorticoids and then receive an ACTH stimulation test 4 to 8 weeks after surgery. **H**

Thyroid-Stimulating Hormone Deficiency

Thyroid-stimulating hormone (TSH) deficiency leads to secondary or central hypothyroidism. Secondary hypothyroidism is clinically identical to primary hypothyroidism (see Disorders of the Thyroid Gland).

Secondary hypothyroidism is diagnosed by demonstrating a simultaneously inappropriately normal or low TSH and low T_4 (free or total). Patients are treated with levothyroxine replacement in the same manner as primary hypothyroidism; however, the serum TSH cannot be used to monitor and assess for adequacy of thyroid hormone replacement dosing. Instead,

Handwritten annotations: cort <3 (am) / stim <20

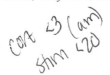

the levothyroxine dose is adjusted based on free T$_4$ levels with the goal of obtaining a value within the normal reference range.

- Patients with secondary cortisol deficiency have isolated glucocorticoid deficiency without mineralocorticoid deficiency; in addition, they do not develop hyperpigmentation or bronzing of the skin because adrenocorticotropic hormone and pro-opiomelanocortin are not hypersecreted.
- Secondary or central hypothyroidism is diagnosed by demonstrating a simultaneously inappropriately normal or low thyroid-stimulating hormone and low thyroxine (T$_4$) (free or total) level.

Gonadotropin Deficiency

The pituitary gland normally secretes LH and FSH in response to GnRH from the hypothalamus. LH and FSH stimulate the secretion of normal male and female sex hormones; LH and FSH deficiency causes hypogonadotropic hypogonadism (see Reproductive Disorders).

Hypogonadotropic hypogonadism may be caused by GnRH deficiency. The most common cause of GnRH deficiency in women is hypothalamic amenorrhea, which is associated with excess exercise, illness, or anorexia. Additional causes of GnRH deficiency include congenital GnRH deficiency and Kallmann syndrome, a condition in which hypothalamic neurons responsible for releasing GnRH fail to migrate into the hypothalamus during embryonic development.

Treatment of hypogonadotropic hypogonadism depends on the goals of therapy and whether the patient desires fertility. Fertility treatment requires replacement of the gonadotropins in men and women. Premenopausal women who do not desire fertility may be treated with estrogen- and progesterone-containing oral contraceptives (after assessment of risk of thromboembolic disease). Treatment of premenopausal hypogonadotropic hypogonadism is recommended to avoid loss of estrogen-dependent bone at a young age, which could lead to osteoporosis. Treatment of postmenopausal hypogonadotropic hypogonadism is not indicated. Men who do not desire fertility may be treated with testosterone replacement therapy (see Reproductive Disorders).

Growth Hormone Deficiency

Growth hormone (GH) is vital for normal linear growth, and deficiency prior to puberty will lead to short stature. At puberty, the epiphyses close, halting linear growth. In adulthood, GH production is necessary for normal physiology but is not as important for growth as during childhood. In adults, GH deficiency causes fatigue, loss of muscle mass, an increased ratio of fatty tissue to lean tissue, and increased risk for osteoporosis.

GH deficiency is often the first hormone deficiency to occur when a patient is developing pituitary insufficiency, but isolated adult-onset GH deficiency is extremely rare, and its clinical significance in adults is debated. Therefore, evaluation for GH deficiency is recommended in patients with at least one known pituitary hormone deficiency. Unfortunately, GH therapy has been used inappropriately as an alternative medication. GH naturally declines with age and does not require replacement. The use of GH does not promote longevity and when used inappropriately can be harmful. Specifically, GH therapy can encourage cancer growth, worsening the disease in a patient with cancer, or promoting growth of an occult, undiagnosed cancer.

Because GH secretion is pulsatile, testing random levels is not diagnostically useful. Therefore, GH deficiency is diagnosed by measurement of IGF-1. A GH deficiency is confirmed by measuring the response of serum GH on a stimulatory test, such as the insulin tolerance test. An insulin tolerance test carries a high risk of severe hypoglycemia, so referral to an endocrinologist for testing is appropriate.

A decision regarding replacement therapy should be made based on that patient's symptoms, goals, and risks in consultation with the patient's endocrinologist. When clinically indicated, GH deficiency is treated with daily subcutaneous GH injections. In an otherwise healthy adult, treatment of GH deficiency can improve quality of life and increase the percentage of lean muscle mass. Also, it can reduce the risk of osteoporosis. However, the risks and benefits of therapy must be carefully considered. Replacement of GH is cost prohibitive for some patients. It is contraindicated in patients with cancer and should not be used in patients with an untreated pituitary tumor due to potential stimulation of tumor growth.

- Isolated adult-onset growth hormone deficiency is extremely rare, and its clinical significance is debated; evaluation for growth hormone deficiency should be reserved for adults with at least one known pituitary hormone deficiency.

Central Diabetes Insipidus

Central diabetes insipidus (DI) results from inadequate production of antidiuretic hormone (ADH) by the posterior pituitary gland. In the presence of ADH, aquaporin water channels are inserted in the collecting tubules and allow water to be reabsorbed. In the absence of ADH, excessive water is excreted by the kidneys. Excretion of more than 3 liters of urine per day is considered polyuric.

The severity of DI varies with the completeness of the deficiency. Patients describe mild to extreme polyuria and corresponding thirst; partial DI is common.

Frank hypernatremia is unusual because patients develop extreme thirst and polydipsia, and with free access to water, can maintain serum sodium in the high normal range. When patients do not drink enough to replace the water lost in the urine, due to poor or absent thirst drive or lack of free access to water, they develop hypernatremia.

In the patient with polyuria, DI is diagnosed with simultaneous laboratory evidence of inability to concentrate urine in the face of elevated serum sodium and osmolality, with inappropriately low urine osmolality. If necessary, a water deprivation test can confirm the diagnosis (see Table 15).

Patients with mild partial DI with an adequate thirst drive and access to water may choose to compensate without hormone replacement therapy, but highly symptomatic polyuria and nocturia that interferes with restful sleep and daily function necessitate treatment. In those requiring treatment, hormone replacement is with desmopressin (1-desamino-8-D-arginine vasopressin, or dDAVP) either intranasally, subcutaneously, or orally. Desmopressin is not absorbed well in the gastrointestinal tract, so oral doses are much higher than intranasal or subcutaneous doses. Most patients with DI require either evening dosing to aid in sleep or twice daily dosing of desmopressin. If ADH is overreplaced, patients will develop water intoxication, volume overload, and hyponatremia. **H**

KEY POINTS

- In the patient with polyuria, diabetes insipidus is diagnosed by clinical symptoms with simultaneous laboratory evidence of inability to concentrate urine with elevated serum sodium and osmolality, and inappropriately low urine osmolality; a water deprivation test can confirm the diagnosis.

- Treatment of central diabetes insipidus is once or twice daily hormone replacement with desmopressin.

Panhypopituitarism

Panhypopituitarism occurs when patients lack all anterior and posterior pituitary hormone production. Panhypopituitarism may be caused by a large or aggressive pituitary tumor or as a complication of surgery. If the pituitary stalk is transected during surgery or as the result of trauma, panhypopituitarism will result acutely. Patients with panhypopituitarism require lifelong replacement of T_4, cortisol, and ADH because these deficiencies can be life-threatening. GH and sex hormones are replaced dependent on each patient's preference, coupled with a discussion of the risks and benefits of therapy. In addition to requiring exogenous gonadotropins to conceive, a reproductive-aged woman with panhypopituitarism will not go into spontaneous labor and will not lactate. These pregnancies are classified as high risk, and obstetric care should be provided by a maternal-fetal specialist.

Patients with panhypopituitarism should wear medical alert identification documenting their panhypopituitarism, specifically noting the need for stress-dose glucocorticoid therapy and desmopressin dosing in emergent situations. **H**

KEY POINT

- Patients with panhypopituitarism require lifelong replacement of thyroxine (T_4), cortisol, and antidiuretic hormone because these deficiencies can be life-threatening.

Pituitary Hormone Excess

Pituitary tumors are called functional when they secrete excessive amounts of hormone. The most common functional pituitary tumor is a prolactinoma. GH and ACTH overproduction by pituitary tumors is important to recognize because the clinical consequences of oversecretion are potentially severe. TSH-secreting tumors cause hyperthyroidism but are extremely rare.

Occasionally, a pituitary tumor can oversecrete more than one hormone, most commonly GH and prolactin, or less commonly, TSH and GH or prolactin.

Hyperprolactinemia and Prolactinoma
Causes
Prolactinomas are pituitary tumors that secrete excessive amounts of prolactin; however, they are not the only cause of hyperprolactinemia (**Table 16**).

The most common cause of hyperprolactinemia is physiologic; prolactin is released during pregnancy and postpartum to cause lactation. Nipple stimulation such as during sex can cause mild hyperprolactinemia (serum prolactin <40 ng/mL [40 µg/L]). Physiologic stress, coitus, and exercise can also increase prolactin levels up to 40 ng/mL (40 µg/L). Nipple piercing can raise prolactin levels above 200 ng/mL (200 µg/L). Clinical breast examination should not raise prolactin levels above the reference range, unless evaluation for milk production is performed, but if desired, palpation of the breast can be deferred until after a serum prolactin level is measured.

Medications are a common cause of hyperprolactinemia (see Table 16). Antipsychotic agents cause hyperprolactinemia due to their antidopaminergic effect that interrupts the inhibition of prolactin by dopamine. Specific agents, such as risperidone or metoclopramide, may raise the prolactin level above 200 ng/mL (200 µg/L). Evaluation for pituitary hypersecretion when a patient is taking a medication known to raise the prolactin level is difficult. When the prolactin level is only mildly elevated (<50 ng/mL [50 µg/L]), it may be reasonable to assume that hyperprolactinemia is a medication side effect. When significantly elevated (>100 ng/mL [100 µg/L]), either the

dopamine inhibits

TABLE 16.	Causes of Hyperprolactinemia	
Physiologic	**Medications**	**Other**
Pregnancy	Antipsychotic agents[a]	Prolactinoma
Lactation	Metoclopramide	Pituitary tumor—stalk compression
Nipple stimulation	Cimetidine	Hypothyroidism
	Verapamil	Cirrhosis
	Methyldopa	Chronic kidney disease
	Opiates	
	Cocaine	

[a]Including risperidone, olanzapine, haloperidol, chlorpromazine, and clomipramine.

medication needs to be withheld to further assess or a pituitary MRI obtained to evaluate for prolactinoma. Caution is warranted when discontinuation of an antipsychotic agent is being considered, and consultation with a psychiatrist is recommended prior to discontinuation.

Another common cause of hyperprolactinemia is primary hypothyroidism. Hypothyroidism can cause diffuse swelling of the pituitary gland that may resemble enlargement due to a pituitary adenoma on imaging. Therefore, a patient with primary hypothyroidism and hyperprolactinemia should be treated with thyroid hormone replacement with retesting of the prolactin level once the TSH has normalized. Further evaluation is indicated if the hyperprolactinemia does not correct when hypothyroidism is treated. If pituitary imaging has noted pituitary enlargement prior to treatment of hypothyroidism, repeat MRI should be obtained when the TSH is normal.

Nonfunctioning pituitary adenomas can also cause hyperprolactinemia by compressing the pituitary stalk and decreasing dopamine inhibition of prolactin secretion. It is important to distinguish between prolactinomas and nonfunctioning pituitary adenomas as the cause of hyperprolactinemia because of different treatment approaches.

Clinical Features and Diagnosis

Physiologically, prolactin induces and regulates lactation. Hence, elevated levels of prolactin cause galactorrhea. Women are more likely to develop galactorrhea than men.

Hyperprolactinemia also causes hypogonadotropic hypogonadism because of negative feedback on GnRH, LH, and FSH by high levels of prolactin. Both men and women present with hypogonadism. Women of reproductive age often present earlier than men because of amenorrhea. They may also have early menopausal symptoms. Symptoms in men are insidious and may go unrecognized for years. Both men and women with hyperprolactinemia are likely to be infertile and are at risk for osteoporosis. Postmenopausal women are already hypogonadal because of ovarian failure; therefore, hyperprolactinemia may have minimal clinical implications in this population. However, the cause of postmenopausal hyperprolactinemia still requires diagnosis because it may be due to a pituitary tumor.

Diagnostic imaging is indicated in situations in which there is unexplained hyperprolactinemia.

The degree of hyperprolactinemia is useful in differentiating prolactinomas from nonfunctioning macroadenomas. In general, large nonfunctioning tumors cause mild serum prolactin elevations (<100 ng/mL [100 μg/L]) from stalk compression. Macroprolactinomas raise serum prolactin levels to greater than 250 ng/mL (250 μg/L). Very large macroprolactinomas may raise prolactin levels greater than 10,000 ng/mL (10,000 μg/L).

Therapy

Patients with microprolactinomas without symptoms of hypogonadism do not require treatment. Symptomatic women with microadenomas may be treated with either oral contraceptive pills (if fertility is not desired) or dopamine agonists. Postmenopausal women with microadenomas do not require treatment. Patients with hypogonadism from medication-induced hyperprolactinemia may be treated with hormone replacement.

Unlike other pituitary tumors, medication rather than surgery is first-line therapy for prolactinomas. Even patients with severe mass effect such as vision loss are treated with medical therapy initially. Rarely, very large tumors or more invasive prolactinomas do not shrink with medical therapy and, also rarely, continue to grow. In these patients, surgery should be considered, followed by radiotherapy if growth recurs or continues. After being debulked, the prolactinoma may respond better to medical therapy.

Prolactinomas are treated with dopamine agonists (DA). The two FDA-approved dopamine agonists are bromocriptine and cabergoline. Dopamine agonists typically decrease the size and hormone production of prolactinomas rapidly. Response to therapy can be monitored by checking serum prolactin levels 1 month after initiating therapy and then every 3 to 4 months. Decreasing serum prolactin usually correlates with decreasing size of the tumor. MRI should be repeated in 1 year for microprolactinomas if the prolactin level normalizes on dopamine agonists. After tumor shrinkage is confirmed, additional MRIs are not necessary unless the serum prolactin level rises. An MRI should be repeated after 3 months of medical therapy for macroprolactinomas, or if prolactin levels are rising on therapy with good medication adherence. MRI should be repeated every 6 to 12 months until the macroprolactinoma is stable on serial studies and the prolactin level is not rising.

Bromocriptine is dosed 1 to 3 times daily, so adherence can be challenging. When initiated, it is associated with orthostasis and lightheadedness, and patients can have dizziness, nausea, and headache during treatment. Cabergoline is much better tolerated and more effective at normalizing prolactin and tumor shrinkage, so it is typically the initial therapy chosen. It is dosed once or twice a week, but typically costs more than bromocriptine.

Therapy may be tapered after the prolactin level has been normal for 2 years, and there is no longer a visible tumor on pituitary MRI. After discontinuing the dopamine agonist, prolactin levels should be followed once a month for 3 months, then every 3 months for the first year, and then annually thereafter; a pituitary MRI should be repeated if the prolactin level rises above normal.

Prolactinomas and Pregnancy

Hyperprolactinemia is a frequent cause of infertility because of the effect on gonadotropin release. DA therapy lowers prolactin, normalizing gonadotropin regulation and allowing normal ovulation. DA therapy should be discontinued when the pregnancy is diagnosed. The pituitary increases in size during normal pregnancy, and prolactinomas can increase in size as well. The risk for significant tumor expansion is negligible in patients with microprolactinomas.

Women with macroprolactinomas are at risk for clinically significant tumor growth or vision compromise during pregnancy. If the tumor is very large or abuts the optic chiasm, patients should be counseled on risk of tumor growth during pregnancy, as well as the risks and benefits of surgical resection of the tumor before pregnancy. DA therapy is sometimes continued during pregnancy if the patient has a history of visual field defect.

Pregnant women with macroprolactinomas should be assessed clinically at least once per trimester and have visual fields tested every trimester or more frequently for vision change. Changes in visual fields or severe headache are indications to proceed with pituitary MRI. If the macroprolactinoma causes mass effect during pregnancy, bromocriptine may be started. If the bromocriptine does not decrease tumor size and reduce symptoms of mass effect, surgical debulking may be necessary.

Normal pregnancy causes hyperprolactinemia, so hyperprolactinemia from prolactinoma does not require treatment during pregnancy. Prolactin levels should not be measured during pregnancy. Postpartum, prolactin levels return to normal within a few months, and lactation becomes nonprolactin mediated.

KEY POINTS

- Prolactinomas, pregnancy and lactation, or medications such as antipsychotic agents are frequent causes of hyperprolactinemia.

- A patient with primary hypothyroidism and hyperprolactinemia should be treated with thyroid hormone replacement with retesting of the prolactin level once the thyroid-stimulating hormone level has normalized.

- Dopamine agonists (bromocriptine and cabergoline) are first-line therapy for symptomatic patients with hyperprolactinemia and prolactinomas.

Acromegaly

Acromegaly is a rare diagnosis that is often missed for years because of the insidious onset and rare presentation in primary care; however, it has very serious implications for a patient's health and longevity and must be diagnosed and treated in as timely a manner as possible.

Causes

Acromegaly is the clinical syndrome that occurs when a pituitary tumor secretes excessive amounts of GH in an adult patient. Prior to puberty, patients with a GH-secreting tumor develop excessive longitudinal growth and gigantism, a term used to indicate excessive growth and height above normal for age. Because epiphyseal growth plates require sex hormones to close, patients with large pituitary tumors causing hypogonadism will not have closure of their growth plates and will continue growth into adulthood.

Clinical Features and Diagnosis in the Adult Patient with Acromegaly

Patients have changes in facial structure such as a prominent brow and jawline, an enlarged skull, a large nose, facial edema, excessive spacing between teeth, and macroglossia. The hands and feet may be disproportionately large. Other manifestations may include arthritis, skin tags, diabetes mellitus, hypertension, colon polyps, thickened skin, and excessive perspiration. Acromegaly can cause severe obstructive sleep apnea because of soft-tissue swelling and macroglossia. Additionally, it can result in heart disease, including left ventricular hypertrophy, cardiomyopathy, valvular heart disease, arrhythmia and diastolic heart failure. Increased rates of cancer are observed in acromegaly, including colon, esophageal, and gastric adenocarcinomas; thyroid cancer; and melanoma. Acromegaly increases mortality, likely due to cardiovascular disease, diabetes, sleep apnea, and cancer. Age-appropriate testing for these conditions should occur for the lifetime of the patient with acromegaly.

Acromegaly is diagnosed biochemically. Because GH is pulsatile throughout the day, it is not useful for diagnosis, so measurement of serum IGF-1 is used instead. Excess GH is confirmed with an oral glucose tolerance test (see Table 15) because glucose normally suppresses GH levels to less than 1 ng/mL (1 µg/L). GH levels greater than 1 ng/mL (1 µg/L) are diagnostic of GH excess. A pituitary MRI should be obtained once GH excess is confirmed biochemically. Consultation with an endocrinologist is recommended if IGF-1 is elevated.

Treatment

Treatment of acromegaly is transsphenoidal tumor resection; surgery is the only treatment that is potentially curative. In many instances, cure with surgery is not possible and additional therapy is necessary to treat the residual GH excess and tumor.

Remission is achieved when IGF-1 levels are within the normal reference range for age and the response of GH to a glucose tolerance test is normal. Patients not achieving remission require medication to decrease GH levels and the long-term effects of GH excess. The initial therapy of choice is injectable somatostatin analogues to inhibit GH secretion. If a patient fails to benefit from somatostatin analogue treatment, high-dose dopamine agonist therapy is marginally effective when the tumor co-secretes prolactin. If IGF-1 remains elevated, pegvisomant, a GH receptor blocker, is used. Pegvisomant effectively lowers IGF-1 levels, but patients on pegvisomant have risk of tumor growth because the medication works in the peripheral tissues as an antagonist to GH and does not decrease GH production by the tumor.

Stereotactic radiosurgery (gamma knife) may be offered to increase the chance of remission or cure. External beam radiation carries a high risk of causing pituitary insufficiency, but the risk is decreased when stereotactic radiosurgery is used.

When acromegaly is in remission, MRI and hormone testing should be completed annually. When the pituitary tumor is stable but the IGF-1 level is elevated, MRI should be repeated annually and treatment should be altered until the IGF-1 declines.

> **KEY POINTS**
> - Acromegaly occurs when a pituitary tumor secretes excessive amounts of growth hormone in an adult patient resulting in changes in facial structure, an enlarged skull, a large nose, facial edema, excessive spacing between teeth, macroglossia, and disproportionately large hands and feet.
> - Treatment of acromegaly is transsphenoidal tumor resection; however, in some patients, adjuvant radiation therapy or medical therapy, such as injectable somatostatin analogues, is needed for residual disease.

Gonadotropin-Producing Adenomas

Gonadotropin-producing pituitary adenomas are typically asymptomatic and are treated similarly to nonfunctioning adenomas because they either do not secrete functional gonadotropins or do not secrete enough FSH or LH to produce a clinical syndrome. Often, the diagnosis is made postoperatively, based on histopathologic staining of surgical pathology specimens.

Thyroid-Stimulating Hormone-Secreting Tumors

TSH-secreting tumors are extremely rare. These tumors may co-secrete TSH and prolactin or GH. TSH-secreting tumors cause hyperthyroidism. Patients with TSH-secreting tumors have either an inappropriately normal or a high TSH level with a simultaneous elevation of T_4 and T_3 levels. They present with identical symptoms associated with non-TSH-mediated thyrotoxicosis (see Disorders of the Thyroid Gland). After biochemical proof of TSH excess is obtained, pituitary imaging is recommended to confirm a pituitary mass. Neurosurgery is first-line therapy, but patients often require additional medical therapy with either somatostatin analogues or dopamine agonists.

Excess Antidiuretic Hormone Secretion

The syndrome of inappropriate ADH secretion (SIADH) causes water retention and hyponatremia. Central nervous system pathology such as stroke, hemorrhage, trauma, or infection can cause SIADH because of the excessive release of hypothalamic and pituitary ADH. Also, transient SIADH is a common complication of pituitary surgery, occurring in about one third of patients approximately 3 to 10 days after surgery (see MKSAP17 Nephrology).

Cushing Disease

Cushing disease is the term used to indicate excess cortisol production due to an ACTH-secreting pituitary adenoma.

Cushing syndrome refers to hypercortisolism from any cause, exogenous or endogenous, ACTH-dependent or not. The most common cause of endogenous Cushing syndrome is Cushing disease. When undiagnosed, Cushing disease is associated with devastating long-term morbidity such as diabetes, morbid obesity, hypertension, infertility, and osteoporosis.

The initial step in evaluation for Cushing disease is to seek biochemical evidence of hypercortisolism (see Disorders of the Adrenal Glands).

Once ACTH-dependent Cushing syndrome is confirmed biochemically, a pituitary MRI should be obtained. If no pituitary tumor or a tumor less than 6 mm is visualized on MRI, an 8-mg dexamethasone suppression test is used to differentiate Cushing disease from an ectopic source of ACTH. Ectopic ACTH production from a nonpituitary tumor (most often lung, pancreas, or thymus carcinomas) is very uncommon.

Dexamethasone is administered at 11 PM, and cortisol is tested at 8 AM. A pituitary source of ACTH will respond to negative feedback from high doses of dexamethasone, suppressing cortisol to less than 5 µg/dL (138 nmol/L), while an ectopic source of ACTH will not have suppressible cortisol. However, this test has low sensitivity (88%) and specificity (57%) for Cushing disease, so intrapetrosal sinus sampling (IPSS) is often recommended before exploratory pituitary surgery. In IPSS, a catheter is threaded through the petrosal sinus, and ACTH levels in the sinus are compared with those in the periphery after the administration of corticotropin-releasing hormone (CRH). A central to peripheral gradient greater than 2.0 before CRH or greater than 3.0 after CRH is diagnostic of Cushing disease (95% sensitivity, 93% specificity). Imaging of the chest and abdomen is indicated in patients with a suspected ectopic source of ACTH.

Treatment

Cushing disease is treated by transsphenoidal pituitary tumor resection, which may be curative. Endogenous ACTH production in the remaining normal pituitary gland will be suppressed after removal of the tumor due to long-standing hypercortisolism, so patients with successful surgical treatment will have acute ACTH deficiency and require glucocorticoid replacement. It may take up to 1 year for endogenous ACTH production to return to normal, and sometimes the hypothalamic-pituitary-adrenal axis does not recover. After successful resection, Cushing disease can recur, and patients must be monitored annually for several years, and then less frequently, or sooner if symptoms of hypercortisolism recur.

If surgical cure is not achieved, patients may be offered pituitary radiation or medical therapy. Medical options include inhibitors of adrenal enzyme synthesis of cortisol, ketoconazole, or metyrapone; the dopamine agonist, cabergoline; or the somatostatin analogue, pasireotide. Medical cure of Cushing disease has a relatively low success rate, but hypercortisolism symptom control is an achievable goal in all patients with endogenous Cushing syndrome.

CONT.

In patients who do not benefit from surgical treatment and who have an inadequate response to medical treatment, bilateral adrenalectomy to remove the target of ACTH stimulation is an option. However, these patients will require lifelong glucocorticoid and mineralocorticoid replacement. **H**

KEY POINTS

- Cushing disease refers to excess cortisol production due to an adrenocorticotropic hormone (ACTH)-secreting pituitary adenoma; Cushing syndrome refers to hypercortisolism from any cause, exogenous or endogenous, ACTH-dependent or not.

- Cushing disease is treated by transsphenoidal pituitary tumor resection; after surgery glucocorticoid replacement therapy will be required at least transiently while the hypothalamic-pituitary-adrenal axis recovers endogenous function.

Disorders of the Adrenal Glands

Adrenal Anatomy and Physiology

Located just superior to each kidney, the paired adrenal glands consist of an outer cortex and an inner medulla that are distinct in embryologic origin and endocrine function. The adrenal cortex is composed of three zones: the zona (outer) glomerulosa, zona (middle) fasciculata, and zona (inner) reticularis. Within these zones corticosteroid hormones are synthesized from cholesterol by cytochrome P450 enzymes. Aldosterone, the principal mineralocorticoid hormone, is produced in the zona glomerulosa. Aldosterone production is triggered by an increase in the extracellular potassium concentration and by activation of aldosterone synthase through the renin-angiotensin-aldosterone pathway. Upon binding to type 1 mineralocorticoid receptors (MR) in the kidney, aldosterone promotes potassium wasting and sodium retention, which leads to an increase in intravascular volume and consequently blood pressure.

The zona fasciculata is the main site of glucocorticoid synthesis. Production of cortisol, the principal glucocorticoid, is stimulated by adrenocorticotropic hormone (ACTH) secretion from the anterior pituitary. Cortisol secretion varies according to the circadian rhythm with relatively little secretion overnight, peak levels in the early morning, and smaller oscillations throughout the day. Cortisol attenuates inflammatory responses and contributes to glucose homeostasis by promoting lipolysis, hepatic gluconeogenesis, and insulin resistance. Physical stress (for example, critical illness) stimulates increased cortisol secretion, which enhances vascular smooth muscle tone and responsiveness to endogenous vasoconstrictors, thereby augmenting blood pressure.

Synthesis of adrenal androgens, dehydroepiandrosterone (DHEA) and its sulfate (DHEAS), and androstenedione, occurs primarily in the zona reticularis and is regulated by ACTH. Although the adrenal androgens themselves have minimal intrinsic androgenic activity, they are converted peripherally to testosterone and dihydrotestosterone. Unlike glucocorticoids and mineralocorticoids, deficiencies of adrenal androgens are not typically recognized due to parallel production of gonadal androgens.

The adrenal medulla and extra-adrenal sites of the sympathetic nervous system consist of chromaffin cells, which synthesize catecholamine hormones from the amino acid tyrosine (**Figure 4**). Catecholamines are stored within chromaffin granules, which release their contents in response to stress. Although catecholamine excess produces disease, hypofunction of the adrenal medulla does not because of redundancy of catecholamine production throughout the sympathetic nervous system. Norepinephrine is synthesized in the adrenal medulla and the extra-adrenal sites of the sympathetic nervous system. It causes vasoconstriction due to preferential binding to α-receptors. Epinephrine is almost exclusively produced in the adrenal medulla. It binds predominantly to β-receptors, and thus has positive effects on cardiac inotropy and chronotropy, produces peripheral vasodilation, and increases plasma glucose levels in response to hypoglycemia.

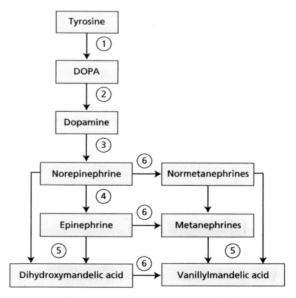

FIGURE 4. Catecholamine hormones are produced in the adrenal medulla and sympathetic ganglia. The pathways of synthesis and degradation are shown. Excessive catecholamine secretion can occur with pheochromocytomas and paraganglionomas.
1 = Tyrosine hydroxylase
2 = DOPA decarboxylase
3 = Dopamine β-hydroxylase
4 = Phenylethanolamine N-methyltransferase (PNMT)
5 = Monoamine oxidase (MAO)
6 = Catechol-O-methyltransferase (COMT)

Adrenal Hormone Excess

Cushing Syndrome

Cushing syndrome (CS) is a rare disorder affecting two to three persons per million per year that results from elevated levels of cortisol. Poor suppressibility of cortisol with dexamethasone and loss of normal diurnal variation in cortisol secretion are seen. Without treatment, it is associated with high morbidity and mortality.

However, iatrogenic hypercortisolism from the administration of exogenous oral, inhaled, intra-articular, or topical glucocorticoids is often seen in clinical practice and is the most common cause of CS overall. The pharmacokinetics and relative potencies of synthetic oral glucocorticoids are shown in **Table 17**. The sustained administration of any synthetic glucocorticoid above the normal physiologic cortisol requirement can result in iatrogenic CS and hypothalamic-pituitary-adrenal (HPA) axis suppression, but is more likely to occur the longer the half-life of the drug. Doses equivalent to prednisone 5 mg/d or less are unlikely to cause clinically significant HPA axis suppression, while those in excess of 10 to 20 mg/d commonly do after 3 weeks or more of consecutive use.

Endogenous CS can result from ACTH-dependent and ACTH-independent causes. Cushing disease, which results from the autonomous secretion of ACTH by a corticotroph adenoma of the pituitary gland, is the cause of CS in more than two thirds of patients (see Disorders of the Pituitary Gland). Ectopic ACTH secretion by carcinomas and carcinoid tumors (usually bronchial origin) is less common, accounting for 10% to 15% of cases, while ectopic corticotropin-releasing hormone (CRH) production is rare. The most common ACTH-independent etiologies of CS are adrenal adenomas and carcinomas, which collectively account for approximately 20% of CS cases.

CS must be differentiated from other disorders and clinical states that are associated with physiologic hypercortisolism (pseudo-Cushing syndrome). Causes of pseudo-Cushing syndrome include severe obesity, polycystic ovary syndrome, pregnancy, anorexia nervosa, depression, alcoholism, and extreme physical stress, as in the setting of infection.

Clinical manifestations of CS are listed in **Table 18**. Clinical findings that are highly specific for CS include centripetal obesity, facial plethora, abnormal fat deposition in the supraclavicular or dorsocervical ("buffalo hump") areas, and wide (>1 cm) violaceous striae (**Figure 5**). It is important to initiate evaluation for CS in patients who have specific signs and symptoms of CS, rather than in patients who are diffusely obese, have nonpathologic striae, and are having trouble losing weight because endogenous CS is such a rare condition with a costly evaluation algorithm.

Biochemical testing is used to establish the diagnosis of CS. It is critical that the biochemical diagnosis is firmly established prior to any imaging studies due to the relatively high prevalence of clinically insignificant pituitary and adrenal nodules. At least two first-line tests should be diagnostically abnormal before the diagnosis is confirmed. Initial tests include the overnight low-dose dexamethasone suppression test (LDST), 24-hour urine free cortisol (UFC), and late-night (LN) salivary cortisol. All three tests have similar diagnostic utility, but the LDST or LN salivary cortisol tests are more convenient. The 24-hour UFC and LN salivary cortisol tests should be performed at least twice to ensure reproducibility of results. Because the secretion of cortisol is pulsatile, measurement of random serum cortisol is neither sensitive nor specific for the diagnosis of CS. An algorithm to establish the diagnosis of CS is shown in **Figure 6**. Referral to an endocrinologist is indicated if two initial tests are abnormal.

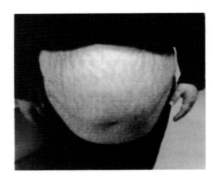

FIGURE 5. Wide violaceous striae are seen on the abdomen of a patient with Cushing syndrome. Striae larger than 1 cm in width are highly specific for hypercortisolism.

TABLE 17. Dose Equivalence and Relative Potencies of Common Synthetic Oral Glucocorticoids				
Synthetic Glucocorticoid	**Equivalent Replacement Dose (mg)[a]**	**Biologic Half-Life (hours)**	**Relative Anti-Inflammatory Potency[b]**	**Relative Mineralocorticoid Potency[c]**
Hydrocortisone	20	8-12	1	1/125
Prednisolone/prednisone	5	18-36	4	1/156
Methylprednisolone	4	18-36	5	0
Dexamethasone	0.75	36-54	25-50	0

[a]Denotes common glucocorticoid dosing for primary adrenal failure equivalent to hydrocortisone, 20 mg.

[b]Anti-inflammatory potency relative to hydrocortisone.

[c]Mineralocorticoid potency relative to fludrocortisone.

TABLE 18. Clinical Features of Cushing Syndrome

Specific Findings	Less Specific Findings	Associated Conditions[a]
Centripetal obesity	Easy bruising	Osteoporosis
Facial plethora	Excessive skin fragility	Hypertension
Supraclavicular fat pads	Proximal muscle weakness	Diabetes mellitus
Dorsocervical fat pads	Impaired memory	Obesity
Wide violaceous striae	Temporal balding[b]	Depression
	Hirsutism (in women)[b]	Hypokalemia
	Menstrual abnormalities[b]	Nephrolithiasis
		VTE/PE

PE = pulmonary embolism; VTE = venous thromboembolism.

[a]Medical disorders that may be seen in association with but are not specific for Cushing syndrome.

[b]Features of androgen excess seen with pituitary corticotroph adenoma or adrenocortical carcinoma.

In the standard LDST, dexamethasone (0.5 mg) is administered every 6 hours for 48 hours and serum cortisol is measured at 9 AM. In the overnight LDST, 1 mg of dexamethasone is administered at 11 PM or midnight, and serum cortisol is measured the next morning at 8 AM. With either test, serum cortisol will typically be suppressed to less than 2 μg/dL (55 nmol/L). Standard assays measure total serum cortisol, or that which is bound to cortisol-binding globulin (CBG) and other proteins. Therefore the LDST should not be performed when CBG is likely to be abnormal, such as with malnutrition, cirrhosis, the nephrotic syndrome, and hyperestrogenemia (oral contraceptive pills or pregnancy). There is no clear association between dexamethasone responses and BMI or weight, and therefore the LDST may be used similarly in the obese population. The LDST is best avoided in patients taking medications that could accelerate dexamethasone metabolism, such as antiepileptic drugs (phenytoin, phenobarbital, and carbamazepine), rifampin, or pioglitazone. Concomitant measurement of serum dexamethasone can confirm altered dexamethasone metabolism and patient adherence.

Measuring 24-hour UFC circumvents problems related to cortisol pulsatility and binding protein abnormalities. The test should be performed at least twice to ensure accuracy. To confirm adequate collection, 24-hour urine creatinine is also measured (normal range, 20-25 mg/kg/24 h [177-221 mmol/kg/24 h] in men; 15-20 mg/kg/24 h [133-177 mmol/L/24 h] in women). A test is considered abnormal when UFC exceeds the upper limit of the normal range of the assay (45 μg/24 h [124 nmol/24 h]), while values greater than 3 times normal are diagnostic of CS. Less marked elevations are seen with pseudo-Cushing syndrome and polyuria. A falsely low UFC can occur in chronic kidney disease and when CS is subclinical or mild.

The LN salivary cortisol test is performed between 11 PM and midnight. The normal evening nadir in cortisol secretion is lost in patients with CS, while it is preserved in patients with pseudo-Cushing syndrome. Both emotional and physical stress (for example, exercise) can cause a physiologic increase of salivary cortisol. False-positive results are seen with

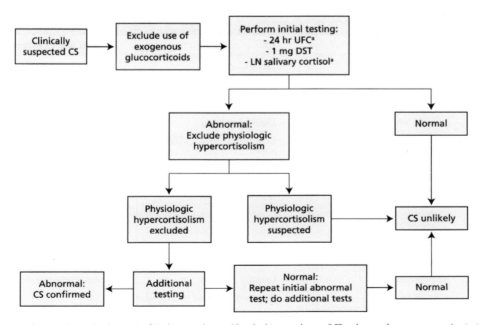

FIGURE 6. Algorithm to confirm or rule out the diagnosis of Cushing syndrome. CS = Cushing syndrome; DST = dexamethasone suppression test; LN salivary cortisol = late-night salivary cortisol; UFC = urine free cortisol.

[a]Must be performed at least twice.

cigarette smoking or use of chewing tobacco. LN salivary cortisol testing should not be performed in patients with erratic sleep schedules (for example, shift-workers).

After CS has been confirmed biochemically, further testing is required to distinguish ACTH-dependent or -independent causes, and consultation with an endocrinologist is recommended. The first step is to measure plasma ACTH on two separate occasions. With adrenal (ACTH-independent) CS, plasma ACTH is usually less than 5 pg/mL (1.1 pmol/L), whereas values greater than 20 pg/mL (4.4 pmol/L) are typically seen with ACTH-dependent causes. Plasma ACTH values of 5 to 20 pg/mL (1.1-4.4 pmol/L) are nondiagnostic but are more likely to be seen with ACTH-dependent disorders. For a discussion of the evaluation and management of ACTH-dependent CS, see Disorders of the Pituitary Gland.

The next step in the evaluation of ACTH-independent CS is with imaging of the adrenal glands, such as dedicated adrenal imaging with thin-section CT or MRI. Both studies have equal sensitivity; however, MRI is more costly. Adrenal adenomas and carcinomas can usually be distinguished from one another radiographically (**Table 19**). Surgery is considered first-line treatment for adrenal adenomas and nonmetastatic adrenocortical carcinomas (ACCs). When surgery is delayed for patients with overt CS, adrenal enzyme inhibitors (metyrapone, ketoconazole, and etomidate) can be used to reduce cortisol levels and decrease the risk of complications, such as opportunistic infections and cardiovascular events. The management of ACC is discussed elsewhere (see Adrenocortical Carcinoma).

Following adrenalectomy, patients with adrenal CS will often develop acute adrenal insufficiency because of HPA axis suppression and contralateral adrenal atrophy from long-standing elevated cortisol levels. All patients should therefore be treated with stress-dose glucocorticoids during the perioperative period and continued on physiologic replacement until HPA axis recovery has been confirmed. Following successful surgery, the physical changes associated with CS can take up to 1 year to resolve.

KEY POINTS

- Cushing syndrome results from endogenous hypercortisolism or exogenous exposure to glucocorticoids; it is associated with poor suppressibility of endogenous cortisol production with oral dexamethasone.

- The most common cause of Cushing syndrome is the administration of exogenous glucocorticoid therapy for another medical condition.

- Initial tests for Cushing syndrome include the overnight low-dose dexamethasone suppression test, 24-hour urine free cortisol, and late-night salivary cortisol.

Pheochromocytomas and Paragangliomas

Paragangliomas are tumors composed of chromaffin cells. Approximately 80% are intra-adrenal (pheochromocytomas); the rest originate from extra-adrenal sympathetic or parasympathetic paraganglia. The most common location for extra-adrenal sympathetic paragangliomas is the abdomen, whereas parasympathetic paragangliomas are usually found in the head and neck. Pheochromocytomas and extra-adrenal sympathetic paragangliomas almost always secrete catecholamines (norepinephrine, epinephrine, dopamine); however, head and neck parasympathetic paragangliomas almost never do.

TABLE 19.	Typical Imaging Characteristics of Adrenal Masses		
Adrenal Mass	**Overall**	**CT**	**MRI Signal Intensity**[a]
Adrenal adenoma	Diameter <4 cm	Density <10 HU	Isointense on T2-weighted images
	Homogeneous enhancement[b]	Contrast washout >50% (10 min)	
	Round, clear margins		
Adrenocortical carcinoma	Usually >4 cm	Density >10 HU	Hyperintense on T2-weighted images
	Heterogeneous enhancement[b]	Contrast washout <50% (10 min)	
	Irregular margins		
	Calcifications, necrosis		
Pheochromocytoma	Variable size	Density >10 HU	Hyperintense on T2-weighted images
	Heterogeneous enhancement[b], cystic areas	Contrast washout <50% (10 min)	
	Round, clear margins		
	Can be bilateral		
Metastases	Variable margins	Density >10 HU	Hyperintense on T2-weighted images
	Can be bilateral	Contrast washout <50% (10 min)	

HU = Hounsfield units (measure of radiodensity compared with water).

[a]Signal intensity as compared with liver.

[b]Enhancement following intravenous contrast administration.

Although catecholamine-secreting tumors are rare overall, they are found in 0.5% of patients with hypertension, and pheochromocytomas account for 5% of adrenal incidentalomas (see Incidentally Noted Adrenal Masses). Most pheochromocytomas secrete norepinephrine, resulting in episodic or sustained hypertension. Orthostatic hypotension can also be seen and likely reflects low plasma volume. In addition to the classic triad of diaphoresis, headache, and tachycardia, common symptoms include palpitations, tremor, pallor, and anxiety. Less common features are papilledema, diabetes mellitus, and cardiomyopathy. Approximately 10% of pheochromocytomas and 20% to 50% of paragangliomas are malignant.

One third of pheochromocytomas and paragangliomas occur in the context of a genetic disorder. Pheochromocytomas are seen with multiple endocrine neoplasia (MEN) syndromes type 2A and 2B (**Table 20**), neurofibromatosis type 1, and von Hippel-Lindau syndrome (VHL). Paragangliomas and, less frequently, pheochromocytomas can occur with familial paraganglioma syndrome mutations, some of which are associated with high rates of malignancy.

The diagnosis of pheochromocytoma and paraganglioma is based on confirmation of the excessive secretion of catecholamines or their metabolites, as measured in the plasma or urine. Evaluation is recommended, if clinically suspected, in the evaluation of an incidentally noted adrenal mass or in the setting of hereditary pheochromocytoma or paraganglioma syndromes. The sensitivity of plasma free metanephrines is the highest of any screening test (96%-100%); however, its specificity is relatively low (85%-89%). Therefore, plasma free metanephrines will reliably exclude a pheochromocytoma when negative, but further testing is needed to confirm the diagnosis unless the result is markedly abnormal (above 4 times the upper limit of normal). The sensitivity and specificity of 24-hour urine fractionated metanephrines and catecholamines are 91% to 98%. Due to the lower frequency of false-positive results, 24-hour urine measurements are recommended when the pre-test probability of disease is relatively low (adrenal mass without typical radiographic appearance), while measurement of plasma free metanephrines is preferred when clinical suspicion is higher (known hereditary syndrome). Referral to an endocrinologist is recommended when biochemical testing is abnormal.

Many medications and other substances cause falsely high levels of plasma and urine catecholamines or metanephrines (**Table 21**); therefore, discontinuation of these agents before testing is recommended. If a catecholamine-secreting tumor is strongly suspected in a critically ill hospitalized patient, CT or MRI of the abdomen is the preferred initial test because biochemical testing cannot be interpreted reliably in this setting.

Following the biochemical diagnosis of pheochromocytoma or catecholamine-secreting paraganglioma, radiographic localization is needed. Because most catecholamine-secreting tumors are located in the abdomen, CT or MRI of the abdomen and pelvis is the best initial study. If negative, iodine 123 (^{123}I)-metaiodobenzylguanidine (MIBG) scanning can be performed. Adjunctive diagnostic tests are CT or MRI of the chest or head and neck region.

When multiple tumors or malignant pheochromocytomas or paragangliomas are suspected, MIBG scanning should be performed preoperatively. However, for identification of metastatic disease, fluorine 18 (^{18}F)-fluorodeoxyglucose (FDG) PET scanning is superior to other diagnostic tests.

Preoperative pharmacologic treatment is mandatory for pheochromocytomas and paragangliomas to prevent life-threatening cardiovascular complications related to the massive release of catecholamines during surgery. Preoperative blockade of α-adrenoceptors, usually with phenoxybenzamine, is first-line medical therapy. The dosage is titrated to achieve a blood pressure below 130/80 mm Hg seated and greater than 90 mm Hg (systolic) standing. Commonly used but non-FDA approved alternatives include calcium channel blockers and selective α$_1$-blockers (terazosin or doxazosin). β-Adrenoceptor blockers (metoprolol or propranolol) are

TABLE 20. Multiple Endocrine Neoplasm Syndromes			
Type	**Mutation**	**Most Common Feature**	**Associated Features**
1	*MEN1* (inheritance of one mutated allele with somatic mutation in other allele leads to neoplasia)	Parathyroid adenoma (often multiple)	Pancreatic islet cell and enteric tumors (gastrinoma, insulinoma most common)
			Pituitary adenoma
			Other (carcinoid tumors, adrenocortical adenoma)
2A	*RET* (exon 11, codon 634[a])	Medullary thyroid carcinoma	Pheochromocytoma (often multifocal)
			Parathyroid hyperplasia
2B	*RET* (exon 16, codon 918[a])	Medullary thyroid carcinoma	Pheochromocytoma (often multifocal)
			Mucosal neuroma
			Gastrointestinal ganglioneuroma
			Marfanoid body habitus

[a]Most common mutation observed.

TABLE 21. Substances Associated with False-Positive Biochemical Testing for Pheochromocytoma

Drug Class	Medication/Substance
Analgesics	Acetaminophen
Antiemetics	Prochlorperazine
Antihypertensives	Phenoxybenzamine[a]
Psychiatric medications	Antipsychotics
	Buspirone
	Monoamine oxidase inhibitors
	Tricyclic antidepressants[a]
Stimulants	Amphetamines
	Cocaine
	Caffeine
Other agents	Levodopa
	Decongestants (pseudoephedrine)
	Reserpine
Withdrawal	Clonidine
	Ethanol
	Illicit drugs

[a]Most likely to cause false-positive results.

added later to treat reflex tachycardia, but should never be started before adequate α-blockade has been achieved due to the risk of hypertensive crisis from unopposed α-receptor stimulation. A heart rate of 60 to 70/min seated and 70 to 80/min standing can be targeted in most patients.

Because it is associated with fewer surgical complications and shorter postoperative hospital stays, laparoscopic adrenalectomy is preferred for pheochromocytoma except in the case of large or malignant tumors, when open adrenalectomy is required. Following the surgical removal of a catecholamine-secreting tumor, large-volume intravenous crystalloid is administered to counter hypotension. Vasopressors (for example, norepinephrine) are sometimes required. Long-term follow-up is needed for pheochromocytomas and paragangliomas due to difficulty distinguishing benign from malignant tumors. Metastases have been reported up to 20 years after diagnosis. In addition to routine clinical surveillance, annual measurement of plasma or urine metanephrines is indicated to assess for recurrent or metastatic disease. Metastatic disease is managed with additional surgery, iodine 131 (^{131}I)-labeled MIBG therapy, chemotherapy, and/or radiotherapy. Cure is not possible unless all disease can be surgically resected.

KEY POINTS

- Pheochromocytomas are seen with multiple endocrine neoplasia (MEN) syndromes type 2A and 2B, neurofibromatosis type 1, and von Hippel-Lindau syndrome.

(Continued)

KEY POINTS *(continued)*

- When clinical suspicion of pheochromocytoma or paraganglioma is low, measurement of 24-hour urine fractionated metanephrines and catecholamines are the tests of choice because of their high specificity (low false-positive rates); when clinical suspicion is high, measuring plasma free metanephrines is preferred due to its greater sensitivity.

- Preoperative α-adrenergic blockade is first-line medical therapy for pheochromocytomas and paragangliomas; β-adrenoceptor blockers (metoprolol or propranolol) are added after α-blockade to treat reflex tachycardia.

- Pheochromocytomas and paragangliomas require lifelong surveillance for recurrence with annual plasma free metanephrine measurement.

Primary Hyperaldosteronism

Primary hyperaldosteronism (PA) results from the autonomous secretion of excessive aldosterone. PA is relatively common, occurring in approximately 10% of patients with hypertension. Additional signs of PA include hypokalemia and metabolic alkalosis. Without treatment, excess cardiovascular morbidity and mortality are seen.

Aldosterone-producing adrenocortical adenomas (APA; aldosteronomas) cause approximately 40% of PA, whereas nearly all other cases are due to bilateral adrenal hyperplasia. Unilateral adrenal hyperplasia and aldosterone-secreting adrenocortical carcinomas (ACCs) are rare. Familial hyperaldosteronism is also uncommon.

Testing for PA should be considered in all patients with difficult to control hypertension. It should also be performed in patients with hypertension and an incidentally noted adrenal mass or spontaneous or diuretic-induced hypokalemia. A number of disorders can mimic PA clinically; however, the results of biochemical testing will differ. Examples include secondary hyperaldosteronism (renal artery stenosis or renin-secreting tumors), autosomal dominant pseudoaldosteronism (Liddle syndrome), CS, certain forms of congenital adrenal hyperplasia (CAH), and licorice-induced hypermineralocorticoidism.

Initial screening for PA is with the simultaneous measurement of midmorning ambulatory plasma renin activity (PRA) and plasma aldosterone concentration (PAC), in a volume replete normokalemic patient. Testing is positive if PAC is frankly elevated (>15 ng/dL [414 pmol/L]), PRA is suppressed, and PAC/PRA ratio is greater than 20. Many medications, including common antihypertensive agents, can affect measurements of PAC, PRA, or both (**Table 22**). However, because patients undergoing screening often have drug-resistant hypertension, discontinuing all potentially offending medications can be unsafe. Stopping mineralocorticoid receptor antagonists (spironolactone and eplerenone) for 4 to 6 weeks prior to testing is recommended. Diuretics should also be discontinued prior to testing to assure euvolemia. Most other medications

TABLE 22. The Effect of Commonly Prescribed Medications on Measurements of Plasma Renin Activity and Plasma Aldosterone Concentration

Effect on Test Results	Medication Class	PRA	PAC	PAC/ PRA
False-Positive	α-Adrenoceptor agonist	↓↓	↓	↑
	β-Adrenoceptor blocker	↓↓	↓	↑
	Direct renin inhibitor	↓	↓	↑
	NSAID	↓↓	↓	↑
False-Negative	ACE inhibitor/ARB	↑↑	↓	↓
	Dihydropyridine CCB	↑	↓	↓
	Diuretic[a]	↑↑	↑	↓
	Mineralocorticoid receptor antagonist	↑↑	↑	↓
	SSRI		↑	↓

ARB = angiotensin receptor antagonist; CCB = calcium channel blocker; PAC = plasma aldosterone concentration; PRA = plasma renin activity; SSRI = selective serotonin reuptake inhibitor.

[a]Both potassium-sparing (amiloride) and potassium-wasting (hydrochlorothiazide) diuretics.

CONT.

can be continued, but results must be interpreted in context. For example, if PRA is suppressed despite treatment with an ACE inhibitor or angiotensin receptor blocker, PA is likely. If results are difficult to interpret, repeat testing after eliminating potential interfering medications is advised. Verapamil, hydralazine, and α-blockers (doxazosin) can be substituted for blood pressure control if necessary. Referral to an endocrinologist is recommended when screening tests are abnormal.

Confirmatory testing is performed except when initial testing is diagnostic for PA, as in cases of spontaneous hypoka-

lemia with undetectable PRA and PAC greater than 30 ng/dL (828 pmol/L). Confirmatory tests include oral and intravenous salt loading and the fludrocortisone suppression and captopril challenge tests (**Table 23**).

Once the diagnosis of PA has been confirmed biochemically, radiographic localization with abdominal CT is indicated. CT is recommended over MRI in most cases due to similar efficacy and lower cost. Adrenal hyperplasia and adenomas can often be visualized and adrenocortical carcinoma can be ruled out. Adrenal vein sampling (AVS) is needed in most patients to determine the source of aldosterone secretion when imaging is unrevealing and to confirm lateralization when imaging demonstrates an adrenal adenoma. AVS is especially important in older patients (40 years and older) because of a higher frequency of nonfunctioning adrenal incidentalomas. AVS should be performed at experienced centers only.

The goals of treatment include improvement in blood pressure (resolution of hypertension is unlikely), normalization of serum potassium (this is very likely), and reduction in plasma aldosterone because hyperaldosteronemia is associated with a blood pressure–independent increase in cardiovascular events. The treatment of choice for PA due to APA or unilateral adrenal hyperplasia is laparoscopic adrenalectomy.

For patients with bilateral adrenal hyperplasia or those with unilateral causes of PA who are not surgical candidates, medical therapy with a mineralocorticoid antagonist is indicated. Spironolactone is the most commonly used medication due to its proven efficacy and cost-effectiveness. Eplerenone is less likely to cause side effects (gynecomastia in men and menstrual irregularities in women) because of greater mineralocorticoid receptor selectivity. Amiloride is a potassium-sparing diuretic that blocks the aldosterone-sensitive sodium channel. Use of amiloride in PA is second-line therapy because of lower efficacy. ▣

TABLE 23. Laboratory Testing Used in the Diagnosis of Hyperaldosteronism

Test	Details	Positive If...
Captopril challenge test	Administer: Captopril 25-50 mg orally after the patient has been seated for 1 hour	PAC remains elevated and PRA suppressed
	Measure: PAC, PRA, and cortisol at 0 and 1 or 2 hours while seated	(Normal response is suppression of PAC by >30%)
Fludrocortisone suppression test	Administer: Fludrocortisone 0.5 mg orally every 6 hours for 4 days along with sodium and potassium supplementation	PAC >6 ng/dL (165.6 pmol/L)
		PRA <1 ng/mL/h (1 μg/L/h)
	Measure: Serum cortisol at 7 and 10 AM, and PAC and PRA at 10 AM on day 4	(Cortisol at 10 AM lower than 7 AM)
Oral salt loading test	Administer: Sodium chloride 6 g orally daily (in divided doses) for 3 days	24-hour urine aldosterone >12 μg
		(Urine Na >200 mEq [220 mmol/L])
	Measure: 24-hour urine aldosterone and urine Na on the third day	
Intravenous salt loading test	Administer: 2 L 0.9% saline intravenously over 4 hours while supine	PAC >10 ng/dL (276.0 pmol/L)
	Measure: PAC, PRA, cortisol, and serum K at 0 and 4 hours	

IM = intramuscular; IV = intravenous; K = potassium; Na = sodium; PAC = plasma aldosterone concentration; PRA = plasma renin activity.

KEY POINTS

- Testing for primary hyperaldosteronism is with the simultaneous measurement of midmorning ambulatory plasma renin activity and plasma aldosterone levels; testing is positive if plasma aldosterone concentration is frankly elevated (>15 ng/dL [414 pmol/L]), plasma renin activity is suppressed, and a ratio of the former over the latter is greater than 20.

- The treatment of choice for primary hyperaldosteronism due to an aldosteronoma or unilateral adrenal hyperplasia is laparoscopic adrenalectomy; for patients with bilateral adrenal hyperplasia or those with unilateral causes of primary hyperaldosteronism who are not candidates for surgery, medical therapy with a mineralocorticoid antagonist such as spironolactone is indicated.

Androgen-Producing Adrenal Tumors

Pure androgen-secreting adrenal neoplasms are very rare. These tumors usually secrete DHEA and DHEAS and/or androstenedione, which are converted peripherally to testosterone. Approximately half of androgen-producing tumors are benign and half are malignant. Manifestations of androgen-producing adrenal tumors are usually absent in adult men, although decreased testicular volume can occur. In women, rapid onset of hirsutism, menstrual irregularities, and virilization can be seen and, if present, should raise suspicion for tumoral hyperandrogenism. Signs of virilization are deepening of the voice, clitoromegaly, and temporal hair loss. The diagnosis of an androgen-producing adrenal tumor is based on demonstrating elevated levels of DHEA and its sulfate (usually greater than 800 µg/dL [21.6 µmol/L]) and/or androstenedione. Although adrenal androgen excess can be seen in 30% to 40% of women with polycystic ovary syndrome, mild elevation of DHEAS (approximately 300 µg/dL [8.1 µmol/L]) is typical. Adrenal imaging with CT or MRI is indicated following biochemical diagnosis of disease to locate the tumor. Treatment is surgical removal of the tumor.

Adrenal Insufficiency

Adrenal insufficiency may be due to failure of the adrenal glands (primary adrenal failure), or there may be inadequate secretion of cortisol from the adrenals due to other causes, including critical illness and pituitary ACTH deficiency (secondary cortisol deficiency). For a discussion of secondary cortisol deficiency, see Disorders of the Pituitary Gland.

Primary Adrenal Failure

Causes and Clinical Features

Primary adrenal failure is a rare disorder resulting from a failure in production of all the hormones of the adrenal cortex. The overall prevalence is 10 to 15 per 100,000 persons. Autoimmune adrenalitis is the most common etiology accounting for 70% to 80% of cases. Up to two thirds of patients have at least one other autoimmune endocrine disorder, and more than 80% have adrenal autoantibodies (21-hydroxylase antibodies). Infiltration of the adrenal glands by tuberculosis (Addison disease) was formerly the most common etiology of primary adrenal failure; now it is responsible for only 7% to 20%. Replacement of the adrenal glands can also occur with metastatic cancer. Genetic causes include autoimmune polyglandular syndromes (APS) type 1 and 2, congenital adrenal hyperplasia, and X-linked adrenoleukodystrophy. Adrenal crisis resulting from bilateral adrenal hemorrhage can occur with the antiphospholipid syndrome, disseminated intravascular coagulation, or systemic anticoagulation.

The clinical presentation of primary adrenal failure depends on disease chronicity and the presence of physical stressors. In autoimmune adrenalitis, the zona glomerulosa is usually affected first, which is manifest by an increase in PRA. With involvement of the zona fasciculata, a diminished cortisol response to ACTH is seen, followed by an increase in basal plasma ACTH, and lastly a decrease in serum cortisol. Patients typically do not have symptoms until hypocortisolemia occurs. **Table 24** shows the clinical and laboratory manifestations of primary adrenal failure. Hyperpigmentation is a clinical hallmark of this disorder that is not seen with secondary cortisol deficiency (see Disorders of the Pituitary Gland for discussion of secondary cortisol deficiency).

Adrenal crisis may occur when onset of adrenal failure is abrupt (bilateral adrenal hemorrhage) or when increased stress occurs in the setting of chronic adrenal failure. Manifestations of adrenal crisis include shock, hypotension, fever, nausea, vomiting, abdominal pain, tachycardia, and even death. Aldosterone is critical to the maintenance of intravascular volume and blood pressure, while cortisol contributes to augmentation of blood pressure mostly during times of increased physical stress (see Adrenal Anatomy and Physiology). Aldosterone deficiency is the major impetus for the development of hypotension and shock in patients with untreated primary adrenal failure. Adrenal crisis is rare in the setting of secondary cortisol deficiency because the renin-angiotensin-aldosterone pathway is intact.

Diagnosis

The diagnosis of primary adrenal failure is based on demonstrating inappropriately low serum cortisol levels. Because most assays measure total cortisol, abnormalities in cortisol-binding protein or albumin can trigger spurious results. An early morning (8 AM) serum cortisol of less than 3 µg/dL (82.8 nmol/L) is consistent with cortisol deficiency, whereas values greater than 15 to 18 µg/dL (414.0-496.8 nmol/L) exclude the diagnosis when binding protein abnormalities and synthetic glucocorticoid exposure are excluded. For patients with nondiagnostic basal cortisol values (5-12 µg/dL [138-331.2 nmol/L]), stimulation testing with synthetic ACTH (cosyntropin) is indicated (see Disorders of the Pituitary Gland). A normal response is a peak serum cortisol level greater than 20 µg/dL (552 nmol/L). ACTH stimulation testing should not be used

TABLE 24. Clinical and Laboratory Manifestations of Primary Adrenal Failure

Hormone Deficiency	Symptoms	Signs	Laboratory Findings
Cortisol	Fatigue Weakness Low-grade fever Weight loss Anorexia Nausea/vomiting Abdominal pain Arthralgia Myalgia	Hyperpigmentation[b] (palmar creases, extensor surfaces, buccal mucosa) Decrease in BP	↓ Serum cortisol ↑ Plasma ACTH ↓ Serum sodium[c] ↓ Plasma glucose[d]
Aldosterone	Salt craving Dizziness	Orthostasis Hypotension	↑ PRA ↓ Serum sodium ↑ Serum potassium
DHEAS	Reduced libido[a]	Decreased axillary or pubic hair[a]	↓ Serum DHEAS

ACTH = adrenocorticotropic hormone; BP = blood pressure; DHEAS = dehydroepiandrosterone sulfate; PRA = plasma renin activity.

[a]Women only.

[b]Occurs exclusively in primary adrenal failure.

[c]Cortisol inhibits the secretion of antidiuretic hormone (ADH), so hypocortisolemia will lead to increased secretion of ADH and hyponatremia.

[d]Rare in adults.

for diagnosis in the critical care setting (see Adrenal Function During Critical Illness).

Once the diagnosis of cortisol deficiency has been established, measurement of 8 AM plasma ACTH will differentiate primary and secondary causes. In primary adrenal failure, ACTH is typically greater than 200 pg/mL (44 pmol/L), whereas it will be low or inappropriately normal in secondary cortisol deficiency. Although not specific for the diagnosis, hyponatremia and hyperkalemia are characteristic of primary adrenal failure and principally result from aldosterone deficiency.

Treatment

Without appropriate treatment, primary adrenal failure is uniformly fatal. Even when treated, the mortality of patients is twice that of the general population. Normal adrenal physiology cannot be reproduced exactly by the administration of exogenous glucocorticoids and mineralocorticoids. Moreover, the administration of doses of glucocorticoid in excess of physiologic replacement can be associated with decreased bone mineral density and features of CS, with increased risk of metabolic syndrome, type 2 diabetes mellitus, hypertension, hyperlipidemia, obesity, and cardiovascular disease. Avoidance of chronic overreplacement is paramount.

Table 25 shows the medical treatment for primary adrenal failure. Most patients require glucocorticoid doses equivalent to 12.5 to 25 mg of hydrocortisone daily. Hydrocortisone is administered 2 to 3 times daily, while once daily dosing of

longer-acting glucocorticoids (prednisone or dexamethasone) is acceptable. All patients with cortisol deficiency need to receive instructions for increasing their cortisol replacement dose during illness ("sick day rules"). Patients should always wear a medical alert identification.

In contrast to patients with secondary cortisol deficiency (see Disorders of the Pituitary Gland), those with primary adrenal failure also require mineralocorticoid replacement. Usual doses are 0.05 to 0.2 mg per day of fludrocortisone. Measurements of serum sodium and potassium help guide dosing. Replacement of DHEA is controversial. It is not indicated for men but can be considered for some women with primary adrenal failure. However, the objective benefit is minimal, and there are concerns regarding the quality and safety of U.S. preparations where DHEA is considered a supplement rather than a pharmaceutical.

Patients who present emergently with suspected adrenal crisis should be treated empirically prior to confirmation of the diagnosis. A blood sample should be drawn for serum cortisol, plasma ACTH, and routine chemistries. The patient should receive immediate treatment with 100 mg of hydrocortisone intravenously and aggressive fluid resuscitation. Hydrocortisone is continued at 100 to 200 mg per day in divided doses (every 6-8 hours) and then tapered to physiologic replacement if cortisol deficiency is confirmed with the above testing. Other synthetic glucocorticoids can also be used for the treatment of adrenal crisis; however, only hydrocortisone in supraphysiologic doses has clinically relevant

TABLE 25. Chronic Medical Treatment of Primary Adrenal Failure

Medication	Basal Dose	Considerations
Glucocorticoid[a] Hydrocortisone Prednisone Prednisolone Dexamethasone	Hydrocortisone Usually 12.5-25 mg/d, divided into 2-3 doses over the day *Alternatives to hydrocortisone:* Prednisone 2.5-5 mg once daily Dexamethasone 0.25-0.75 mg once daily *How to dose:* Titrate to clinical response with goal of no signs or symptoms of cortisol deficiency or excess (increase dose if symptoms of cortisol deficiency remain; decrease if CS signs and symptoms are present)	*"Sick Day Rules":* patient follows at home For minor physiologic stress (upper respiratory infection, fever, minor surgery under local anesthesia) 2-3 times basal dose for 2-3 days *Stress Dosing:* health care providers follow while patient is in the hospital For moderate physiologic stress (minor or moderate surgery with general anesthesia) Hydrocortisone 45-75 mg/d orally or IV in 3-4 divided doses for 2-3 days *Alternatives:* Prednisone 10-20 mg or dexamethasone 2-3 mg/d in 1-2 divided doses For major physiologic stress (major surgery, trauma, critical illness, or childbirth) Hydrocortisone 150-200 mg/day IV in 3-4 divided doses; 100 mg/day the next day; taper to baseline in 3-5 days *Alternative:* Dexamethasone 6-8 mg/d IV in 2-3 divided doses
Mineralocorticoid Fludrocortisone	0.05-0.2 mg once daily in the morning *How to dose:* Titrate to 1. Normal BP 2. Normal serum Na, K	Fludrocortisone is not required if hydrocortisone dose >50 mg/d
Adrenal androgen DHEA	25-50 mg once daily	Consider DHEA for women with impaired mood or sense of well-being when glucocorticoid replacement has been optimized.

BP = blood pressure; CS = Cushing syndrome; DHEA = dehydroepiandrosterone; IV = intravenous; Na = sodium; K = potassium.

[a]Shorter acting glucocorticoids may be preferred over longer acting agents due to lower risk of glucocorticoid excess. Longer-acting preparations have the advantage of once daily dosing (see Table 17).

CONT.

mineralocorticoid activity. If present, electrolyte abnormalities and hypoglycemia should be treated, and precipitants of adrenal crisis (for example, infection) should be sought and treated.

It is critical that patients with suspected primary or secondary cortisol deficiency and concomitant hypothyroidism be treated with glucocorticoids first because correcting thyroid hormone deficiency will accelerate the clearance of cortisol and can precipitate acute adrenal crisis.

In the nonmedical literature, the term "adrenal fatigue" has been used to describe a constellation of symptoms, including difficulty sleeping, fatigue, and salt and sugar craving, hypothetically from long-term emotional or physical stress having a deleterious effect on the adrenal glands, resulting in a simultaneous excess and deficiency of cortisol. However, there is no scientific evidence to support this claim, and the term "adrenal fatigue" should not be used. Proponents of adrenal fatigue prescribe synthetic glucocorticoids and supplements containing adrenal, pituitary, or hypothalamic extracts that can cause iatrogenic CS, as well as mineralocorticoid supplements that can lead to hypertension. Patients should receive appropriate evaluation for their symptoms and be educated to avoid taking hormonal replacements for which there has not been a demonstrated biochemical need.

Adrenal Function During Critical Illness

Glucocorticoid deficiency related to critical illness is an entity that has not been well characterized. It has been postulated that critical illness may lead to transient primary or secondary cortisol deficiency (ACTH deficiency) or an increase in tissue resistance to cortisol. The American College of Critical Care Medicine recommends considering this diagnosis in patients with hypotension who have responded insufficiently to fluids and vasopressor therapy. A maximum increase in serum cortisol of 9 µg/dL (248.4 nmol/L) or less following the administration of synthetic ACTH has been associated with increased mortality from septic shock; however, results of testing do predict benefit from glucocorticoid therapy. In the setting of critical illness, both CBG and albumin concentrations decrease resulting in lower total cortisol. Free cortisol levels, either directly measured or calculated based on total cortisol and CBG, may be more reliable in critically ill patients with hypoalbuminemia. It is not known if free cortisol levels provide useful prognostic information. The administration of glucocorticoids has not been shown to benefit critically ill patients who do not have shock, and the results of placebo-controlled randomized trials in patients with septic shock are conflicting. Further research is needed to clarify if there is a population of critically ill patients who can objectively benefit from glucocorticoid therapy. **H**

Adrenal Masses

Incidentally Noted Adrenal Masses

Adrenal masses are often discovered incidentally when abdominal imaging is performed for another reason. These adrenal incidentalomas are seen on 4% of all CT scans and 7% of those performed in patients 70 years of age and older. The differential diagnosis includes benign and malignant neoplasia of adrenal cortex or medulla, adrenal cysts, adrenal hyperplasia, metastatic tumors of nonadrenal origin, and infections and infiltrative disorders. The most common cause of an adrenal mass is an adrenal adenoma, and adrenal metastasis is the next most common. The two main goals in the evaluation of an incidentally noted adrenal mass are to identify adrenal masses that are likely to be malignant and those that are associated with hormonal hypersecretion so that targeted treatment can

be undertaken promptly. An algorithm for the evaluation and follow up of an adrenal mass is shown in **Figure 7**.

The risk of malignancy varies according to size. Only 2% of adrenal masses smaller than 4 cm are cancerous; however, 25% of those larger than 6 cm are malignant. An adrenal mass's risk of malignancy can be clarified based on its appearance on CT or MRI (see Table 19 for the typical radiographic features of adrenal masses).

Adrenal metastases account for about half of adrenal masses in patients with known nonadrenal malignancies. Cancers that metastasize to the adrenal glands include lymphomas, carcinomas, and melanomas. Percutaneous biopsy is indicated to confirm the diagnosis of adrenal metastasis; however, this should never be performed prior to ruling out pheochromocytoma biochemically. Biopsy is not recommended when adrenocortical carcinoma (ACC) is suspected because it cannot reliably distinguish benign from malignant adrenocortical neoplasia. The evaluation and management of ACC are covered in the Adrenocortical Carcinoma section.

One quarter of incidentally noted adrenal masses autonomously secrete hormones (cortisol 6%-10%; catecholamines

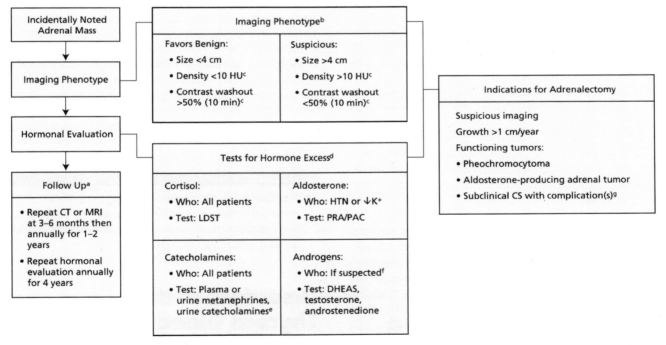

FIGURE 7. Algorithm for the initial diagnostic evaluation and follow up of an incidentally noted adrenal mass. CS = Cushing syndrome; DHEAS = dehydroepiandrosterone sulfate; HTN = hypertension; HU = Hounsfield units; K = potassium; LDST = low-dose (1-mg) dexamethasone suppression test; PAC = plasma aldosterone concentration; PRA = plasma renin activity.

[a]Repeat imaging and hormone testing are indicated for adrenal masses not meeting criteria for surgery at initial diagnosis.

[b]Refer to Table 19 for more CT and MRI findings. If imaging is suspicious in a patient with known malignancy, biopsy should be considered to confirm adrenal metastasis after screening for pheochromocytoma is completed.

[c]CT scan findings.

[d]Positive screening tests usually require further biochemical evaluation to confirm the diagnosis (see text).

[e]Measure plasma metanephrines if radiographic appearance is typical for a pheochromocytoma; otherwise measure 24-hour urine metanephrines and catecholamines.

[f]Hormonal evaluation for an androgen-producing adrenal tumor is indicated only if clinically suspected based on the presence of hirsutism, virilization, or menstrual irregularities in women.

[g]Adrenalectomy is considered for confirmed cases of subclinical CS associated with recent onset of diabetes, hypertension, obesity, or low bone mass.

5%; aldosterone 1%). Excess cortisol secretion is most common; however, the majority of patients have subclinical disease without classic stigmata of CS. Despite this, important complications may be seen, including osteoporosis, hypertension, diabetes mellitus, and cardiovascular events. The LDST is the initial screening test of choice. A serum cortisol value greater than 5 μg/dL (138 nmol/L) is considered positive; however, some advocate using a cut-off of 1.8 μg/dL (49.7 nmol/L) to increase diagnostic sensitivity if CS is suggested by history or physical examination. Because the specificity of the LDST is only approximately 90%, the diagnosis of subclinical CS should be confirmed with additional testing. For a review, see the Cushing Syndrome section.

Aldosteronomas are usually smaller than 2 cm. Case detection for PA is performed in all patients with hypertension or those on antihypertensive medications. Testing for autonomous secretion of adrenal androgens is performed if clinically suspected following careful history and physical examination. All patients with an incidental adrenal mass should be tested for pheochromocytoma. Measurement of 24-hour urine metanephrines and catecholamines is the preferred first test in most asymptomatic patients, due to the lower incidence of false-positive test results. However, if the radiographic appearance of the adrenal mass is suspicious for a pheochromocytoma (see Table 19) or the patient is symptomatic, then plasma free metanephrines should be measured (see Primary Hyperaldosteronism, Androgen-Producing Adrenal Tumors, and Pheochromocytomas and Paragangliomas).

Adrenal masses that are larger than 4 cm, those with worrisome radiographic findings, and pheochromocytomas should be removed surgically. Surgery is also indicated for unilateral aldosteronomas and is considered for patients with subclinical CS associated with the recent onset of diabetes, hypertension, obesity, or low bone mass. For nonfunctioning adrenal masses, if imaging favors a benign lesion, repeat radiographic evaluation is recommended in 3 to 6 months, and then annually for 1 to 2 years. Adenomas usually will not grow more than 1 cm over 12 months. More rapid growth should prompt adrenalectomy. Screening for hormonal hypersecretion is repeated annually for 4 years, as in the rare instance that the mass becomes functional, it is likely to occur in the first 4 years following its discovery. A recent study documented subclinical CS on follow-up testing in approximately 8% of patients who were thought to have nonfunctioning adenomas at initial screening.

KEY POINTS

- The two main goals of evaluation of adrenal incidentalomas are to identify adrenal masses that are likely to be malignant and those that are associated with hormonal hypersecretion so that targeted treatment can be undertaken promptly.

- Adrenal masses that are larger than 4 cm, those with worrisome radiographic findings, and pheochromocytomas should be removed surgically.

Adrenocortical Carcinoma

ACC is a rare malignancy affecting 0.5 to 2 persons per million per year that is often associated with the excessive production of adrenal hormones. Patients with ACC most frequently present with signs and symptoms related to hormonal excess. They may also experience symptoms related to local tumor growth (abdominal fullness, nausea, or back pain) or metastasis. ACC is sometimes detected incidentally when abdominal imaging is performed for another reason (see Incidentally Noted Adrenal Masses).

Autonomous secretion of adrenal hormones or their biologically inactive precursors is seen in more than 80% of patients with ACC (cortisol 50%; multiple hormones 20%; androgens 5% to 10%; aldosterone rarely). The pathologic diagnosis of ACC is challenging, such that with low-risk pathology but large tumor size or concerning imaging findings (see Table 19) close interval radiographic follow up is needed after surgery.

The prognosis of ACC is very poor with an overall mortality rate of 67% to 94%. Management depends on the extent of disease at presentation. Open surgical resection is first-line treatment for early disease. Adjuvant radiotherapy to the tumor bed is used when resection is incomplete. Adjuvant medical therapy with mitotane, an adrenolytic drug, is recommended for patients with known or suspected residual or metastatic disease. Cytotoxic chemotherapy has poor efficacy. In addition to mitotane, inhibitors of adrenal steroidogenesis (metyrapone, ketoconazole, and etomidate) are used to treat CS, if present. Surgery for metastatic ACC is indicated if symptoms related to hormonal hypersecretion cannot be controlled with medical therapy alone. Percutaneous radiofrequency ablation may also be used to treat unresectable primary tumors or metastases when needed.

KEY POINT

- Adrenocortical carcinoma is marked by signs and symptoms related to hormonal excess as well as symptoms related to local tumor growth (abdominal fullness, nausea, or back pain) or metastasis.

Disorders of the Thyroid Gland

Thyroid Anatomy and Physiology

In healthy adults in the United States, each thyroid lobe normally measures up to 5 cm in length, 2 cm in width, and 2 cm in depth; the entire gland weighs 10 to 20 grams. The isthmus, a thin band of thyroid tissue that connects the two lobes, is 1 to 4 mm in thickness and is typically not palpable. Diffuse thyroid disorders, such as lymphocytic thyroiditis, may result in enlargement of the isthmus to 5 mm or more, which may be palpable and give the clinician the false sense that the entire thyroid is enlarged.

There are two forms of active thyroid hormone: thyroxine (T_4) and triiodothyronine (T_3). Iodine is necessary for the formation of thyroid hormone. Deficiency may result in hypothyroidism. The hypothalamic-pituitary-thyroid axis responds to the subsequent hormone deficiency by increasing thyroid-stimulating hormone (TSH) secretion, resulting in development of a goiter. Iodine is typically obtained through diet; it is present in seafood, dairy products, and iodized salt. Although iodine deficiency is a worldwide health problem, it is relatively rare in the United States with the incorporation of iodine into salt.

Thyroid hormone production is controlled by two main forces: secretion of TSH (thyrotropin) and regulation of peripheral conversion of T_4 to T_3. TSH release from the anterior pituitary is stimulated by decreases in concentrations of serum T_4 and T_3 and secretion of thyrotropin-releasing hormone (TRH) from the hypothalamus. The T_3 and T_4, in turn, decrease secretion of TSH from the anterior pituitary as part of a negative feedback loop. Additionally, T_3 inhibits further secretion of TRH from the hypothalamus.

Although the thyroid gland produces both T_3 and T_4, the ratio of T_4 to T_3 secretion is nearly 20:1, with most T_3 (80%) resulting from 5'-deiodination of T_4 in peripheral tissues.

The vast majority of both hormones are bound to circulating proteins, including thyroxine-binding globulin, transthyretin, albumin, and lipoproteins. The function of these proteins is to increase the circulating pool of hormone by delaying clearance and maintaining a reservoir of hormone available for use. Only a small percentage of total circulating thyroid hormone is free (unbound); this fraction is readily available for cellular uptake and determines the biologic activity of the hormone.

KEY POINT

- Thyroid hormone production is controlled by two main forces: secretion of thyroid-stimulating hormone (thyrotropin) and regulation of peripheral conversion of thyroxine (T_4) to triiodothyronine (T_3).

Evaluation of Thyroid Function

In patients with an intact hypothalamic-pituitary axis, the initial laboratory test of thyroid activity is TSH measurement, which is exquisitely sensitive for detection of disorders of thyroid dysfunction. In patients for whom there is a high suspicion of thyroid or pituitary dysfunction, a concomitant thyroid hormone (T_4) level should be assessed with the TSH level to evaluate for central hypothyroidism. The TSH level may reflect hypofunction (high TSH), hyperfunction (low TSH), or a normal range.

The normal reference range for TSH is variable among laboratories but is generally between 0.5 and 5 μU/mL (0.5-5 mU/L), and determinations of normal TSH levels should be made based on the reference range of the laboratory being used. There are three very important exceptions to this general

range. During pregnancy, the range shifts lower and varies by trimester (see Thyroid Function and Disease in Pregnancy). The second important exception is in the elderly. With aging, the reference range shifts higher; the upper limit of normal extends to 7 μU/mL (7 mU/L) in patients older than 70 years. The third exception is in patients with known pituitary dysfunction or a risk of pituitary dysfunction (history of cranial irradiation, pituitary surgery, or massive head trauma).

If the serum TSH level is frankly abnormal, additional evaluation of thyroid function should be considered to determine the extent of the dysfunction. This is accomplished by measuring T_4 when the TSH is elevated and by measuring T_4 and T_3 when the TSH is suppressed.

When indicated by an abnormal TSH, the circulating level of thyroid hormone should be assessed using total or free T_4 levels. Total T_4 is a reflection of the bound and unbound fractions of the hormone and is a reasonable method of assessing overall thyroid hormone levels in most patients. However, in patients with disorders of protein metabolism, such as kidney or liver disease, measurement of free T_4 ensures a more accurate representation of the hormone concentrations. Additionally, conditions that raise serum total protein level, such as in patients taking estrogen or during pregnancy, may result in a higher total T_4 concentration, and measuring the free T_4 is indicated. The same rules apply to T_3 as to T_4 regarding protein levels, but free T_3 has a very short half-life and levels fluctuate more and are less reliable; therefore, it is controversial whether total or free T_3 should be measured in patients at risk for protein abnormalities.

Measurement of serum T_3 is necessary if the patient has a suppressed TSH level because, in some patients with thyrotoxicosis, T_3 may be preferentially secreted over T_4 (T_3 toxicosis). In patients with an elevated TSH level, indicating hypothyroidism, measurement of serum T_3 is not helpful because it will be maintained in the normal range even in those with significant disease.

Thyroid autoantibody measurement may be helpful under certain clinical circumstances. In patients with a personal history of autoimmune disease (such as type 1 diabetes mellitus, systemic lupus erythematosus, or celiac disease) or a strong family history of thyroid dysfunction, measuring thyroid autoantibodies may indicate the cause of the thyroid dysfunction or whether a patient is at risk for developing thyroid autoimmune disease if the TSH is normal. There is no clinical indication for serial measurement of thyroid antibody titers to determine the need for or to guide therapy. There are three forms of thyroid autoantibodies: thyroid peroxidase (TPO), thyrotropin receptor (TRAb), and thyroglobulin (TgAb). Elevated titers of TPO antibodies are associated with autoimmune hypothyroidism, or Hashimoto disease. Patients with TPO antibodies and normal thyroid function tests are at an increased risk of developing overt thyroid failure (2%-4% per year). Thyrotropin receptor antibodies (TRAb) are divided into three types: blocking (also called thyrotropin-binding inhibitory immunoglobulins), stimulating (also called thyroid-stimulating immunoglobulins or TSI), and neutral. The presence of TSI autoantibodies is responsible for the development of Graves disease. TSI autoantibodies should be measured if autoimmune hyperthyroidism is suspected. Thyroglobulin (Tg) is a glycoprotein located within the colloid on which thyroid hormones are synthesized and stored. Serum Tg and TgAb measurements are used to monitor patients with thyroid cancer; serum Tg is a highly sensitive and specific marker of residual thyroid tissue. After total thyroidectomy and radioactive iodine ablation, the persistence of a detectable serum Tg is a possible indicator of residual or recurrent disease. Thyroglobulin antibodies are present in up to 30% of patients. Their presence in the serum is only significant in patients with thyroid cancer, as they can falsely lower the serum Tg. Therefore, TgAb titers should always be assessed simultaneously with the Tg; if antibodies are present, the Tg level may not be reliable.

Calcitonin, secreted by the C cells of the thyroid, is most frequently used as a tumor marker in patients with a history of medullary thyroid carcinoma. Serum calcitonin levels can help increase the sensitivity of detection of medullary thyroid carcinoma when used in conjunction with fine-needle aspiration (FNA). However, it is not recommended as a screening test in all patients with thyroid nodules because it lacks the requisite specificity. Instead, measurement of calcitonin should be considered if a patient with thyroid nodular disease has a history of hyperparathyroidism or a family history of medullary thyroid carcinoma or multiple endocrine neoplasia type 2, or if there is clinical suspicion for these disorders.

Radioactive iodine uptake (RAIU) is a measure of iodine uptake by the thyroid over a pre-specified time frame, typically 24 hours. RAIU is used to evaluate the cause of hyperthyroidism; it is not indicated in patients with normal or elevated TSH levels. The degree of uptake is useful for distinguishing the various causes of hyperthyroidism. RAIU percentage is typically very high in patients with Graves disease (diffusely increased uptake) and only moderately elevated in those with toxic multinodular goiter (patchy uptake in areas of nodules with relative suppression of normal tissue). In contrast, the RAIU is very low in those with thyroiditis or exposure to exogenous thyroid hormone. The presence of a "cold" nodule on isotope scanning is an indication for ultrasonography to help determine if FNA is indicated. RAIU is contraindicated during pregnancy and while breastfeeding.

KEY POINTS

- The initial laboratory test of thyroid activity is thyroid-stimulating hormone measurement; in patients with an intact anterior pituitary, measurement of thyroid-stimulating hormone is exquisitely sensitive for detection of disorders of thyroid hypofunction (high thyroid-stimulating hormone) and hyperfunction (low thyroid-stimulating hormone).

(Continued)

KEY POINTS *(continued)*

- If central hypothyroidism is suspected, a concomitant thyroid hormone (thyroxine [T_4]) level should be assessed in conjunction with the thyroid-stimulating hormone level.

- If the thyroid-stimulating hormone level is frankly abnormal, additional evaluation of thyroid function should be considered to determine the extent of the dysfunction; measure thyroxine (T_4) when the thyroid-stimulating hormone is elevated and measure both thyroxine (T_4) and triiodothyronine (T_3) when the thyroid-stimulating hormone is suppressed.   **HVC**

- There is no clinical indication for serial measurement of thyroid antibody titers to determine the need for or to guide therapy except to monitor for residual disease in patients treated for thyroid cancer.   **HVC**

- Radioactive iodine uptake is a measure of iodine uptake by the thyroid over 24 hours; it is used to evaluate the cause of hyperthyroidism and is not indicated in patients with normal or elevated thyroid-stimulating hormone levels.   **HVC**

Functional Thyroid Disorders
Thyrotoxicosis
Evaluation

Thyrotoxicosis is a term used to describe thyroid hormone excess from all sources, whereas hyperthyroidism is the more specific term to describe thyroid gland overactivity. Thyrotoxicosis may result from endogenous thyroid disorders, pituitary tumors, and exogenous levothyroxine. The most common causes of hyperthyroidism are Graves disease and toxic adenoma(s).

The symptoms of thyrotoxicosis include heat intolerance, palpitations, dyspnea, tremulousness, menstrual irregularities, hyperdefecation, weight loss, increased appetite, proximal muscle weakness, fatigue, insomnia, and mood disturbances. The severity of symptoms may not correlate with the level of thyroid hormone derangement. In older patients, many of the classic symptoms of thyroid hormone excess may be absent, and the only presenting symptom may be atrial fibrillation or heart failure; this is known as apathetic hyperthyroidism.

The initial evaluation based on clinical signs and/or symptoms of thyrotoxicosis should be measurement of serum TSH alone, followed by measurement of T_4 and T_3 levels if TSH is suppressed. The typical pattern of hyperthyroidism is TSH suppression with an elevated T_4 and/or T_3. A normal serum TSH in the setting of an elevated T_4 and/or T_3 concentration suggests the presence of a TSH-secreting pituitary adenoma; these tumors are extremely rare and are managed differently from other causes of thyrotoxicosis (see later discussion).

KEY POINT

- The typical pattern of laboratory studies in hyperthyroidism is thyroid-stimulating hormone suppression with an elevated thyroxine (T_4) and/or triiodothyronine (T_3) level.

Management

Although the specific intervention used is usually determined by the underlying cause and patient and physician preference, control of the thyrotoxic state may be achieved by one of three treatment modalities: thionamides, radioactive iodine ablation, or surgery.

Rapid control of adrenergic symptoms with a β-blocker is indicated in most patients with thyrotoxicosis. Although propranolol is frequently used for its added effect of inhibition of peripheral conversion of T_4 to T_3, cardioselective β-blockers, such as atenolol, are preferred owing to the additional benefits of decreased central nervous system side effects and improved adherence with once-daily dosing.

Methimazole and propylthiouracil (PTU) are the two thionamides available in the United States. Methimazole is the preferred agent because it has a higher intrathyroidal retention (potency), a preferable dosing regimen (typically once daily), and a reduced side-effect profile. Antithyroid medications reduce T_3 and T_4 levels within a few days of initiation, but the full effect may take several weeks. Normalization of a previously suppressed TSH level may take several months. It is critical, therefore, to monitor T_4 and T_3 levels during treatment of hyperthyroidism because the TSH may not be an accurate reflection of the thyroidal status.

Thionamides may be used to prepare patients for thyroidectomy or radioiodine treatment, or they may be used as the primary therapy. Thionamides may be used for 1 to 2 years in patients with Graves disease in the hope of achieving remission; more definitive therapy with radioactive iodine or surgery may then be sought after that timeframe if hyperthyroidism persists. Although thionamides are generally well tolerated, it is important to be familiar with their side-effect profile. The most common reaction to antithyroid medications is a rash, seen in up to 10% of patients. Additionally, PTU may cause elevations of aminotransferase levels. Rare cases of fatal hepatotoxicity have been described with PTU. Therefore, its use is reserved for patients who cannot tolerate methimazole and during the first trimester of pregnancy, when methimazole has a possible teratogenic effect. A cholestatic pattern of liver test abnormalities may also be seen with methimazole, but it is typically temporary and milder than that seen with PTU. Both drugs may be associated with reversible agranulocytosis in approximately 1 in 500 patients. Baseline liver chemistry studies and complete blood count with differential are recommended before initiation of antithyroid medications, with serial monitoring of the complete blood count during therapy. If patients taking a thionamide develop a fever, rash, severe sore throat, jaundice, or other symptoms of serious illness, they should be assessed promptly for an adverse reaction to the medication.

The goal of radioactive iodine ablation is to render the patient hypothyroid, which can typically be accomplished in 90% of patients with the first treatment. Although a minority of patients may develop acute anterior neck pain from radiation thyroiditis, radioactive iodine ablation is typically well tolerated. It may take several months for the development of hypothyroidism, so it is important to monitor thyroid function tests monthly after therapy. In a patient with severe thyrotoxicosis, radioactive iodine may provide additional substrate to the hyperfunctioning gland, resulting in exacerbation of the hyperthyroid state. Consequently, it may be reasonable to initiate a thionamide prior to ablation to lower the thyroid hormone levels.

Surgery is rarely first-line therapy, given the inherent risks with any surgery. Patients in whom control cannot be achieved with thionamides and those who are not comfortable with radioiodine therapy are typically referred for surgery. Because of the increased intrathyroidal vascularity, the procedure can be technically more difficult than a typical thyroidectomy. Additionally, restoration of the euthyroid state before surgery with thionamides is important to improve hemodynamics during general anesthesia and decrease the patient's risk of thyroid storm.

KEY POINT

- Control of hyperthyroidism may be achieved by one of three treatment modalities: thionamides, radioactive iodine ablation, or surgery; modality choice depends on the underlying cause and patient preference.

Graves Disease

Graves disease is a multiorgan system autoimmune disorder that can affect the thyroid, eyes, and skin. It is frequently seen in women between the ages of 20 and 50 years and is the most common cause of hyperthyroidism in the United States. Antibodies against the TSH receptor (TSI or TRAb) stimulate autonomous production of T_4 and T_3. Patients frequently report a family history of Graves disease, Hashimoto thyroiditis, or other autoimmune conditions.

On physical examination, patients have elevated systolic blood pressure with a widened pulse pressure, tachycardia, and a diffusely enlarged thyroid. Further inspection of the thyroid may reveal a bruit. Careful examination of the skin may reveal pretibial myxedema, an infiltrative process that is typically patchy with a peau d'orange appearance to the skin.

Diagnosis of Graves disease is made clinically in most instances, and measurement of TSI antibodies is reserved for patients who are not markedly thyrotoxic on examination and do not have a classic smooth, rubbery, diffuse goiter. In those patients, TSI antibodies may help determine the cause of the hyperthyroidism. RAIU and scan will show markedly increased uptake with diffuse activity on the scan.

If ophthalmopathy is present, the patient may exhibit lid retraction (lid lag), whereby contraction of the levator palpebrae muscles of the eyelids results in immobility of the upper eyelid with downward rotation of the eye. Additionally, patients may have proptosis, scleral injection, and periorbital edema.

Because thionamide drugs also have an immunomodulatory effect that reduces autoantibody titers, antithyroid drugs are often first-line treatment for Graves disease. Up to 50% of patients may go into remission within 24 months, and some may maintain a euthyroid state without further therapy after an initial treatment with thionamides. If the patient does not go into remission or if disease recurs, definitive therapy with radioactive iodine ablation or surgery is recommended. However, in patients with Graves ophthalmopathy, there is an acute escalation of thyroid autoantibody titers following radioiodine therapy that may exacerbate ocular symptoms. Such patients may be better treated with thionamides and/or surgery.

Toxic Adenoma and Multinodular Goiter

Activating mutations in the TSH receptor gene are responsible for the autonomous production of thyroid hormone in a toxic nodule (adenoma) or in multiple hyperfunctioning nodules in a toxic multinodular goiter. Because of this loss of normal regulation of thyroid hormone production, patients are at risk for developing acute thyrotoxicosis when exposed to iodine excess, particularly after a contrast load for medical testing (Jod-Basedow phenomenon), such as in cardiac catheterization and contrast-enhanced CT scans. Although patients with a toxic adenoma or multinodular goiter may exhibit the typical symptoms of thyrotoxicosis, they can be relatively asymptomatic. On physical examination, a nodule may be palpable or there may be a diffusely enlarged goiter with a nodular contour but no discrete palpable nodules.

If a patient is suspected of having a toxic nodule, thyroid scintigraphy should be performed to determine if the nodule is autonomous. The thyroid uptake scan will reveal increased activity in the "hot" nodule with relative suppression of the remaining thyroid tissue. These results should then be correlated with the ultrasonographic findings to determine if any additional nodules exist, which will require further investigation with FNA.

Radioactive iodine ablation or surgery is the most common treatment for toxic nodules. Thionamides can be used to decrease hormone production in the short term, but unlike Graves disease, this condition has no chance of spontaneous remission and would require lifelong medical therapy, which is not recommended. Radioiodine therapy will ideally ablate only the autonomous areas. In elderly patients, those with coronary disease, those who are highly symptomatic, and those with severe thyrotoxicosis, thionamides are recommended to normalize thyroid hormone levels prior to radioactive iodine; this is done to avoid exacerbation of the thyrotoxicosis due to release of preformed hormone from the gland acutely after radioactive iodine ablation. Thionamides

should be withheld for 5 to 7 days before the administration of radioactive iodine therapy. If a patient has a particularly large goiter with compressive symptoms or if there is concern for malignancy, surgery is recommended as first-line therapy.

KEY POINT

- Radioactive iodine ablation or surgery is the most common treatment for toxic thyroid nodules; indications for surgery include a large goiter with compression symptoms or concern for malignancy.

Destructive Thyroiditis

Thyroiditis is a self-limited inflammatory condition of the thyroid resulting in the release of preformed thyroid hormone into the circulation. The duration of the thyrotoxic phase is typically 2 to 6 weeks, during which patients may exhibit classic symptoms of thyrotoxicosis. Following the release of preformed hormone, the damaged thyroid ceases production of T_3 and T_4 during the recovery phase; consequently, administration of thionamides will not be effective in treating elevated hormone levels. The patient may then become clinically hypothyroid, a condition that may require temporary levothyroxine therapy. The length of the hypothyroid phase can vary but classically is 6 to 12 weeks.

There are two categories of thyroiditis: painful and painless. The causes of painful thyroiditis are inflammatory (de Quervain or subacute granulomatous thyroiditis), infectious (suppurative), and radiation-induced. The pain, typically only present during the thyrotoxic phase, can be quite intense. Treatment is aimed at controlling inflammation with NSAIDs or systemic glucocorticoids if severe. Subacute thyroiditis is the most common form and is presumably caused by a postviral inflammatory process; many patients report a recent history of upper respiratory illness preceding the thyroiditis. Radiation thyroiditis may occur 5 to 10 days after treatment with radioactive iodine. This may be associated with transient exacerbation of the hyperthyroidism. The accompanying pain is usually mild and lasts for up to 1 week. Infectious thyroiditis is rare but may be seen in an immunocompromised patient; the most common causative organisms are *Staphylococcus* and *Streptococcus* species.

Painless thyroiditis is more commonly seen than painful thyroiditis and has several causes, including postpartum thyroiditis, silent thyroiditis, and drug-induced thyroiditis. Postpartum thyroiditis may occur up to 1 year after delivery; the frequency is variably reported but may occur in up to 10% of pregnancies. The presence of TPO antibodies is nearly universal, and the likelihood of subsequent permanent hypothyroidism is very high. Thyroiditis is also likely to recur in later pregnancies.

KEY POINT

- Thyroiditis is a self-limited inflammatory condition of the thyroid resulting in the release of preformed thyroid hormone into the circulation; the duration of the thyrotoxic phase is typically 2 to 6 weeks, which is followed by a hypothyroid phase typically lasting 6 to 12 weeks.

Central Hyperthyroidism

TSH-secreting pituitary adenomas are extremely rare. In this condition, serum TSH is detectable or normal in the setting of an elevated T_4 and/or T_3 concentration. A dedicated pituitary MRI will demonstrate an adenoma. Treatment should focus on removal of the pituitary tumor; thyroid-targeted therapy is ineffective (see Disorders of the Pituitary Gland).

Subclinical Hyperthyroidism

Subclinical hyperthyroidism is a laboratory-based diagnosis, defined as the presence of a suppressed TSH level with normal T_3 and T_4 levels. Repeat assessment of thyroid function should be performed 6 to 12 weeks after the initial tests, as the values will normalize in up to 30% of patients. Symptoms of thyrotoxicosis are typically mild; most patients are asymptomatic.

Which patients will benefit most from normalization of the TSH level is not universally agreed on, but consensus opinion recommends treatment for patients with a TSH level below 0.1 µU/mL (0.1 mU/L). The benefits of treatment for asymptomatic patients with a TSH level between 0.1 µU/mL (0.1 mU/L) and the lower limit of the normal reference range are less clear. Emerging data suggest that chronic subclinical hyperthyroidism has a negative effect on cardiac function, the central nervous system, and bone mass. The risk of atrial fibrillation is significantly increased when the TSH level is below 0.3 µU/mL (0.3 mU/L), so patients over the age of 65 years and those with a history of coronary artery disease or tachyarrhythmias, as well as patients with osteoporosis, may benefit from normalization of the TSH level. Radioiodine is the preferred treatment, but often the gland does not have sufficient iodine avidity and methimazole must be used.

KEY POINTS

HVC
- In patients with subclinical hyperthyroidism, repeat assessment of thyroid function should be performed 6 to 12 weeks after the initial tests, as the values will normalize in up to 30% of patients.

- Treatment for subclinical hyperthyroidism is recommended when the thyroid-stimulating hormone level is less than 0.1 µU/mL (0.1 mU/L).

Thyroid Hormone Deficiency
Hypothyroidism
Evaluation

Hypothyroidism refers to low circulating thyroid hormone levels. Hypothyroidism is more prevalent in women than men (2% versus 0.2%) and in those with other autoimmune diseases. The most frequent cause is Hashimoto thyroiditis, also known as chronic lymphocytic thyroiditis. Iatrogenic causes include surgery, radioiodine therapy, and external beam radiation therapy to the neck. Hypothyroidism may also be medication induced; the most common causative agents include lithium, amiodarone, interferons, interleukin-2, and tyrosine kinase inhibitors. Rarely, pituitary tumors, severe head trauma, pituitary surgery, or cranial radiation can cause central hypothyroidism.

The clinical manifestations of hypothyroidism include fatigue, cold intolerance, constipation, heavy menses, weight gain, impaired concentration, dry skin, edema, depression, mood changes, muscle cramps, myalgia, and reduced fertility. The physical examination findings may include reduction in basal temperature, diastolic hypertension, bradycardia, dry skin, brittle hair, hoarseness, delayed relaxation phase of the deep tendon reflexes, and an enlarged thyroid.

An elevated serum TSH level indicates the diagnosis of primary hypothyroidism. In patients with an elevated TSH that is less than 10 µU/mL (10 mU/L), a low serum T_4 measurement is helpful, as a frankly low value indicates that thyroid hormone replacement is necessary. The presence of TPO antibodies suggests that Hashimoto thyroiditis is the underlying cause. Thyroid imaging is not indicated unless there is concern for a nodule on physical examination.

KEY POINTS

- An elevated serum thyroid-stimulating hormone level indicates the diagnosis of primary hypothyroidism; thyroid imaging is not indicated unless there is concern for a nodule on physical examination. **HVC**

- The most frequent cause of primary hypothyroidism is Hashimoto thyroiditis (chronic lymphocytic thyroiditis); the presence of TPO antibodies is suggestive of Hashimoto thyroiditis.

Management

In patients with a TSH level greater than 10 µU/mL (10 mU/L), daily thyroid hormone replacement is recommended.

Thyroid hormone replacement with levothyroxine alone is recommended. The goal of thyroid hormone replacement therapy is normalization of the TSH. The starting dose can be weight-based at 1.67 µg/kg/d, using ideal body weight. In patients with prevalent cardiac disease, tachyarrhythmias, or multiple comorbidities, or in those who are older than 65 years, the dose should not be based on weight but rather should be 25 to 50 µg/d. The dose should be titrated based on TSH levels measured 6 to 8 weeks after any dose change. To improve gastrointestinal absorption, levothyroxine should be taken on an empty stomach, 1 hour before or 2 to 3 hours after ingestion of food or medications that would interfere with absorption, such as calcium- or iron-containing supplements. Patients with celiac disease may require higher levothyroxine doses because of impaired absorption.

There has been significant debate regarding the need for supplementation of T_3 (liothyronine) in patients with hypothyroidism. The short half-life of T_3 triggers acute spikes in serum T_3 levels, which are of significant concern for elderly patients or those with preexisting cardiac issues. Additionally, numerous studies have failed to show a clear benefit of a T_4/T_3 combination over T_4 alone; therefore, this is not generally recommended.

KEY POINT

- In patients with a thyroid-stimulating hormone level greater than 10 μU/mL (10 mU/L), daily thyroid hormone replacement is recommended and should be taken on an empty stomach; the dose should be titrated based on thyroid-stimulating hormone levels measures 6 to 8 weeks after any dose change.

Subclinical Hypothyroidism

Subclinical hypothyroidism is defined as an elevated serum TSH level with a normal T_4 level. The potential causes are the same as for overt hypothyroidism. Repeat measurement of the TSH level is recommended, particularly in an asymptomatic patient, as it will normalize in up to 30% of patients by 6 weeks.

Patients typically have mild or no symptoms of hypothyroidism. Subclinical hypothyroidism may be associated with several laboratory abnormalities including elevated total cholesterol, LDL cholesterol, and C-reactive protein levels. Large studies suggest that these laboratory abnormalities translate into an increased risk of atherosclerosis and cardiac events. However, supplementation with levothyroxine has not been shown to mitigate this risk. Treatment is generally recommended for those with a TSH level greater than 10 μU/mL (10 mU/L), but levothyroxine treatment should be considered in patients who have positive TPO antibodies or a large goiter, as these patients are at risk for progression to overt hypothyroidism at rates of 3% to 8% per year. A goal TSH level less than or equal to 2.5 μU/mL (2.5 mU/L) is recommended for women with subclinical hypothyroidism and positive TPO antibody status who are planning to conceive.

KEY POINT

HVC

- In patients with suspected subclinical hypothyroidism, repeat measurement of the thyroid-stimulating hormone level is recommended, as it will normalize in up to 30% of patients by 6 weeks.

Drug-Induced Thyroid Dysfunction

Various medications can affect thyroid function and are listed in **Table 26** based on their mechanism of action.

Amiodarone may have a potentially toxic effect on the thyroid. The iodine content of amiodarone is 37% by weight. It is stored in fat, myocardium, liver, lung, and thyroid tissues, with a half-life exceeding 50 days. This long half-life, coupled with the high iodine content, renders it a potentially toxic compound to the thyroid. The two types of amiodarone thyroid toxicity are changes in thyroid function studies seen in all patients (obligatory effects), and those seen in only a subset of patients (facultative effects).

The obligatory effects result from the increased circulating iodine after initiation of the drug. Adaptation to the acute iodine excess causes a reduction in organification of iodine and reduced production of thyroid hormone (Wolff-Chaikoff

effect). The result is a temporary reduction in circulating T_3 and T_4 levels with a minor rise in the TSH level; these changes typically reverse within the first 3 months of treatment and require no intervention.

Facultative effects, seen in up to 15% of patients, may cause either hypo- or hyperthyroidism. In areas of iodine sufficiency, hypothyroidism is the more common toxicity. Those at highest risk are women with preexisting TPO antibody positivity. Amiodarone-induced thyrotoxicosis (AIT) is more commonly seen in males and in those living in iodine-deficient areas. Type 1 AIT is the result of exposure to excess iodine and occurs in those with preexisting thyroid conditions, such as latent Graves disease or nodular goiter, in which the iodine increases unregulated thyroid hormone production. Type 2 AIT is the result of the cytotoxic effects of amiodarone on thyroid tissue, producing a clinical picture of painless thyroiditis, with abnormal release of thyroid hormone. The treatments differ with each type, but distinguishing between the two forms of AIT often can be challenging and may require the aid of an endocrinologist. The time to recovery of normal thyroid function may be several months, even with prompt diagnosis and treatment. Discontinuation of amiodarone is typically necessary, particularly in those patients with type 1 AIT.

KEY POINTS

- In the majority of patients, amiodarone causes a temporary reduction in circulating triiodothyronine (T_3) and thyroxine (T_4) and levels with a minor rise in the thyroid-stimulating hormone that reverses within first 3 months of treatment and requires no intervention.

- In 15% of patients, amiodarone may cause either hypo- or hyperthyroidism; those at highest risk for amiodarone-induced hypothyroidism are women with preexisting thyroid peroxidase antibody positivity.

Thyroid Function and Disease in Pregnancy

Significant changes in thyroid function occur during pregnancy; understanding the normal physiology during gestation is critical for a correct interpretation of thyroid laboratory studies. Abnormalities of thyroid function can have a dramatic effect on the health of the mother and the fetus. A diagram of the physiologic changes in thyroid function during each trimester is shown in **Figure 8**.

Increased estrogen levels cause a rise in thyroxine-binding globulin. To maintain a stable free T_4 and T_3, thyroid hormone production is increased and TSH remains within the normal reference range for the patient's trimester (see later discussion for trimester-specific ranges). Routine screening of TSH is not indicated for every pregnant woman. TSH screening is indicated in women with a risk of thyroid gland dysfunction, including those already on thyroid hormone replacement therapy; those with autoimmune disorders, goiter, previous

TABLE 26. Medications that Affect Thyroid Function

Mechanism of Action	Drugs	Comments
Decreased absorption or enterohepatic circulation	Calcium	It is recommended that levothyroxine ingestion be separated from these medications by several hours
	Proton pump inhibitors	
	Iron	
	Cholestyramine	
	Aluminum hydroxide	
	Soybean oil	
	Sucralfate	
	Psyllium	
Increased metabolism of levothyroxine	Phenytoin	Higher levothyroxine doses may be required to maintain levothyroxine in the normal range
	Carbamazepine	
	Rifampin	
	Phenobarbital	
	Sertraline	
Thyroiditis	Amiodarone	May cause hypo- or hyperthyroidism
	Lithium	
	Interferon alfa	
	Interleukin-2	
	Tyrosine kinase inhibitors	
De novo development of antithyroid antibodies	Interferon alfa	May develop Hashimoto thyroiditis, Graves disease, or painless thyroiditis
Inhibition of TSH synthesis or release	Glucocorticoids	
	Dopamine	
	Dobutamine	
	Octreotide	
Increased thyroxine-binding globulin	Estrogen	False elevation of total T_3, total T_4 levels; free T_3, T_4 may be more accurate reflection of hormone levels
	Tamoxifen	
	Methadone	
Decreased thyroxine-binding globulin	Androgen therapy	False lowering of total T_3, total T_4 levels; free T_3, T_4 may be more accurate reflection of hormone levels
	Glucocorticoids	
	Niacin	

T_3 = triiodothyronine; T_4 = thyroxine; TSH = thyroid-stimulating hormone.

head/neck irradiation, previous thyroid surgery, known positive TPO antibodies or positive TSI antibodies, or a strong family history of thyroid dysfunction; those who live in iodine-deficient areas; or those older than 30 years. In patients on levothyroxine replacement, the dose of the medication may need to be increased, on average by 30% to 50%, and patients should have their TSH level checked as soon as a pregnancy test is positive.

Fetal thyroid tissue is not functional until 10 to 12 weeks' gestation, necessitating maternal thyroid hormone transfer through the placenta. Thyroid hormone deficiency can negatively affect fetal neurocognitive development. It is critical to maintain a euthyroid state during pregnancy in these patients. TSH testing should be performed every 6 weeks throughout

pregnancy, with adjustments in thyroid hormone replacement dosing as needed to maintain the TSH within the trimester-specific normal range. The largest dose escalations typically occur in the first trimester, with more dose stability later in pregnancy.

Diagnosing possible hyperthyroidism during pregnancy may be challenging because some physiologic changes during gestation may overlap with symptoms of thyrotoxicosis, such as tachycardia, fatigue, and heat intolerance. Serum TSH and human chorionic gonadotropin have a common α-subunit, allowing cross-reactivity at the TSH receptor. Consequently, TSH declines during the first trimester; the reference range shifts down to 0.03 to 2.5 μU/mL (0.03-2.5 mU/L). During the second and third trimesters the upper limit of TSH rises to

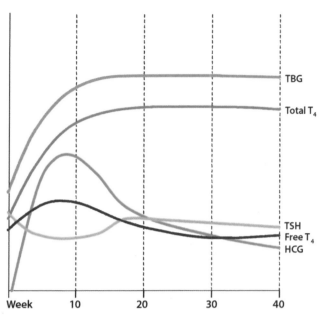

FIGURE 8. Thyroid function in pregnancy. HCG = human chorionic gonadotropin; T_4 = thyroxine; TBG = thyroid-binding globulin; TSH = thyroid-stimulating hormone.

3.0 µU/mL (3.0 mU/L). An additional complicating factor is that radioiodine scanning is contraindicated during pregnancy because of the risk for fetal thyroid exposure to radiation. Instead, several clinical clues may be used to help determine if the patient has thyrotoxicosis, including the presence of a goiter, ophthalmopathy, or TSI antibodies, all of which are suggestive of Graves disease.

The use of thionamides is considered safe during pregnancy, but PTU is preferred during the first trimester because of potential teratogenic effects from methimazole during organogenesis. Although rarely indicated, surgery may be performed during the second trimester. It should be reserved for those who are unable to tolerate thionamides or who have inadequate control on medical therapy. Radioiodine therapy is contraindicated during pregnancy and while breastfeeding. Treatment goals with thionamides are a detectable TSH in the lower end of the pregnancy reference range and a free T_4 in the upper end of the reference range.

KEY POINT

- In pregnant patients on levothyroxine replacement, the dose may need to be increased, on average by 30% to 50%; patients should have their thyroid-stimulating hormone level checked as soon as a pregnancy test is positive.

Euthyroid Sick Syndrome

Euthyroid sick syndrome (ESS), nonthyroidal illness syndrome, or low T_3 syndrome are various names that have been assigned to the changes seen in thyroid function test results during critical illness. Although not a true syndrome, there are significant

perturbations of the hypothalamic-pituitary-thyroid (HPT) axis that occur in up to 75% of hospitalized patients. The underlying cause of the critical illness may influence the pattern of thyroid function abnormalities. Drugs that are frequently used in critically ill patients can have a significant effect on the HPT axis (see Table 26). The typical pattern is initially a low T_3 level, followed by a decline in the T_4 level. As the patient becomes more critically ill, the TSH level may also decline, creating a clinical picture that is difficult to discern from central hypothyroidism. Rarely, TSH can be elevated in ESS.

Two general guidelines are important in evaluating a critically ill patient. First, measurement of TSH alone should be obtained only if there is a high clinical suspicion of thyroid dysfunction. If TSH is abnormal, the previously described recommendations for additional laboratory studies should be followed. If the TSH is greater than 20 µU/mL (20 mU/L) or is undetectable, ESS is less likely to be the cause and overt thyroid dysfunction should be strongly considered. If the TSH falls between these two values, historical clues and examination findings are very important for identifying patients with true thyroid dysfunction.

After discharge from the hospital, thyroid function abnormalities may persist for several weeks. The typical pattern is a mildly elevated TSH level and slightly low T_4 and T_3 levels. In a clinically euthyroid patient, thyroid function tests should be repeated 6 weeks after hospitalization to confirm overt thyroid dysfunction with persistent TSH abnormality or confirm ESS with normalization of TSH.

KEY POINTS

- Critical illness can cause changes in thyroid function tests in up to 75% of hospitalized patients, known as euthyroid sick syndrome; measurement of TSH should only be obtained in the hospital when there is a high clinical suspicion of thyroid dysfunction.

- The typical pattern of euthyroid sick syndrome, nonthyroidal illness syndrome, or low triiodothyronine (T_3) syndrome is a mildly elevated thyroid-stimulating hormone level and slightly low thyroxine (T_4) and triiodothyronine (T_3) levels. **HVC**

- After patients with euthyroid sick syndrome are discharged from the hospital, thyroid function abnormalities may persist for several weeks so follow-up thyroid function tests should not be repeated until 6 weeks after discharge. **HVC**

Thyroid Emergencies

Although most thyroid conditions are not urgent, thyroid storm and myxedema coma represent true medical emergencies requiring critical care. Failure to make a timely diagnosis and institute treatment is associated with a high mortality rate.

Thyroid Storm

Thyroid storm is a severe manifestation of thyrotoxicosis with life-threatening secondary systemic decompensation (shock).

CONT.

The cardinal features for diagnosis include elevated temperature, significant tachycardia, heart failure, gastrointestinal dysfunction (nausea, vomiting, diarrhea, and/or jaundice), and neurologic disturbances. The range of central nervous system manifestations includes increasing agitation, emotional lability, confusion, paranoia, psychosis, or coma. Although thyroid storm has been reported with many causes of thyrotoxicosis, it occurs most commonly with Graves disease. Thyroid storm may be precipitated by another event such as infection, surgery, myocardial infarction, trauma, or parturition. Administration of radioactive iodine therapy to a patient with untreated or uncontrolled hyperthyroidism can trigger thyroid storm.

The diagnosis is based on clinical presentation but can generally be ruled out if T_4 and T_3 levels are within normal limits.

Treatment of thyroid storm should be directed toward reduction of thyroid hormone production, decreasing peripheral conversion of T_4 to T_3, addressing adrenergic symptoms and thermoregulatory changes, searching for and treating precipitating factors, and reversing systemic decompensation. Thionamides and β-blockers are the mainstay of treatment to reduce thyroid hormone production and control adrenergic symptoms. PTU and propranolol are the preferred agents because they have the added benefit of blocking peripheral conversion of T_4 to T_3. Additionally, high-dose glucocorticoids reduce T_4 conversion to bioactive T_3. At least 1 hour after the first dose of a thionamide, iodine drops should be administered to inhibit further release of thyroid hormone from the gland. Acetaminophen and cooling blankets may be used to control the hyperthermia. However, even with aggressive therapy and supportive measures, mortality rates are as high as 15% to 20%.

KEY POINTS

- Thyroid storm is a severe manifestation of thyrotoxicosis with life-threatening secondary systemic decompensation (shock); it occurs most commonly with underlying Graves disease coupled with a precipitating factor such as infection, surgery, myocardial infarction, or parturition and mortality is 15% to 20%.

- In addition to supportive care and treating the participating cause, thionamides and β-blockers are the mainstay of treatment to reduce thyroid hormone production and are often combined with iodine drops and high-dose glucocorticoids to treat thyroid storm.

Myxedema Coma

Myxedema coma is an extreme but rare manifestation of hypothyroidism, resulting in life-threatening secondary systemic decompensation. Without a frankly low T_4 level, myxedema coma is unlikely, regardless of the degree of TSH elevation. It has a very high mortality rate if there is a delay in treatment. Myxedema coma is more common in elderly women; it may occur in those with a history of hypothyroidism or no antecedent illness. Precipitating events are frequent, such as myocardial infarction, infection, stroke, trauma, gastrointestinal bleeding, or metabolic derangements. Cold exposure appears to be a risk factor, as this condition is more commonly seen in the winter months.

Mental status changes and hypothermia are the most common clinical manifestations. The spectrum of mental status changes includes lethargy, stupor, coma, depression, or even psychosis. Hypothermia (temperature less than 34.4 °C [94.0 °F]) is present in nearly all patients; lower temperatures are associated with a worse prognosis. Ventilatory drive is decreased, resulting in hypoxemia and hypercapnia. Additional signs include bradycardia, hypoglycemia, hyponatremia, and/or hypotension. A significant percentage of patients experience seizures, which may be related to the coexisting metabolic derangements.

If myxedema coma is suspected, the serum TSH and T_4 levels should be tested immediately. Diagnosis is made based on the clinical presentation and the coexisting metabolic abnormalities. The serum cortisol level should be checked as soon as possible to evaluate for concomitant adrenal insufficiency prior to initiation of thyroid hormone replacement. While awaiting the results of the serum cortisol measurement, it is generally advisable to empirically initiate high-dose glucocorticoid therapy. This therapy may be discontinued if the serum cortisol level is found to be normal or high.

The treatment of myxedema coma is aimed at restoration of the euthyroid state with thyroid hormone therapy, supportive care (mechanical ventilation, vasopressors, and glucocorticoids), warmed intravenous fluids, warming blankets, and management of the underlying precipitating event. The exact dose and preparation of thyroid hormone to administer is controversial; minimal clinical trial information is available to ascertain the optimal treatment regimen. It is important to balance the need for rapid reinstatement of a euthyroid state with the risk of precipitating a fatal cardiac event due to increased cardiac work with administration of thyroid hormone. Generally, intravenous levothyroxine therapy is administered, initially as an intravenous bolus of 200 to 500 μg, followed by daily doses of 50 to 100 μg intravenously until transition to an oral formulation is feasible. Treatment with T_3 is not recommended.

Even with aggressive therapy, the mortality rate for myxedema coma is 20% to 25%.

KEY POINTS

- Myxedema coma is an extreme but rare manifestation of hypothyroidism, resulting in life-threatening secondary systemic decompensation and a mortality rate of 20% to 25%.

- The treatment of myxedema coma is aimed at restoration of the euthyroid state with thyroid hormone therapy, supportive care (mechanical ventilation, vasopressors, and glucocorticoids), warmed intravenous fluids, warming blankets, and management of the underlying precipitating event.

Structural Disorders of the Thyroid Gland

Thyroid Nodules

Nodularity of the thyroid is extremely common; large population studies suggest that up to 5% of women and 1% of men have a clinically evident nodule. The prevalence increases with age. In autopsy series and screening ultrasound studies, nodules may be seen in up to 60%.

The differential diagnosis for a nodule in the thyroid is varied and includes both primary thyroid disorders and metastatic spread from other primary malignancies (**Table 27**). Most thyroid nodules are benign, with only approximately 10% harboring a malignancy. Ultrasonography is an inexpensive and highly effective method for stratification of malignancy risk. All patients with a suspected thyroid nodule should have a neck ultrasound that includes evaluation of the thyroid and cervical lymph nodes.

Nodules are frequently detected incidentally on imaging studies performed for other reasons. The diagnostic evaluation of incidentally discovered thyroid nodules is identical to those that are clinically detected, with the same rate of malignancy. Nodules incidentally identified on fluorodeoxyglucose-PET (FDG-PET) scanning, however, have a malignancy rate of 30% to 50%. Consequently, FDG-avid nodules found on PET scans require heightened suspicion and a lower threshold for intervention or diagnostic evaluation.

A careful history should be performed in patients with a thyroid nodule. Increased risk of malignancy is found in patients with history of radiation exposure to the head or neck, a family history of thyroid cancer, or a personal history of thyroid cancer. Additional factors that increase the risk for malignancy in a nodule include male sex, extremes of age (<20 or >60 years), rapid nodule growth, and hoarseness. On physical examination, the nodule should be assessed for texture, mobility, and associated lymphadenopathy. If the nodule is hard, fixed to surrounding tissue (nonmobile with swallowing), and/or there is associated cervical lymphadenopathy, the risk of malignancy is greater. Pain is an uncommon finding with thyroid nodules, but when present it is usually associated with benign conditions.

A serum TSH measurement is the initial laboratory test in a patient with a thyroid nodule. If the TSH is suppressed, measurement of T_4 and T_3 should be performed, and a radionuclide scan should be considered (**Figure 9**). The objective of the scan is to identify "hot" or functioning nodules, which have a very low likelihood of malignancy and typically do not require FNA. In contrast, if the TSH is high or normal, the radionuclide scan is unnecessary as it is unlikely to reveal a hot

TABLE 27. Types of Thyroid Nodules	
Benign	**Malignant**
Multinodular goiter (colloid adenoma)	Papillary thyroid cancer
Hashimoto (chronic lymphocytic) thyroiditis	Follicular thyroid cancer
Colloid cyst	Medullary thyroid cancer
Hemorrhagic cyst	Anaplastic thyroid cancer
Follicular adenoma	Primary thyroid lymphoma
Hürthle cell adenoma	Metastatic cancer
	Breast
	Melanoma
	Renal cell

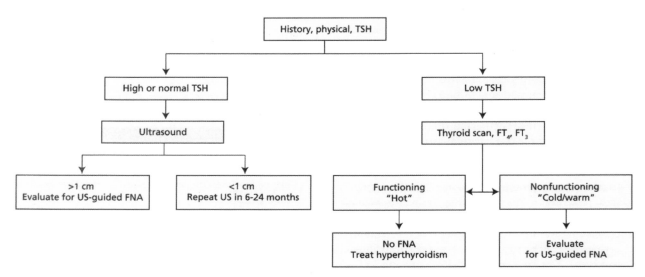

FIGURE 9. Initial evaluation of a thyroid nodule. There are size thresholds for FNA based on US appearance. A less suspicious lesion may not need FNA until it is larger than 2 cm, suspicious nodules if larger than 1 cm. FNA = fine-needle aspiration; FT_3 = free triiodothyronine; FT_4 = free thyroxine; TSH = thyroid-stimulating hormone; US = ultrasound.

nodule; the evaluation should proceed with an ultrasound and possible FNA. As thyroid nodular disease can be altered by normalization of the TSH, ultrasound and FNA should be postponed in patients with elevated TSH until TSH is normal, unless there is marked concern for malignancy. One-time measurement of thyroid antibodies may be appropriate if autoimmune thyroid disease is suspected or if multinodular goiter is identified by ultrasound to stratify the patient's future risk of developing overt thyroid failure. Serum thyroglobulin measurement is not useful and is not recommended.

FNA, performed under ultrasound guidance, is the optimal test to determine whether a nodule is malignant. When performed by an experienced clinician, FNA is safe and relatively simple to perform. The sensitivity of FNA cytology is 90% to 95%, and the false-negative rate is 3% to 5%. FNA of a nodule is generally recommended for those nodules larger than 1 cm that are solid and hypoechoic. The threshold for FNA of nodules that are partially cystic and lacking suspicious ultrasound features is 2 cm in size or greater. Aspirating a nodule of 5 mm or more may be considered if a patient has risk factors such as a personal or family history of thyroid cancer or prior radiation exposure.

The sonographic appearance of a nodule may be used to assess the risk of malignancy and thereby guide the decision of which nodules require biopsy. Features concerning for malignancy include microcalcifications, marked hypoechogenicity, irregular borders, and taller-than-wide shape. Such findings are nearly 70% specific for cancer, but their poor sensitivity cannot exclude the presence of malignancy.

The various diagnoses obtained on FNA and the associated risks of malignancy are listed in **Table 28**.

TABLE 28. Diagnoses Obtained by Fine-Needle Aspiration of Thyroid Nodules and Risk for Malignancy

FNA Diagnosis	Risk for Malignancy	Management
Benign	<3%	Serial ultrasound examinations for growth
Atypia of uncertain significance/follicular lesion of uncertain significance	5%-10%	Repeat FNA
Suspicious for follicular lesion	20%-30%	Hemithyroidectomy
Suspicious for malignancy	50%-75%	Hemithyroidectomy or total thyroidectomy
Malignant	97%-100%	Total thyroidectomy
Nondiagnostic	0%-50%	Repeat FNA; if two nondiagnostic FNAs, surgery

Modified from: Cibas ES, Ali SZ; NCI Thyroid FNA State of the Science Conference. The Bethesda System For Reporting Thyroid Cytopathology. Am J Clin Pathol. 2009 Nov;132(5):658-65. [PMID: 19846805]

FNA = fine-needle aspiration.

Nodules that are benign by FNA should be followed with repeat ultrasound examination in 6 to 18 months to assess for significant changes. If the nodule is stable on repeat imaging and lacks suspicious features, clinical examination and repeat ultrasound can be extended to longer intervals, such as 3 to 5 years. Greater than 50% change in nodule volume or interval development of concerning ultrasound characteristics should prompt a repeat FNA to evaluate for a false-negative initial biopsy.

Malignant nodules and those that are suspicious for malignancy require prompt excision; this is typically done with total thyroidectomy, but hemithyroidectomy may be preferable for patients younger than 45 years of age with a tumor smaller than 4 cm. A nondiagnostic FNA warrants a repeat attempt. In a solid nodule with two unsatisfactory biopsies, diagnostic hemithyroidectomy is indicated. Surgical complications include hypoparathyroidism and recurrent laryngeal nerve paresis; although typically temporary, either complication may be permanent in up to 3% of patients.

KEY POINTS

- Thyroid nodules are found in 1% to 5% of the population; most thyroid nodules are benign, with only approximately 10% harboring a malignancy.

- A serum thyroid-stimulating hormone measurement is the initial laboratory test in a patient with a thyroid nodule; if the thyroid-stimulating hormone is suppressed, then measurement of thyroxine (T_4) and triiodothyronine (T_3) should be performed, and a radionuclide scan should be considered to identify "hot" or functioning nodules, which have a very low likelihood of malignancy and typically do not require fine-needle aspiration. **HVC**

- If the thyroid-stimulating hormone level is high or normal, the radionuclide scan is unnecessary as it is unlikely to reveal a hot nodule and ultrasonography is an inexpensive and highly effective method for stratification of malignancy risk for nonfunctioning thyroid nodules. **HVC**

- Fine-needle aspiration of a nodule is generally recommended for those nodules larger than 1 cm (0.4 in) that are solid and hypoechoic and is the optimal test to determine whether a nodule is malignant.

Goiters

Multinodular Goiter

Multinodular goiters occur more frequently with advancing age, low iodine intake, or Hashimoto disease. The risk for malignancy is the same for multiple nodules as it is for a solitary nodule; therefore, the evaluation and management are identical. Biopsy should be performed on the three or four nodules (larger than 1 cm) with the most suspicious ultrasound features. In the absence of suspicious features, the largest nodules should be chosen for aspiration.

A large multinodular goiter may be associated with compressive symptoms such as dysphagia, hoarseness, or positional dyspnea. To assess the extent of mass effect, additional testing and imaging, including noncontrast CT of the neck/chest, barium swallow, direct laryngoscopy, and/or spirometry with flow-volume loops, may be indicated. Levothyroxine therapy to suppress TSH secretion and reduce goiter size is generally not helpful, poses a risk of thyrotoxicosis, and is not recommended. Radioactive iodine ablation is not an option for euthyroid and hypothyroid patients. Surgical removal is the treatment of choice if the compressive symptoms are significant, if malignancy is suspected, or if the patient desires cosmetic intervention.

KEY POINTS

- In patients with a multinodular goiter, the risk for malignancy is the same for multiple nodules as it is for a solitary nodule; therefore, the evaluation and management are identical.

- Surgical removal of a large multinodular goiter is the treatment of choice if the compressive symptoms are significant, if malignancy is suspected, or if the patient desires cosmetic intervention.

Simple Goiter

A simple goiter is defined as an enlargement of the thyroid gland without the presence of nodules. It may be seen in conditions of dyshormonogenesis, autoimmune thyroid disease, or primary thyroid lymphoma. Primary thyroid lymphoma is a rare condition that typically occurs in elderly women with a history of Hashimoto thyroiditis. The clinical presentation is a symptomatic, rapidly enlarging goiter with a very firm texture. Patients may also have systemic lymphoma symptoms and lateral cervical lymphadenopathy. The diagnosis can be made by FNA. Treatment typically involves chemotherapy and/or radiation therapy. Surgery generally is not indicated, but it can be used to aid in diagnosis when FNA is not informative.

Thyroid Cancer

The incidence of thyroid cancer is rising at a faster rate than any other type of malignancy; the incidence has more than doubled in the last 30 years. This increase is due solely to papillary cancers, with the highest rate of rise occurring in tumors measuring less than 2 cm. Meanwhile, the survival rate for thyroid cancer has remained stable or slightly improved. Autopsy series reveal that occult thyroid cancers measuring less than 1 cm may be identified in as many as 20% of dissected specimens. This finding, coupled with the improving survival rate, has led some investigators to conclude that the change in incidence of thyroid cancer is due solely to increased incidental detection of indolent tumors because of greater use of imaging modalities. Although there is little doubt that escalated detection of otherwise occult tumors has contributed to

the trend, there is evidence that larger tumors are increasingly being discovered.

The vast majority of patients with thyroid cancer have well-differentiated thyroid cancer, with excellent long-term survival. The major forms and their relative frequency are listed in **Figure 10**. The most common well-differentiated thyroid cancers are papillary, papillary-follicular variant, and follicular. There are rare, less well-differentiated variants of papillary thyroid cancer (columnar, tall cell, insular, oxyphilic, clear cell, diffuse sclerosing) that are more aggressive and carry a worse prognosis. Anaplastic thyroid cancer is undifferentiated and is the most aggressive form of thyroid cancer; 1-year survival rates range from 20% to 30%.

Staging and prognosis of well-differentiated thyroid cancers (papillary and follicular) are based on the American Joint Committee on Cancer criteria, which include age (<45 or ≥45 years), primary tumor size, local and distant metastases, and capsular and lymphovascular invasion. However, because the majority of patients have excellent survival, T (tumor) N (node) M (metastasis) staging plays a minimal role in the management of thyroid cancers. Instead, decisions regarding treatment are aimed at lowering the likelihood of recurrent disease.

Treatment of well-differentiated thyroid cancer includes a combination of surgery, radioactive iodine, and levothyroxine suppression. The extent of surgery is largely based on the tumor size; solitary tumors smaller than 1 cm may be sufficiently managed with lobectomy alone. Patients with larger tumors, multifocal disease, nodal metastases, or a history of irradiation are best treated with total or near-total thyroidectomy. For patients younger than 45 years of age with a tumor smaller than 4 cm and no evidence of nodal or distant metastases, hemithyroidectomy may be a reasonable alternative to total thyroidectomy. The decision to administer radioactive iodine is based on two factors: improvement in mortality rates and/or reduction in recurrence risk. Patients with distant metastases have improved survival with successful radioiodine

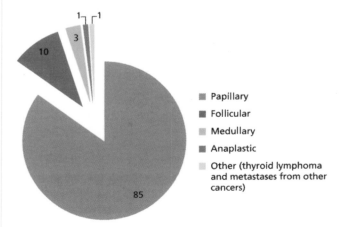

FIGURE 10. Relative frequency of the types of thyroid cancer.

Data from Hundahl SA, Fleming ID, Fremgen AM, Menck HR. A National Cancer Data Base report on 53,856 cases of thyroid carcinoma treated in the U.S., 1985-1995. Cancer. 1998 Dec 15;83(12):2638-48. [PMID: 9874472]

therapy, whereas administration of radioactive iodine may decrease the likelihood of recurrent disease in those patients with nodal metastases. Suppression of TSH with levothyroxine therapy may also be used to improve morbidity and reduce mortality, particularly in patients with persistent disease or distant metastases. The necessary degree of TSH suppression varies according to the risk of cancer progression and comorbidities of the patient. Patients with persistent disease typically require lowering of their TSH level to less than 0.1 µU/mL (0.1 mU/L), whereas those who are free of disease but have a high risk for recurrence should have a target TSH level of 0.1 to 0.5 µU/mL (0.1-0.5 mU/L) for 5 to 10 years. Those patients who are disease-free with a low risk of recurrence should maintain a TSH level of 0.3 to 2.0 µU/mL (0.3-2.0 mU/L).

Medullary thyroid cancer represents less than 10% of all thyroid cancers. Approximately 25% of medullary thyroid cancers are hereditary; all patients with medullary thyroid cancer should be screened with *RET* proto-oncogene sequencing. Medullary thyroid cancer may be associated with several syndromes, including multiple endocrine neoplasia type 2A (MEN2A) (which may include pheochromocytoma and hyperparathyroidism), MEN2B (marfanoid habitus and mucosal ganglioneuromas), or familial medullary thyroid cancer (medullary thyroid cancer alone). Biochemical screening for pheochromocytoma with measurement of plasma fractionated metanephrine levels should be done in all patients with an *RET* mutation prior to thyroidectomy.

KEY POINTS

- The vast majority of patients with well-differentiated thyroid cancer have excellent long-term survival.

- Treatment of well-differentiated thyroid cancer includes a combination of surgery, radioactive iodine, and levothyroxine suppression of thyroid-stimulating hormone for patients with persistent disease or high risk of recurrence.

Reproductive Disorders
Physiology of Female Reproduction

A regular, predictable menstrual cycle requires coordination of inhibition and stimulation between the hypothalamus (secreting gonadotropin-releasing hormone [GnRH]), the pituitary (secreting follicle-stimulating hormone [FSH] and luteinizing hormone [LH]), and the ovaries (secreting estradiol and progesterone). The coordination of these signals is referred to as the hypothalamic-pituitary-ovarian axis. The GnRH pulse frequency varies throughout the menstrual cycle to promote follicular development and ovulation (**Figure 11**). The phases of the menstrual cycle are referred to in reference to the activity of the ovary (follicular and luteal phases).

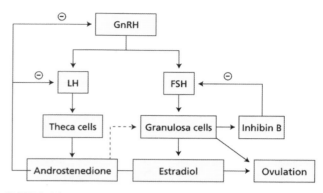

FIGURE 11. Female reproductive axis. Pulses of GnRH drive LH and FSH production. LH acts on theca cells to stimulate androgen (principally androstenedione) production. Androstenedione is metabolized to estradiol in granulosa cells. FSH acts on granulosa cells to enhance follicle maturation. Granulosa cells produce inhibin B as a feedback regulator of FSH production. FSH = follicle-stimulating hormone; GnRH = gonadotropin-releasing hormone; LH = luteinizing hormone; – (circled) = negative feedback.

FSH, under control of pulsatile GnRH secretion, rises in the early menstrual cycle to promote recruitment and growth of a follicle containing a microscopic oocyte (follicular phase). Granulosa cells lining the follicle secrete estradiol, which contributes to negative feedback inhibition of FSH secretion and resultant monofollicular development in the majority of women. Estradiol also stimulates endometrial proliferation. Further into the follicular phase, estradiol levels peak and exert acute positive feedback on the pituitary gland, which elicits an LH surge. This LH surge results in ovulation and initiates the luteal phase of the menstrual cycle. LH stimulates androgen production by the theca cells, which also line the follicle; androgen is subsequently aromatized to estrogen in the granulosa cells via aromatase enzyme. After the LH surge and ovulation, the follicle develops into the corpus luteum, which secretes both estradiol and progesterone and causes the secretory phase of the endometrium in preparation for implantation of a fertilized oocyte. With implantation, the early embryo produces human chorionic gonadotropin, which maintains the corpus luteum. However, when a fertilized embryo is not present, progesterone levels decline, leading to the menstrual phase of the endometrium and menstrual bleeding.

An average menstrual cycle ranges from 25 to 35 days in length. The follicular phase may vary in each woman but is typically from 14 to 21 days. Variability in a menstrual cycle is typically the result of a shortened or lengthened follicular phase, more commonly seen during the first 5 years of menstruation. A decrease in follicular phase length occurs commonly in perimenopause. The luteal phase is usually 14 days and is constant. In women younger than 40 years of age, menstrual cycles less than 25 days or greater than 35 days are likely anovulatory.

KEY POINT

- In women younger than 40 years of age, menstrual cycles less than 25 days or greater than 35 days are likely anovulatory.

Amenorrhea

Clinical Features

Primary Amenorrhea

Primary amenorrhea is the absence of menses by age 16 years accompanied by normal sexual hair pattern and normal breast development. Primary amenorrhea with absence of thelarche (breast development at the beginning of puberty) and/or adrenarche (androgen production increase that typically occurs at age 8 or 9 years) prior to 14 years of age should be evaluated. Pregnancy must be ruled out in any patient with primary amenorrhea before additional evaluation occurs. Causes of primary amenorrhea may be genetic, hormonal, or structural. Fifty percent of patients with primary amenorrhea have a chromosomal abnormality, such as Turner syndrome (45,XO) (gonadal dysgenesis), although some patients with Turner mosaicism may have secondary amenorrhea (see Secondary Amenorrhea).

Turner syndrome is commonly characterized by other clinical manifestations such as short stature, neck webbing, recurrent otitis media with hearing loss, aortic coarctation, and bicuspid aortic valve. The diagnosis of Turner syndrome may be made with a karyotype.

Approximately 15% of patients presenting with primary amenorrhea may have an anatomic abnormality of the uterus, cervix, or vagina such as müllerian agenesis, transverse vaginal septum, or imperforate hymen. Digital vaginal examination, transvaginal ultrasound, or MRI may help to identify outflow tract anomalies.

KEY POINT

- Fifty percent of patients with primary amenorrhea have a chromosomal abnormality, such as Turner syndrome (45,XO) (gonadal dysgenesis); 15% of patients presenting with primary amenorrhea may have an anatomic abnormality of the uterus, cervix, or vagina.

Secondary Amenorrhea

Secondary amenorrhea is the absence of a menstrual cycle for three cycles or 6 months in previously menstruating women. The most common cause of secondary amenorrhea is pregnancy. A potential structural cause of secondary amenorrhea, such as Asherman syndrome, should be considered. Asherman syndrome is an uncommon complication of dilation and curettage, intrauterine device placement, or surgical procedures such as hysteroscopic myomectomy; it is caused by lack of basal endometrium proliferation and formation of adhesions (synechiae). Diagnosis should be considered in any woman with amenorrhea and past exposure to uterine instrumentation. The classic presentation is amenorrhea or scant bleeding during periods (hypomenorrhea) with ovulatory symptoms (cervical mucous changes, adnexal tenderness associated with follicle formation) or premenstrual symptoms (mood changes or breast tenderness). Some patients will maintain small functional pockets of active endometrium with outflow obstruction by synechia closer to the cervix, resulting in cyclic pain and hematometrium identifiable on ultrasound.

After structural causes and pregnancy are excluded, the hormonal status should be assessed. Low estradiol and inappropriately normal FSH and LH levels indicate hypogonadotropic hypogonadism and point to a central cause (hypothalamic-pituitary). Low estradiol in the setting of elevated FSH and LH levels indicates hypergonadotropic hypogonadism and points to ovarian insufficiency.

The most common hormonal cause of secondary amenorrhea is polycystic ovary syndrome (PCOS) (see Hirsutism and Polycystic Ovary Syndrome), which accounts for 40% of cases. Additional hormonal causes of secondary amenorrhea include hypothalamic amenorrhea (hypogonadotropic hypogonadism), hyperprolactinemia, thyroid disease, and premature ovarian insufficiency (POI) (hypergonadotropic hypogonadism).

Hypogonadotropic hypogonadism caused by hypothalamic amenorrhea (HA) or functional hypothalamic amenorrhea (FHA) affects 3% of women between the ages of 18 and 40 years. Risk factors include low BMI and low body fat percentage, rapid and substantial weight loss or weight gain, eating disorders, excessive exercise, severe emotional stress, or acute and chronic illness. FSH and LH levels are inappropriately low in HA but may be inappropriately normal in FHA. Estradiol levels are typically low, and patients may experience vasomotor symptoms and sleep disturbance. If left untreated, patients are at increased risk for osteoporosis owing to this low-estrogen state. Recovery of menses may occur if BMI returns to normal. Cognitive-behavioral therapy for cases caused by emotional stress has been shown to be effective.

Hyperprolactinemia causes secondary amenorrhea through direct inhibition of GnRH secretion. Treatment of the cause of hyperprolactinemia typically results in restoration of menses. Hypothyroidism may cause secondary amenorrhea through increased thyrotropin-releasing hormone levels, which causes stimulation of prolactin secretion.

Hypergonadotropic hypogonadism as a result of POI is defined as amenorrhea before age 40 years in the setting of two elevated FSH levels (>40 mU/mL [40 U/L]) more than 1 month apart. Possible causes include Turner mosaicism (in which secondary amenorrhea may occur due to POI), fragile X premutation, chemotherapy or radiation, and autoimmune oophoritis. In patients in whom an autoimmune cause is diagnosed, evaluation of other endocrine organs (thyroid, parathyroid, pancreas, and adrenal) is recommended at the time of diagnosis and annually thereafter.

Estrogen replacement is necessary in patients with hypergonadotropic hypogonadism to prevent bone mass loss until the average age of natural menopause (50-51 years). Estrogen replacement preparations are available in oral, transdermal, subcutaneous, and vaginal routes of administration. The dose of estrogen required by young women is titrated to prevent vasomotor symptoms and vaginal dryness and may be higher than that used in an older age group. Because spontaneous ovulation may occur (although it is infrequent), counseling on contraceptive options should also be provided for sexually active women not desiring pregnancy. Cyclic progesterone exposure should be considered in patients with an intact uterus to prevent excessive unopposed endometrial proliferation. Oocyte donation may be considered for fertility options for this patient population.

KEY POINT

- The most common causes of secondary amenorrhea are pregnancy, structural abnormalities, and polycystic ovary syndrome.

Evaluation of Amenorrhea

A thorough history and physical examination, including a pelvic examination, are needed to evaluate both primary (no history of menstruation) and secondary amenorrhea (cessation of menstruation after menarche). Urine or serum human chorionic gonadotropin (HCG) testing should be done first to exclude pregnancy, as this is the most common cause of amenorrhea. In patients with primary amenorrhea, a karyotype is recommended if a pregnancy test is negative. Serum levels of prolactin, FSH, LH, estradiol, and thyroid-stimulating hormone (TSH) should then be obtained in the evaluation of primary and secondary amenorrhea. Abnormal levels of prolactin and/or TSH support a nonovarian cause of amenorrhea. Elevations of FSH and LH levels in the presence of a low estradiol level support the diagnosis of POI.

If no elevations in these hormones are found, a progesterone challenge test (oral medroxyprogesterone acetate, 10 mg for 7-10 days) may be used to determine if the amenorrhea is due to estrogen deficiency. If the patient has menstrual bleeding within 1 week of completing 7 to 10 days of medroxyprogesterone, estrogen deficiency is not the cause. In this case PCOS (or a similar diagnosis) should be considered. If no menstrual bleeding occurs, the patient has a low-estrogen state, and hypogonadotropic hypogonadism is the diagnosis (see Disorders of the Pituitary Gland).

Pelvic ultrasound is helpful to identify structural causes of amenorrhea such as müllerian agenesis and intrauterine synechiae. Saline-infusion sonohysterogram can identify intrauterine synechiae, and transvaginal or transabdominal ultrasound can identify absence of a uterus in patients with müllerian agenesis. Endocrinology consultation for further evaluation and testing of patients with findings suspicious for a genetic cause of amenorrhea may be appropriate. A pituitary MRI may be indicated to exclude other intracranial causes of hypogonadotropic hypogonadism when diagnosing HA or FHA, and consultation with an endocrinologist is recommended before imaging is pursued.

KEY POINTS

- After excluding pregnancy, the laboratory evaluation of primary and secondary amenorrhea includes measurements of prolactin, follicle-stimulating hormone, luteinizing hormone, estradiol, and thyroid-stimulating hormone.

- If hormonal evaluation for amenorrhea is negative, the next step is a progesterone challenge test; if the patient bleeds within 1 week of completing 7 to 10 days of progesterone, estrogen deficiency is not the cause and PCOS should be considered

Hyperandrogenism Syndromes
Hirsutism and Polycystic Ovary Syndrome

When hirsutism is present, the patient should be assessed for virilization, or development of male characteristics. Rapid onset and progression of deepening of the voice, severe acne, clitoromegaly, and male pattern balding are signs of virilization and are concerning for an ovarian or adrenal tumor. Age of onset after 30 years is also a risk factor for an androgen-secreting tumor.

In patients with hirsutism or virilization, recommended initial laboratory tests include measurement of plasma dehydroepiandrosterone sulfate (DHEAS) level and serum levels of TSH, prolactin, total testosterone, and follicular-phase 17-hydroxyprogesterone. Normal levels exclude adrenal tumors, hypothyroidism, hyperprolactinemia, and ovarian tumor. Common forms of late-onset congenital adrenal hyperplasia, often mistaken for PCOS, can be excluded with a normal 17-hydroxyprogesterone level. Pelvic ultrasound and adrenal CT should be performed to exclude an ovarian or adrenal neoplasm if the serum total testosterone level is greater than 200 ng/dL (6.9 nmol/L). Adrenal CT is necessary to exclude an adrenal cortisol-secreting and/or androgen-secreting neoplasm if the plasma DHEAS level is greater than 700 µg/mL (18.9 µmol/L). Hirsutism is typically a benign condition, most commonly from PCOS. A marked elevation of total testosterone or DHEAS is not compatible with a diagnosis of PCOS.

PCOS has a prevalence of 7% to 10% and is one of the most common endocrine disorders in young women. Two sets of diagnostic criteria are commonly used. The 2003 American Society for Reproductive Medicine and the European Society of Human Reproduction criteria for PCOS require two of the following three findings in the absence of other endocrine disorders: (1) oligo-ovulation or anovulation, (2) clinical or biochemical evidence of hyperandrogenism (such as hirsutism or acne), or (3) ultrasound findings of polycystic ovarian morphology in at least one ovary. The 1990 criteria from the National Institutes of Health and the National Institute of Child Health and Human Development require all of the following for diagnosis of PCOS: oligo-ovulation, signs of androgen excess (clinical or biochemical), exclusion of other disorders that can result in menstrual irregularity, and hyperandrogenism.

A constant stagnant follicular stage is seen in PCOS, resulting in unopposed estradiol secretion from small ovarian follicles. Owing to disordered secretion of LH by the anterior pituitary, intraovarian androgen production is also increased in PCOS, resulting in the hyperandrogenism associated with the disorder. Women with PCOS typically have elevated resting LH levels. In patients trying to conceive, this can lead to false-positive indication of the ovulatory LH surge on home urinary LH kits for ovulation.

Estradiol secretion results in proliferation of the endometrium in the absence of progesterone secretion from a corpus luteum. This predisposes patients to endometrial hyperplasia and heavy menstrual bleeding as a result of anovulatory bleeding. Oligo-ovulation and anovulation result in infertility but are typically correctable with clomiphene citrate or letrozole for ovulation induction if fertility is desired. If fertility is not desired, oral contraceptives should be considered if not contraindicated. Addition of oral contraceptives will increase secretion of sex hormone–binding globulin (SHBG) and decrease circulating levels of free testosterone. If a patient has a contraindication to oral contraceptives, a progestin-secreting intrauterine device or cyclic oral or vaginal progesterone should be given to prevent prolonged unopposed estrogen exposure.

Hyperandrogenism may present as hirsutism, acne, or androgenic alopecia. In patients with hirsutism desiring treatment, existing terminal hairs will need to be removed with depilatory methods, but the rate of hair growth while on treatment will decrease. Spironolactone, an aldosterone and androgen inhibitor, may be added after 6 months if acne and hirsutism are still cosmetically bothersome. Before initiation of therapy, the patient should be counseled about teratogenic effects on a male fetus, and contraceptive counseling should be provided.

Both obese and lean women with PCOS also have insulin resistance, and studies have identified an increased incidence of metabolic syndrome, obesity, impaired glucose tolerance, and type 2 diabetes mellitus in these women. Although insulin resistance may improve with weight loss, the use of insulin-sensitizing agents such as metformin is associated with a decrease in serum androgens; however, it is not very effective as a single agent for ovulation induction.

Evaluation of patients with PCOS should include assessment for signs of sleep apnea, hypercholesterolemia, and fatty liver. In women with a thickened endometrium or menometrorrhagia, endometrial sampling with endometrial biopsy should be considered to evaluate for endometrial hyperplasia. Weight loss and exercise should be emphasized.

KEY POINTS

- Polycystic ovary syndrome has a prevalence of 7% to 10% and is one of the most common endocrine disorders in young women; it is often associated with insulin resistance, metabolic syndrome, obesity and type 2 diabetes mellitus.

(Continued)

KEY POINTS *(continued)*

- Polycystic ovary syndrome can be diagnosed if two of the following three findings are present: (1) oligo-ovulation or anovulation, (2) clinical or biochemical evidence of hyperandrogenism (such as hirsutism or acne), or (3) ultrasound findings of polycystic ovarian morphology in at least one ovary.

- The 1990 criteria from the National Institutes of Health and the National Institute of Child Health and Human Development require all of the following for diagnosis of PCOS: oligo-ovulation, signs of androgen excess (clinical or biochemical), exclusion of other disorders that can result in menstrual irregularity, and hyperandrogenism.

Androgen Abuse in Women

Anabolic steroids may be abused by some women to enhance their athletic performance or physique. Such exogenous administration may result in absence of GnRH pulsatility and resultant hypogonadotropic hypogonadism and amenorrhea. Adverse effects may include hirsutism, acne, deepening of the voice, decreased breast size, and clitoromegaly. Withdrawal of exogenous androgens does not result in severe hypogonadism as it does in men, and most women return to regular menstrual cycles.

Female Infertility

Infertility is defined as the absence of conception after 1 year of unprotected intercourse (on average twice weekly) in a woman younger than 35 years of age. Investigation should begin after 6 months if no conception has occurred in a woman 35 years of age or older. Infertility evaluation should include a careful medical history of both partners with special focus on menstrual history, previous exposure to sexually transmitted infections, pelvic surgery, and previous obstetric complications such as miscarriage or cesarean delivery. If a report of oligomenorrhea is elicited, measurement of serum TSH and prolactin levels is appropriate to exclude thyroid disease and hyperprolactinemia as causes of oligo-ovulation.

Further evaluation of infertility causes typically includes semen analysis of the male partner, confirmation of ovulation with measurement of midluteal progesterone level (>3 ng/mL [9.5 nmol/L]), and because Fallopian tubes may be obstructed due to infection such as pelvic inflammatory disease, tubal patency evaluation with hysterosalpingogram. A common cause of tubal occlusion and resultant infertility is past pelvic inflammatory disease. Laparoscopy for evaluation of pelvic adhesions or mild endometriosis may be warranted in patients with dysmenorrhea, previous exposure to sexually transmitted infections, or previous pelvic surgery.

If no abnormalities are found, treatment to enhance endogenous gonadotropin release and increase the numbers of oocytes ovulated monthly may be warranted. Some studies support moving directly to in vitro fertilization treatment for women with infertility at age 40 years. In women treated with ovarian stimulation, oral medications such as clomiphene citrate or letrozole are typically used. This therapy is not appropriate in patients with POI. Patients should be counseled about the 5% to 8% risk of multiple gestation with these therapies. Referral to a reproductive endocrinologist is recommended.

KEY POINT

- Infertility evaluation in women should include a medical history of both partners with special focus on menstrual history, previous exposure to sexually transmitted infections, pelvic surgery, and previous obstetric complications such as miscarriage or cesarean delivery.

Physiology of Male Reproduction

Control of spermatogenesis and testosterone production depends on the pulsatile secretion of GnRH from the hypothalamus as well as subsequent downstream stimulation of the anterior pituitary and male gonads. In the testicle, FSH stimulates Sertoli cell spermatogenesis, and LH stimulates Leydig cell testosterone production. Negative feedback from testosterone production inhibits FSH and LH secretion at the level of the anterior pituitary as well as pulsatile hypothalamic GnRH secretion. Inhibin B, produced by the Sertoli cells, also inhibits FSH (**Figure 12**).

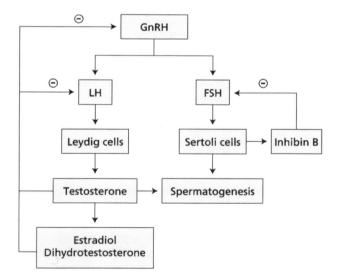

FIGURE 12. Male reproductive axis. Pulses of GnRH elicit pulses of LH and FSH. FSH acts on Sertoli cells, which assist sperm maturation and produce inhibin B, the major negative regulator of basal FSH production. The Leydig cells produce testosterone, which feeds back to inhibit GnRH and LH release. Some testosterone is irreversibly converted to dihydrotestosterone or estradiol, which are both more potent than testosterone in suppressing GnRH and LH. FSH = follicle-stimulating hormone; GnRH = gonadotropin-releasing hormone; LH = luteinizing hormone; – (circled) = negative feedback.

Leydig cell production of testosterone occurs in a diurnal pattern, with the highest concentration observed in the morning. A large percentage of circulating testosterone is bound either to SHBG or albumin. A serum total testosterone level measured in the early morning is generally considered to be an accurate measurement of a patient's androgen status, but it does not account for decreased SHBG as seen in obesity (see Evaluation of Male Hypogonadism).

Hypogonadism
Primary Hypogonadism

Primary hypogonadism, or testicular failure, represents a decrease in testosterone or sperm production. Primary hypogonadism is uncommon and may have congenital or acquired causes. Klinefelter syndrome is the most common cause of congenital primary hypogonadism. Klinefelter syndrome is a common cause of hypergonadotropic hypogonadism and azoospermia, resulting in infertility. A 47,XXY karyotype is diagnostic of Klinefelter syndrome. Mosaic variants of this condition exist but typically present with oligoasthenospermia, testicular failure or hypogonadism. Concomitant symptoms often include sexual dysfunction and generalized fatigue. Tall stature is a common finding. Patients with Klinefelter syndrome may fail to achieve puberty or may present after sexual maturation with azoospermia. Exposure to chemotherapy or radiation may also result in primary testicular failure. Local injury as a result of torsion, orchitis, or trauma may result in ischemia and necrosis of testicular tissues.

Secondary Hypogonadism

Typically secondary hypogonadism is a result of insufficient GnRH production by the hypothalamus or deficient LH/FSH secretion by the anterior pituitary. Causes may be congenital or acquired. Idiopathic hypogonadotropic hypogonadism, with anosmia (Kallmann syndrome) or without anosmia, is the most common cause of congenital secondary hypogonadism. Acquired secondary hypogonadism is most commonly iatrogenic due to exogenous testosterone administration. Untreated sleep apnea and obesity are other common causes. Other acquired causes include hyperprolactinemia, chronic opioid use, glucocorticoid use, or infiltrative disease (lymphoma or hemochromatosis).

Androgen Deficiency in the Aging Male

The natural progression of male aging involves testosterone level decline. Most men will not become hypogonadal, and the decline in testosterone production is highly variable with each person. "Low T" has become a part of the popular vernacular, owing to aggressive direct-to-consumer marketing, and describes many symptoms that may or may not be associated with a low serum testosterone level in men. Both prescription and over-the-counter testosterone and derivative sales have surged in the United States and many other countries. With the increased sales of testosterone formulations to treat aging men, questions have emerged about the potential adverse effects of exogenous testosterone therapy, particularly in men who have no biochemical evidence of testosterone deficiency. Potential adverse effects include increased risk of cardiovascular disease and death, venous thromboembolism, and prostate cancer.

Evaluation of Male Hypogonadism

A thorough history and physical examination are essential in the evaluation of hypogonadism. A sleep history is especially helpful. A large constellation of nonspecific symptoms is associated with male hypogonadism, which makes diagnosis and treatment based on symptoms alone not advisable. Nonspecific symptoms include fatigue, decreased muscle strength, decreased libido, amotivational state, or decreased robustness or frequency of erections. Testosterone measurements are not recommended if only nonspecific symptoms are present; rather, investigation of other causes of the patient's symptoms is appropriate. More specific symptoms include gynecomastia, diminished testicular volumes, and absence of morning erections. Measurement of testosterone levels is not recommended if a patient is having regular morning erections, does not have true gynecomastia on examination, and has a normal testicular examination, as it is highly unlikely that he has testosterone deficiency.

Testosterone deficiency is diagnosed with two early morning serum total testosterone levels below the reference range. Because illness and strenuous activity can falsely lower testosterone levels, measurement should occur in healthy men who have avoided strenuous activity for several days. Measurements of the testosterone level occurring later in the morning or in the afternoon are not useful for interpretation. Consultation with an endocrinologist should be considered if two early morning total testosterone levels are low. In certain clinical scenarios, such as morbid obesity, total testosterone may be low but free testosterone may be normal. Free testosterone assays can be unreliable, and routine measurement of free testosterone is not recommended. Free testosterone by equilibrium dialysis is the gold-standard assay.

Once confirmed, the cause of hypogonadism (primary or secondary) should be further investigated prior to initiation of testosterone replacement. Serum LH, FSH, prolactin, and TSH levels should be measured. Primary testosterone deficiency (hypergonadotropic hypogonadism) is diagnosed when FSH and LH levels are frankly elevated in the presence of a simultaneously low testosterone level. Low or inappropriately normal FSH and LH levels in the presence of simultaneous low testosterone levels are diagnostic of secondary hypogonadism (hypogonadotropic hypogonadism).

A hypergonadotropic state (elevated LH and FSH levels) should be further investigated with a karyotype if no history of gonadotoxic therapy or testicular insult is elicited. If a hypogonadotropic state is revealed, transferrin saturation and ferritin levels should be evaluated to exclude hemochromatosis. MRI of the pituitary should be performed to evaluate for hypothalamic or pituitary masses as the cause of the hypogonadotropic state if no confounding medications or reversible secondary causes are discovered. **Figure 13** shows an algorithm for evaluating male hypogonadism.

KEY POINTS

- Measurement of testosterone levels is not recommended **HVC** if a patient is having regular morning erections, does not have true gynecomastia on examination, and has a normal testicular examination, as it is highly unlikely that he has testosterone deficiency.

- Testosterone deficiency is diagnosed with two early morning total testosterone levels below the reference range.

- Once testosterone deficiency is confirmed, the cause should be further investigated prior to initiation of testosterone replacement.

Testosterone Replacement Therapy

Testosterone replacement therapy is a widely used treatment for men with hypogonadism. Possible benefits seen with testosterone replacement therapy, such as improved libido, energy level, and bone density, have been described but remain controversial. Testosterone therapy has been associated with increased hemoglobin and hematocrit levels, worsened obstructive sleep apnea, and a decrease in HDL cholesterol levels. LDL cholesterol levels do not appear to be affected.

Although hypogonadism remains an independent risk factor for mortality, recent studies have examined the association between testosterone therapy and cardiovascular risk. The association between testosterone therapy and mortality has remained controversial. Physicians prescribing testosterone therapy to elderly men with biochemically proven testosterone deficiency and comorbidities should use it prudently with close follow-up. Cardiovascular disease risk as well as risk for thrombosis should be discussed with patients before pursuing therapy. Prescribing testosterone therapy in the absence of biochemically proven testosterone deficiency puts the patient at risk for iatrogenic hyperandrogenism with subsequent increased risk of myocardial infarction, stroke, death, venous thromboembolism, polycythemia, and obstructive sleep apnea. Prescribing testosterone therapy in the absence of a full evaluation may delay treatment for secondary causes such as prolactinoma, hemochromatosis, or intracranial mass.

Although implantable pellets and injectable testosterone preparations are available, the most popular testosterone preparations currently are topical (most commonly hydroalcoholic

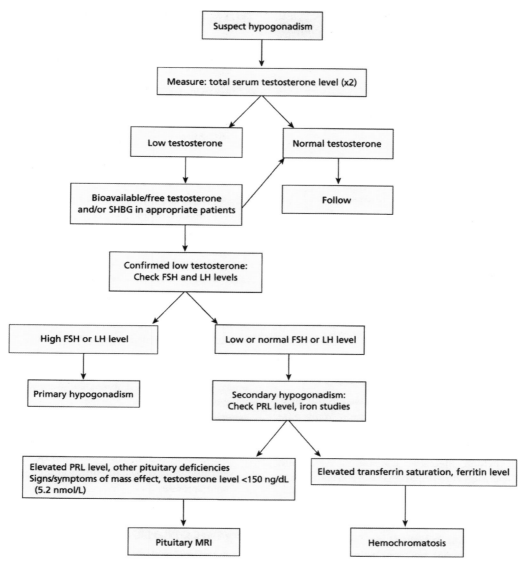

FIGURE 13. Algorithm for evaluating male hypogonadism. FSH = follicle-stimulating hormone; LH = luteinizing hormone; PRL = prolactin; SHBG = sex hormone–binding globulin; ×2 = two separate measurements.

gels). They require daily use and may incur significant cost to the patient, but the steady level of testosterone achieved within 30 minutes of application is an appealing feature. Inadvertent absorption by patient contacts may occur; users should be informed that virilization of contacts is not uncommon and premature puberty can occur in exposed children. The patient should also be counseled that decline in endogenous testosterone production and spermatogenesis may occur. If fertility is desired, testosterone therapy should be avoided, and consultation with a reproductive endocrinologist is recommended.

Patients requiring testosterone replacement therapy should have testosterone levels monitored at 3 and 6 months after initiation and annually thereafter; the goal total testoste-

rone level should be in the mid-normal range. Monitoring of the prostate specific antigen and hematocrit level should follow Endocrine Society guidelines (**Table 29**).

KEY POINTS

- Testosterone deficiency should be diagnosed biochemically, and its cause should be definitively determined before initiation of testosterone replacement therapy.

- Patients requiring testosterone replacement therapy should have testosterone, prostate specific antigen, and hematocrit levels monitored.

- Goal total testosterone level should be in the mid-normal range for patients requiring testosterone therapy.

TABLE 29. Endocrine Society Clinical Guidelines for Monitoring Adverse Effects of Testosterone Replacement Therapy

Parameter	Recommended Screening Schedule	Alerts
Hematocrit	Value obtained at baseline and then at 3 months and 6 months after therapy initiation, followed by yearly measurements	Value >54%
PSA level	For patients >40 years of age with a baseline value >0.6 ng/mL (0.6 µg/L), DRE and PSA level (determined at 3 and 6 months after therapy initiation followed by regular screening)	Increase >1.4 ng/mL (1.4 µg/L) in 1 year or >0.4 ng/mL (0.4 µg/L) after 6 months of use; abnormal results on DRE; AUA prostate symptoms score/ IPSS >19

AUA = American Urological Association; DRE = digital rectal examination; IPSS = International Prostate Symptom Score; PSA = prostate-specific antigen.

Data from Bhasin S, Cunningham GR, Hayes FJ, et al. Testosterone therapy in men with androgen deficiency syndromes: an Endocrine Society Clinical Practice Guideline. J Clin Endocrinol Metab. 2010;95(6):2550. [PMID: 20525905]

Anabolic Steroid Abuse in Men

Testicular testosterone production is suppressed in the presence of exogenous testosterone administration. Many elite athletes abuse androgens in injectable form, and herbal preparations of oral testosterone are readily available. Commonly used androgens include injectable testosterone esters and oral alkylated testosterone preparations. HCG injections mimic LH stimulation to the Leydig cells and result in elevated testosterone levels. Although this therapy is appropriate in men with hypogonadotropic hypogonadism, it may also be abused. Aromatase inhibitors are frequently used concurrently with exogenous testosterone preparations to prevent adipose conversion of estrogens to androgens and development of gynecomastia. Androstenedione supplements are commonly abused.

Excessive muscle bulk, acne, gynecomastia, and decreased testicular volume may be found on physical examination in patients using anabolic steroids. Irreversible hypogonadism may result and often presents as male infertility with oligospermia or azoospermia on sperm analysis. Permanent inability to produce endogenous testosterone may occur. Extratesticular effects may also be noted, including low HDL cholesterol level, hepatotoxicity, erythrocytosis, and increased risk of obstructive sleep apnea. Mood disorders are common in anabolic steroid users.

Laboratory studies showing low or normal gonadotropin levels and a low testosterone level with clinical evidence of hyperandrogenism are consistent with use of a non–testosterone-containing product, such as one containing androstenedione, or cessation of long-standing (typically greater than 1 year) anabolic steroid use, with failure to recover endogenous testosterone function.

KEY POINTS

- Excessive muscle bulk, acne, gynecomastia, and decreased testicular volume may be seen on physical examination in male patients using anabolic steroids.

- Exogenous testosterone use may result in irreversible decline in spermatogenesis and resultant infertility, as well as permanent inability to produce endogenous testosterone.

Male Infertility

Physical examination should include assessment for the presence or absence of the vas deferens, evaluation for congenital bilateral absence of the vas deferens (as seen in cystic fibrosis), assessment of testicular volume, and evaluation for the presence of hernia, varicocele, or tumor. Semen analysis obtained after 48 to 72 hours of abstinence from sexual activity is the best test to assess male fertility. For accurate results, analysis of the sample should occur within 1 hour of ejaculation. Extended abstinence periods may diminish fructose in the ejaculate and artificially lower sperm motility. If the physical examination is abnormal, evaluation by a urologist may be appropriate. If semen analysis results are abnormal, the test should be repeated, and referral, if abnormal, to a reproductive endocrinologist is warranted.

KEY POINT

- Semen analysis obtained after 48 to 72 hours of abstinence from sexual activity is the best test to assess male fertility; if abnormal, the test should be repeated for confirmation.

Gynecomastia

Gynecomastia is glandular breast tissue enlargement in men due to imbalance in the levels or activity of testosterone and estrogen. This imbalance results in an increased estrogen-to-testosterone ratio, which in turn results in decreased inhibitory action of testosterone on the breast tissue. The less testosterone and/or more estrogen the breast tissue is exposed to, the more likely gynecomastia will develop. Although abnormal in the postpubertal man, it is usually benign. It is typically bilateral but not always symmetric. Unilateral gynecomastia is uncommon and should be evaluated with mammogram as soon as possible owing to risk of breast cancer.

There are many causes of gynecomastia, ranging from drug-induced (marijuana, alcohol, 5α-reductase inhibitors, H₂-receptor antagonists, spironolactone, digoxin, ketoconazole, calcium channel blockers, ACE inhibitors, antiretroviral agents, tricyclic antidepressants, selective serotonin reuptake inhibitors) and hypogonadism (primary, secondary) to chronic illness (hepatic cirrhosis, chronic kidney disease) and endocrine disorders (hyperprolactinemia, acromegaly, hyperthyroidism, Cushing syndrome). Obesity and aging are associated with gynecomastia owing to increased aromatase activity in the periphery. Estrogen-secreting tumors (such as Leydig or Sertoli cell tumors or adrenal cortical carcinoma) and HCG-secreting tumors (such as germ cell tumors and hepatic carcinomas) are associated with gynecomastia.

A thorough history should be obtained. The breasts should be examined for glandular enlargement, which typically extends concentrically from under the areolae, and is firm, mobile, and rubbery. The breasts may be tender if the time course is acute. Pseudogynecomastia is subareolar adipose tissue, without glandular proliferation, that is associated with obesity. True gynecomastia typically distorts the normally flat contour of the male nipple, causing it to protrude owing to the mass of glandular tissue beneath it. In pseudogynecomastia, the nipple is typically still flat but soft, and nondescript subcutaneous fat tissue is present in the breast area.

Mild, chronic, asymptomatic gynecomastia does not warrant evaluation. Evaluation of gynecomastia that is asymmetric or concerning for malignancy (bloody nipple discharge, hard and fixed, associated with regional lymphadenopathy), of rapid and recent onset, or larger than 2 cm (>5 cm in obese men owing to the known increase in aromatase activity in obesity), should include measurement of total testosterone, LH, FSH, and TSH levels, as well as assessment of liver and kidney function. If indicated by findings on history and/or physical examination, measurement of prolactin, estradiol, and HCG may also be indicated. If the biochemical evaluation demonstrates abnormalities, further evaluation with testicular ultrasound, adrenal CT, or pituitary MRI may be indicated; consultation with an endocrinologist is recommended before imaging is ordered.

KEY POINTS

- Unilateral gynecomastia in the male patient is concerning for malignancy and warrants immediate evaluation with a mammogram.

HVC
- Mild, chronic, asymptomatic gynecomastia in the male patient does not warrant evaluation.

Calcium and Bone Disorders

Calcium Homeostasis and Bone Physiology

Serum calcium levels are tightly regulated on a moment-to-moment basis by the actions of vitamin D and parathyroid hormone (PTH). The amount of calcium that is albumin bound can be affected by hydration and nutritional status. If albumin levels decrease, total serum calcium levels may appear low (pseudohypocalcemia). Conversely, if albumin levels increase, total calcium levels will appear elevated (pseudohypercalcemia).

In both cases, ionized calcium should be measured. It will usually be normal, indicating normal circulating free levels of calcium. There are also instances of artificially increased calcium levels due to high protein states as in multiple myeloma (elevated monoclonal immunoglobulins), hyperalbuminemia, Waldenström macroglobulinemia, and thrombocytosis. In these patients, ionized calcium would be normal with elevated total serum calcium.

Vitamin D is a fat-soluble vitamin, and body sources include de novo production from the skin, through forms found in food, and through supplementation (**Table 30**). There are two forms of vitamin D supplementation: vitamin D_2 (ergocalciferol) and vitamin D_3 (cholecalciferol). Although both forms are useful in raising vitamin D levels, vitamin D_3 may be more beneficial because of tighter bonding to vitamin D receptors, longer shelf life, greater potency than vitamin D_2, and being identical to the vitamin D that naturally occurs in humans after ultraviolet light exposure.

Regardless of the method of ingestion, vitamin D_3 and D_2 are both inactive forms that must be hydroxylated twice before becoming active. The first occurs in the liver and converts vitamin D to 25-hydroxyvitamin D [25(OH)D], also known as calcidiol. The second occurs primarily in the kidney and forms

TABLE 30.	Sources of Vitamin D	
Sources	**Type of Vitamin D**	**Amount of Vitamin D**
Food Sources		
Cod liver oil	Cholecalciferol	400-1000 U/teaspoon
Salmon, wild caught	Cholecalciferol	600-1000 U/4 oz
Salmon, canned	Cholecalciferol	300 U/4 oz
Mackerel, canned	Cholecalciferol	250 U/4 oz
Sundried shitake mushrooms	Ergocalciferol	1600 U/4 oz
Egg yolk	Ergocalciferol	20 U/yolk
Sunlight (one minimal erythermal dose)		20,000 U in bathing suit
Fortified Foods		
Milk	Cholecalciferol	
Orange juice	Cholecalciferol	
Infant formula	Cholecalciferol	
Pharmaceutical Sources		
Vitamin D_2	Ergocalciferol	50,000 U/capsule
Liquid vitamin D_2	Ergocalciferol	8000 U/capsule
Multivitamin	Ergocalciferol and cholecalciferol	400, 500, or 1000 U/capsule
Vitamin D_3	Cholecalciferol	400, 800, 1000, 2000, 5000, 10,000, 50,000 U/capsule

the physiologically active 1,25-dihydroxyvitamin D [1,25(OH)₂D], also known as calcitriol (**Figure 14**).

Because 25-hydroxyvitamin D has a relatively long half-life of several weeks, it is the best indicator of whole body vitamin D status. Active vitamin D acts on three organ systems to achieve and maintain normal serum calcium: bone, intestine, and kidney. With adequate vitamin D, bone resorption is increased, intestinal uptake of dietary calcium is increased, and excretion of calcium through the kidney is decreased. PTH is secreted to increase the calcium in the blood in response to even the slightest degree of hypocalcemia; it acts on the kidney to increase production of active vitamin D and promote calcium reabsorption in the distal convoluted tubule and loop of Henle, and increased resorption in bones, thereby increasing release of calcium into the blood.

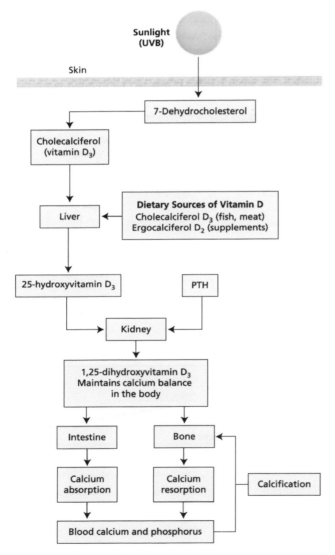

FIGURE 14. Production of vitamin D. PTH = parathyroid hormone; UVB = ultraviolet B.

Hypercalcemia
Clinical Features of Hypercalcemia

Hypercalcemia is marked by serum calcium levels above the normal range, usually greater than 10.5 mg/dL (2.6 mmol/L). Most patients are asymptomatic, and hypercalcemia may be noted incidentally on laboratory tests obtained for other reasons. Symptoms may occur with any degree of hypercalcemia but are more likely when serum calcium levels exceed 12 mg/dL (3 mmol/L). Classic symptoms of polyuria, polydipsia, and nocturia sometimes occur with elevated calcium levels of 11 mg/dL (2.8 mmol/L) or less. Other symptoms such as anorexia, nausea, abdominal pain, constipation, increased creatinine levels, and mild mental status changes are more likely to occur with levels greater than 11 mg/dL (2.8 mmol/L). As serum calcium levels continue to increase beyond 12 mg/dL (3 mmol/L), symptoms become more severe such as profound mental status changes, obtundation, acute kidney injury due to profound dehydration, and increased creatinine concentration.

KEY POINTS

- Classic symptoms of hypercalcemia are polyuria, polydipsia, anorexia, nausea, abdominal pain, constipation, and mental status changes; as serum calcium levels increase and/or the rate of change increases, symptoms become more severe, with profound mental status changes, obtundation, and acute kidney injury.

- 25-Hydroxyvitamin D has a relatively long half-life of several weeks, is the best indicator of whole body vitamin D status, and is the recommended test for vitamin D deficiency.

HVC

Diagnosis and Causes of Hypercalcemia

When serum calcium elevation is incidentally noted, repeat measurement of serum calcium is indicated, and if a second hypercalcemic level is noted, further evaluation is warranted to determine the cause (**Table 31**). The next step is determining if the hypercalcemia is PTH- or non-PTH–mediated by simultaneous measurement of serum calcium and intact PTH levels (**Figure 15**). Ionized calcium may be used in evaluating hypercalcemia, but it is rarely helpful in diagnosing hypercalcemia in patients with normal albumin levels or no acid-base disturbances.

Parathyroid Hormone–Mediated Hypercalcemia
Primary Hyperparathyroidism

Primary hyperparathyroidism is the most common cause of PTH-mediated hypercalcemia, and is diagnosed with a simultaneously elevated serum calcium level, with an inappropriately normal or elevated intact PTH level. The incidence peaks in the seventh decade and affects mostly women (75%). Before the age of 45 years, rates are similar in men and women. Approximately 80% of patients will have elevated PTH levels with simultaneously elevated calcium levels. Most commonly,

TABLE 31. Causes of Hypercalcemia
Parathyroid Hormone-Mediated Hypercalcemia
Primary hyperparathyroidism (adenoma, hyperplasia)
Parathyroid cancer
Tertiary hyperparathyroidism
Familial hypocalciuric hypercalcemia
Normocalcemic primary hyperparathyroidism
Non-Parathyroid-Mediated Hypercalcemia
Hypercalcemia of malignancy (humoral and local osteolytic)
Vitamin D toxicity
Vitamin A toxicity
Milk alkali syndrome
Thyrotoxicosis
Prolonged immobilization
Granulomatous diseases (sarcoidosis, tuberculosis)
Lymphomas
Total parenteral nutrition

primary hyperparathyroidism is due to a single parathyroid adenoma; however, rarely it may be attributed to multigland hyperplasia (typical in patients with end-stage kidney disease or multiple endocrine neoplasia syndromes) or parathyroid gland carcinoma (calcium is typically >14 mg/dL [3.5 mmol/L] and intact PTH levels >250 pg/mL [250 ng/L] on presentation; diagnosis is made histopathologically given the overlap with benign primary hyperparathyroidism).

Once diagnosed, measurement of serum phosphorus, 24-hour urine calcium, and serum 25-hydroxyvitamin D levels

may facilitate management. Serum phosphorus levels are typically low or low-normal in these patients. In contrast, phosphorus levels will be elevated in patients with vitamin D toxicity. Approximately 50% of patients with primary hyperparathyroidism will have elevated urine calcium levels, and the other 50% will have normal levels. Occasionally, urine calcium can be low in those patients with concomitant primary hyperparathyroidism and vitamin D deficiency. Additionally, patients with vitamin D deficiency convert more 25-hydroxyvitamin D to 1,25-dihydroxyvitamin D so they may have elevated levels of 1,25-dihydroxyvitamin D.

Parathyroidectomy is the treatment for primary hyperparathyroidism. Surgical management is curative in roughly 90% of patients, but evidence that the benefit outweighs the risk of the surgical procedure is present under only certain circumstances. There have been several long-term observational studies that found stability in biochemical markers and bone density in patients who do not meet the surgical intervention criteria listed in **Table 32**. When one or more of these criteria are met, surgery is recommended. Surgery can be considered when surgical criteria are not met, but patients should be cautioned that there are no robust data to support that intervention.

It is critical that an experienced surgeon perform the surgery to avoid increased risk of postoperative hypoparathyroidism and damage to the recurrent laryngeal nerve. Historically, a bilateral neck dissection was done to identify parathyroid glands that appeared to have irregular appearance or increased size. With the increased use of sestamibi scans, high-definition ultrasound, and intraoperative measurement of PTH levels, the minimally invasive technique is now preferred. Minimally invasive surgery allows for a smaller incision and a shortened surgical duration.

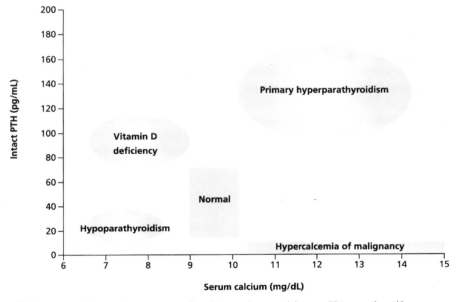

FIGURE 15. Relationship of calcium, PTH, and vitamin D status in normal conditions and in several diseases. PTH = parathyroid hormone.

TABLE 32. Indications for Surgical Intervention in Patients with Primary Hyperparathyroidism

Increase in serum calcium level ≥1 mg/dL (0.25 mmol/L) above upper limit of normal[a]

Creatinine clearance must be <60 mL/min (0.06 L/min)[a]

T-score (on DEXA scan) of −2.5 or worse at the lumbar spine, total hip, femoral neck, or distal radius[a]

Age 50 years or younger[a]

Surgery also indicated in patients in whom medical surveillance is neither desired nor possible, including those with significant bone, kidney, gastrointestinal, or neuromuscular symptoms typical of primary hyperparathyroidism

DEXA = dual-energy x-ray absorptiometry.

[a]In otherwise asymptomatic patients.

Recommendations from Bilezikian JP, Khan AA, Potts JT Jr. Third International Workshop on the Management of Asymptomatic Primary Hyperparathyroidism. Guidelines for the management of asymptomatic primary hyperparathyroidism: summary statement from the Third International Workshop. J Clin Endocrinol Metab. 2009 Feb;94(2):335-9. [PMID: 19193908]

In patients with osteoporosis who are poor surgical candidates or refuse surgery, intravenous bisphosphonate therapy will slow bone resorption and temporarily decrease serum calcium levels. Intravenous bisphosphonate should be redosed when hypercalcemia recurs.

In patients who do not meet the criteria for surgery, surveillance is recommended. Patients should have annual measurement of serum calcium and creatinine levels. A three-site dual-energy x-ray absorptiometry (DEXA) scan should be performed every 1 to 2 years to evaluate bone mineral density of the lumbar spine, hip, and distal radius. The frequency of DEXA scanning should increase to yearly when any treatment has been initiated for bone health or other medications have been added that may affect bone health (antiandrogen, antiestrogen, antiseizure medications, or glucocorticoids).

In patients with asymptomatic primary hyperparathyroidism, other precautions can be taken to prevent disease-related complications. These patients should maintain adequate vitamin D (400-600 U daily) intake to prevent further PTH stimulation. In patients with concomitant vitamin D deficiency, repletion is recommended to replete patients whose levels are below 30 ng/dL (75 nmol/L) with careful attention to urine calcium excretion and serum calcium once values are greater than 30 ng/dL (75 nmol/L). A large study did not show worsening calcium levels when repleting vitamin D in patients with levels less than 30 ng/dL (75 nmol/L). Adequate physical activity to prevent bone resorption and adequate hydration to prevent kidney damage are imperative.

Parathyroid Carcinoma

Parathyroid carcinoma is very rare, accounting for less than 1% of all persons with primary hyperparathyroidism. Mutations in the *HRPT2* gene are thought to be the major genetic link in parathyroid carcinoma, and inactivation of this gene leads to familial hyperparathyroidism as well. When compared with benign primary hyperparathyroidism, parathyroid carcinoma is equally prevalent in both sexes, more commonly presents with kidney and bone involvement and a neck mass, and frequently is associated with a total serum calcium level greater than 14 mg/dL (3.5 mmol/L) and very high parathyroid hormone levels, typically greater than four times the upper limit of normal. Most patients present with single gland involvement. Because parathyroid carcinomas may not appear histologically different from benign adenomas, local spread from the capsule, distant metastasis, or lymph node involvement must be present for carcinoma diagnosis. In these patients, surgical resection is the treatment of choice with calcimimetics used for residual disease or in patients who are poor surgical candidates. Any patient found to have parathyroid carcinoma should be screened for the *HRPT2* gene, and if positive, family members should be screened as well.

Tertiary Hyperparathyroidism

Tertiary hyperparathyroidism is the result of the prolonged PTH stimulation needed to maintain normocalcemia resulting from decreased 1,25-dihydroxyvitamin D levels from kidney impairment. This prolonged stimulation results in increased calcium levels and severe hyperparathyroid hyperplasia and elevated PTH levels that do not respond to phosphate binders and calcitriol therapy. Severe bone loss and other symptoms make surgical resection the treatment of choice.

Normocalcemic Primary Hyperparathyroidism

Normocalcemic primary hyperparathyroidism is defined as increased PTH levels in the absence of elevated calcium levels. This is a diagnosis of exclusion used in patients being evaluated for low bone density in which all secondary causes have been ruled out, including vitamin D deficiency. Approximately 20% of these patients will develop hypercalcemia within 3 years, so they should be monitored closely.

Familial Hypocalciuric Hypercalcemia

The most common form of familial hypercalcemia is familial hypocalciuric hypercalcemia (FHH). It is a rare autosomal dominant condition with a high penetrance that often occurs in childhood. These patients are frequently asymptomatic, but in rare cases the calcium–sensing receptor (*CASR*) gene mutation can increase the risk of pancreatitis. Elevated serum calcium levels are caused by a mutation in the G-coupled protein *CASR* gene. These receptors are in the parathyroid glands and the kidneys. The sensor mutation results in a shift upward in the "normal" range of calcium that the receptor recognizes, resulting in a mildly elevated serum calcium level (usually less than 11.0 mg/dL [2.8 mmol/L]) and high normal or mildly elevated PTH level. An elevated PTH level is more commonly seen in patients with concomitant vitamin D deficiency. The diagnosis is made by measuring 24-hour urine calcium excretion levels. Typically, patients with FHH will have a 24-hour urine calcium level less than 200 mg/24 h (5.0 mmol/24 h). The preferred standard is the calcium-creatinine clearance ratio, using the following formula:

Ca/Cr clearance ratio = [24-hour urine Ca × serum Cr] ÷ [serum Ca × 24-hour urine Cr]. A ratio less than 0.01 confirms the diagnosis if all other causes of hypocalciuria (thiazides, lithium, vitamin D deficiency) have been excluded. FHH is usually a benign condition that requires no intervention but should be recognized to prevent unnecessary parathyroidectomy.

Other Familial Hypercalcemias
Familial hyperparathyroidism is another rare cause of hypercalcemia. The disease presentation is almost identical to sporadic primary hyperparathyroidism, and a careful family history will suggest the diagnosis. Once a diagnosis of primary hyperparathyroidism is made, screening for familial causes should be done if the patient (1) is younger than 30 years of age at the time of diagnosis, (2) has a family history of hypercalcemia, or (3) has a medical history of other endocrinopathies. These patients should be tested for multiple endocrine neoplasia syndrome types 1 and 2 (MEN1 and MEN2).

MEN1 is characterized by functional pituitary adenoma, functional pancreatic tumors, and primary hyperparathyroidism. MEN2A is characterized by medullary thyroid cancer, pheochromocytoma, and parathyroid gland hyperplasia with the associated *RET* oncogene mutation. Patients with MEN would follow similar guidelines for surgical removal of parathyroid glands.

Medications Causing Hypercalcemia
Thiazide diuretics decrease the reabsorption of calcium in the kidney and result in elevated levels. Primary hyperparathyroidism, however, should also be considered if the patient remains hypercalcemic despite the discontinuation of the thiazide diuretic. In these patients, the thiazide may have been masking the PTH-mediated hypercalcemia.

Lithium decreases the parathyroid glands' sensitivity to calcium and may also reduce urine calcium excretion.

Non–Parathyroid Hormone–Mediated Hypercalcemia

In contrast to PTH-mediated hypercalcemia, non–PTH-mediated hypercalcemia is associated with very low PTH levels, typically less than 10 to 15 pg/dL (10-15 ng/L).

Malignancy-Associated Hypercalcemia
There are two mechanisms of hypercalcemia of malignancy: local osteolytic and humoral. When lytic bone metastases are present, hypercalcemia is the result of increased mobilization of calcium from the bone. Humoral hypercalcemia is less common and occurs when the tumor itself produces parathyroid-related protein (PTHrP) that binds to and activates the parathyroid receptor, raising serum calcium levels. Squamous cell carcinomas, breast cancers, and renal cell carcinomas are the tumors most commonly associated with hypercalcemia of malignancy. In multiple myeloma, the hypercalcemia is caused by the release of factors that stimulate osteoclast activity.

Other Causes
Non–PTH-mediated hypercalcemia can be caused by several other mechanisms. Thyrotoxicosis can lead to mild hypercalcemia through increased bone resorption. Resolution of the thyrotoxicosis should lead to normalization of calcium levels. Prolonged immobilization and increased vitamin A levels can lead to increased bone resorption. Increased levels of calcium absorption from the gut can be from markedly high vitamin D levels or increased intake of calcium carbonate products (milk-alkali syndrome). Granulomatous diseases, such as sarcoidosis and Wegener granulomatosis, and malignant lymphomas cause hypercalcemia through increased 1-α-hydroxylation activity that increases 1,25-dihydroxyvitamin D levels and calcium reabsorption in the gastrointestinal tract.

Treatment of Hypercalcemia

The treatment of hypercalcemia should focus on decreasing the serum calcium level by increasing calcium excretion and decreasing bone resorption or intestinal calcium absorption, as well as volume repletion. Polyuria, due to the decreased concentration ability of the distal tubule, is the main cause of dehydration in these patients. Although many patients do not require hospitalization, those with marked mental status changes, acute kidney injury, or calcium levels greater than 12 mg/dL (3 mmol/L) should be hospitalized for treatment. First-line therapy is aggressive intravenous fluid resuscitation. Once the patient is volume replete, an intravenous loop diuretic should be added if the calcium level has not normalized. Intravenous bisphosphonate therapy is usually given for longer-term control of hypercalcemia. Caution should be exercised with these agents in the setting of kidney dysfunction. Zoledronic acid, while more expensive, is a more effective therapy for patients with malignancy-related hypercalcemia. In patients resistant to or intolerant of bisphosphonate therapy, off-label use of denosumab, which also reduces osteoclast-mediated bone resorption can be used. Attention should be turned as quickly as possible to treatment of the underlying cause of the patient's hypercalcemia to ensure long-term maintenance of normocalcemia. If the underlying cause is increased 1,25-dihydroxyvitamin D hydroxylation, glucocorticoids can be effective therapy but may need to be dosed on a regular basis. For patients who present with serum calcium levels greater than 18 mg/dL (4.5 mmol/L) with neurologic symptoms or compromised kidney function, hemodialysis is an appropriate choice to quickly reduce calcium levels.

KEY POINTS

- Primary hyperparathyroidism is the most common cause of parathyroid hormone-mediated hypercalcemia and is diagnosed with simultaneously elevated serum calcium levels, with an inappropriately normal or elevated intact parathyroid hormone level.

- Parathyroidectomy is curative in approximately 90% of patients with primary hyperparathyroidism, but should be performed by an experienced surgeon using minimally invasive techniques.

(Continued)

KEY POINTS *(continued)*

- In contrast to parathyroid hormone-mediated hypercalcemia, nonparathyroid hormone-mediated hypercalcemia is associated with very low parathyroid hormone levels, typically less than 10 to 15 pg/dL (10-15 ng/L).

- The acute treatment of hypercalcemia focuses on decreasing the serum calcium level by increasing calcium excretion with vigorous volume replacement, decreasing bone resorption with bisphosphonates.

Hypocalcemia

Clinical Features of Hypocalcemia

Hypocalcemia, defined by serum calcium levels below the normal range, may be asymptomatic if mild. As calcium levels decrease, particularly below 8.0 mg/dL (2.0 mmol/L), symptoms may develop, including paresthesias (numbness/tingling around the mouth, tingling in fingers and toes), muscle cramping (Trousseau and Chvostek signs), decreased muscle strength, electrocardiogram changes (prolonged Q/T interval), tetany, and seizures.

Diagnosis and Causes of Hypocalcemia

Asymptomatic hypocalcemia may be noted incidentally on routine laboratory tests. When this occurs, the calcium level should be repeated in conjunction with a serum albumin level. If hypocalcemia is confirmed, simultaneous intact PTH and serum calcium must be measured to confirm if PTH is responding appropriately. The appropriate physiologic response to lower calcium levels is an elevation in PTH levels.

Hypoparathyroidism

Hypoparathyroidism, commonly due to trauma during neck surgery (thyroidectomy or parathyroidectomy), is the most common cause of hypocalcemia. During head and neck surgeries, the parathyroid glands can be inadvertently removed or parathyroid hormone production can be transiently decreased due to disruption of blood supply. Only serial measurements of calcium levels will determine whether the damage is transient. Hypoparathyroidism can also be caused by damage from radiation exposure, parathyroid gland infarction, infiltrative diseases (hemochromatosis, Wilson disease, granulomas), or autoimmune hypoparathyroidism. [H]

Other Causes of Hypocalcemia

Other, less common causes of hypocalcemia include poor calcium intake, activating mutations in the *CASR* gene, PTH resistance, increased phosphate binding in vascular space (rhabdomyolysis or tumor lysis syndrome), increased citrate chelation with large volume blood transfusions, sepsis, vitamin D deficiency, and hypomagnesemia. Low levels of magnesium (due to alcohol abuse or malnutrition) activate G-proteins that stimulate calcium-sensing receptors and decrease PTH secretion.

KEY POINT

- The most common cause of hypocalcemia is hypoparathyroidism, which is most often due to trauma during surgery to the neck.

Treatment of Hypocalcemia

Mild, asymptomatic hypocalcemia (serum calcium 8.0-8.5 mg/dL [2.0-2.1 mmol/L]), is a common finding and does not require treatment.

Calcium carbonate and calcium citrate are the most common oral calcium formulations. Calcium carbonate requires an acidic environment to be absorbed; therefore, all patients who are on proton pump inhibitors should be prescribed calcium citrate. Adequate levels of both 25-hydroxyvitamin D and 1,25-dihydroxyvitamin D are also essential. In the acute phase of repletion, 1,25-dihydroxyvitamin D is more effective than 25-hydroxyvitamin D. If the patient is symptomatic or if the hypocalcemia is acute, calcium gluconate and calcium citrate are both available in intravenous form. Goal calcium is 7.0 to 7.5 mg/dL (1.8-1.9 mmol/L) with intravenous repletion, and oral forms can be used once that goal is achieved. The overall goal of repletion is the low to low-normal range (serum calcium 8.0-8.5 mg/dL [2.0-2.1 mmol/L]).

If a patient requires chronic replacement, usually due to hypoparathyroidism, care must be taken to avoid hypercalciuria as calcium nephrolithiasis and decreased glomerular filtration rate can occur. Chronic replacement typically includes calcitriol, calcium, and occasionally magnesium. Calcitriol is the vitamin D source of choice because PTH is needed for optimal conversion of 25-hydroxyvitamin D to 1,25-dihydroxyvitamin D. Serum calcium, magnesium, creatinine, and urine calcium levels should be measured at each follow-up visit. The goal calcium levels should be low-normal without hypercalciuria. The magnesium level should ideally be greater than 2 mg/dL (0.83 mmol/L) and creatinine levels should remain in the normal range. If the urine calcium level is greater than 300 mg/24 h (hypercalciuria), calcium and/or vitamin D replacement needs to be decreased. Calcium is usually decreased first if the vitamin D levels are within the normal sufficiency range.

KEY POINT

- If hypoparathyroidism is the cause of hypocalcemia, correction of any coexisting hypomagnesemia to serum magnesium 2 mg/dL (0.8 mmol/L) or higher is necessary.

Metabolic Bone Disease

Osteopenia and Osteoporosis

Physiology

Bone mineral density begins to increase with puberty, and peak bone mass is achieved in early adulthood. Sex hormones, estrogen and testosterone, are crucial to increasing bone mineral density in women and men, respectively. Specifically, estrogen has impact on osteoclast and osteoblast activity in both men and women. Towards the end of puberty, estrogen halts bone resorption and signals the closure of epiphyseal plates. Bone mass begins to decline in women after menopause, with decreased estrogen levels, and in men over age 50 years. In men, the loss of testosterone typically accelerates bone loss after 70 years of age. Early cessation of sex hormone production in either sex, for any reason, may accelerate the loss of bone mineral density. Bone loss occurs when the removal of old bone (osteoclastic activity) exceeds the replacement with new bone (osteoblastic activity). Accelerated bone loss can often be attributed to hypogonadism or medications that promote bone loss.

Risk Assessment and Screening Guidelines

Declining bone mineral density is associated with future fracture risk and therefore is an important component of fracture risk assessment. Individual peak bone mass is determined by genetic factors, nutrition, changes in hormone (estrogen, testosterone, thyroxine) levels, concomitant health conditions, and physical activity level.

The National Osteoporosis Foundation recommends that all postmenopausal women and men older than 50 years of age be evaluated for osteoporosis. This evaluation includes a thorough history for potential risk factors and physical examination. This preliminary screening will determine if bone mineral density (BMD) or vertebral imaging is necessary. **Table 33** lists several common risk factors for osteoporosis. If a patient is deemed high risk, a study of BMD with DEXA may help further assess fracture risk. The DEXA is designed to measure BMD and establish risk of fracture in postmenopausal women. In young men and premenopausal women, assessment of BMD for fracture risk is not advised or validated. **Table 34** lists the U.S. Preventive Services Task Force recommendations for BMD testing.

Diagnosis

The diagnosis of osteopenia is based on BMD testing. Osteoporosis, however, can be diagnosed by BMD testing or clinically in the patient with history of fragility fracture, hip fracture, or vertebral compression fracture.

DEXA assesses the density of the vertebral and hip bones compared with healthy young-adult sex-matched reference values. The distal one-third of the radius can be used in patients when the hip or vertebral BMD cannot be measured. The score is based on the number of standard deviations above or below the mean reference value and is known as the T-score. Those patients with T-scores at -1.0 and above have normal bone density. A T-score between -1.0 and -2.5 is defined as low bone mass (osteopenia). Osteoporosis is defined as a T-score below -2.5. Severe osteoporosis is defined as a T-score of -2.5 or below with one or more fractures. In women and men younger than 50 years, the International Society for Clinical Densitometry recommends that ethnic- or race-adjusted Z-scores be used. The Z-score compares a patient's BMD with others of their same age and ethnicity, and osteoporosis/osteopenia cannot be diagnosed in these patients. A Z-score of -2.0 or lower should be described as "low bone mineral density for chronologic age" or "below the expected range for age." Patients with Z-scores above -2.0 are "within the expected range for age."

In 2008, the World Health Organization (WHO) created the Fracture Risk Assessment Tool (FRAX) calculator that further defines the 10-year fracture risk for patients with osteopenia, defined as a T-score between -1.0 to -2.5 on DEXA. The FRAX score notes the probability of major osteoporotic fracture and hip fracture in the next 10 years. If the risk of major osteoporotic fracture is greater than or equal to 20% or the risk of hip

TABLE 33. Low Bone Mineral Density Associations				
Lifestyle	**Comorbid Illness**	**Hormonal States**	**Medications**	**Nonmodifiable Risk Factors**
Alcohol use	Vitamin D insufficiency	Premature menopause	Anticonvulsants	Race
BMI <17	Hypercalciuria	Premature ovarian insufficiency	Glucocorticoids (≥5 mg/d of prednisone or equivalent for ≥3 months)	Age
Low calcium intake	Osteogenesis imperfect	Panhypopituitarism		Gender
Smoking	Homocystinuria	Hyperprolactinemia	GnRH antagonists and agonists	First-degree relative with low bone mineral density
Immobilization	Hemochromatosis	Androgen insufficiency	SSRIs	
Weight loss	Glycogen storage disease	Thyrotoxicosis	Thiazolidinediones	
Malabsorptive bariatric surgery	Cystic fibrosis		Aromatase inibitors	
Gastric bypass surgery	Celiac disease		Anticoagulants	
Recurrent falls	Cushing syndrome		Lithium	
	Inflammatory bowel disease			
	Diabetes mellitus (types 1 and 2)			

GnRH = gonadotropin-releasing hormone; SSRI = selective serotonin reuptake inhibitor.

TABLE 34. U.S. Preventive Services Task Force Recommendations for Measurement of Bone Mineral Density and Vertebral Imaging

Bone Mineral Density Testing[a]

Women age 65 and older and men age 70 and older

Postmenopausal women and men age 50 to 69, based on risk factor profile

Those who have had a fracture, to determine degree of disease severity

Radiographic findings suggestive of osteoporosis or vertebral deformity

Glucocorticoid therapy for more than 3 months

Primary hyperparathyroidism

Treatment for osteoporosis (to monitor therapeutic response)

Vertebral Imaging[b]

Women ≥70 and men ≥80 if T-score at the spine, total hip, or femoral neck is ≤ −1.0

Women aged 65-69 and men aged 75-79 if T-score at the spine, total hip, or femoral neck is ≤1.5

In postmenopausal women age 50-64 and men aged 50-69 with the following risk factors:

Low-trauma fractures

Historic height loss of 1.5 in or more (4 cm)

Height loss of 0.8 inches or more (2 cm)

Recent or ongoing long-term glucocorticoid treatment

[a]BMD testing should be performed at DEXA facilities using accepted quality assurance measures.

[b]Vertebral imaging should be repeated when a new loss of height is noted or new back pain is reported.

fracture is greater than or equal to 3%, the patient's benefit from therapy exceeds the risk, and treatment should be offered.

The FRAX was validated for use in persons 40 to 90 years of age who are not currently or previously treated with pharmacotherapy for osteoporosis. The WHO has a web site that offers an online FRAX calculator at www.shef.ac.uk/FRAX.

In additional to BMD testing, vertebral imaging using radiographs is recommended in high-risk groups since many vertebral fractures are asymptomatic. The presence of a vertebral compression fracture establishes the clinical diagnosis of osteoporosis, regardless of T-score on DEXA, and treatment is recommended. Once a vertebral image is obtained, it only needs to be repeated if there is noted height loss or new back pain.

Evaluation of Secondary Causes of Bone Mineral Density Loss

Most cases of osteoporosis are due to declining levels of sex hormones which are non-modifiable, such as age, sex, menopause, height, and build. Some patients, however, have osteoporosis caused by secondary causes. Measurement of complete blood count (for malignancy), complete metabolic panel (for calcium levels and kidney function), thyroid-stimulating hormone, 25-hydroxyvitamin D, and urine calcium (screening for

hypercalciuria) is an appropriate set of laboratory tests to screen for secondary causes of BMD loss. These are modifiable conditions that, if corrected, will result in increased BMD. These patients are typically young with either markedly low BMD for age or a new fracture or patients of any age with multiple fractures.

With all secondary causes of decreased BMD, reversal of the cause should be the first line of therapy and subsequent DEXA should be performed. If the BMD has not improved or the FRAX score suggests increased risk of fracture, treatment should be started. In the event of a fracture, the underlying cause should still be addressed in addition to initiating pharmacologic therapy for osteoporosis.

Pharmacologic Treatment Options

Currently there are six categories of pharmacologic agents that are FDA approved for the treatment of postmenopausal osteoporosis. These medications are bisphosphonates, calcitonin, estrogens, estrogen agonists, parathyroid hormone, and the receptor activator of nuclear factor κB (RANK) ligand inhibitor family. Bisphosphonates are usually first-line therapy unless there is a compelling reason why another therapy should be used. The other modalities are typically used after a bisphosphonate failure or inability to use the medication. Most of these medications can also be used for prevention of osteoporosis. Prevention therapy may be used in patients with osteopenia who do not meet FRAX standards for therapy but have multiple risk factors such as high-risk medications (glucocorticoids or antiestrogen, antiandrogen, or antiseizure medications) in combination with a strong family history of osteoporosis.

Bisphosphonates

Bisphosphonate medications work by inhibiting osteoclastic activity. Before starting any bisphosphonate therapy, vitamin D status and calcium levels should be evaluated, as bisphosphonates can lead to hypocalcemia. For oral bisphosphonates, integrity of the esophageal lining and ability to swallow pills are important. Kidney function should be assessed as bisphosphonates are contraindicated in patients with an estimated glomerular filtration rate less than 35 mL/min/1.73 m^2. Although rare, osteonecrosis of the jaw has been reported with bisphosphonate usage, particularly with high-dose intravenous administration and increased duration of the bisphosphonate. Additionally, atypical femur fractures have been reported with long-term usage. Regular questioning about pain in the thigh or groin area is recommended for patients on bisphosphonates. If patients report discomfort, a radiograph should be obtained. To reduce the risk of these side effects, a drug holiday has been suggested in patients with low-risk osteoporosis (T-score greater than −2.5 or single fractures) who have been on therapy for 3 to 5 years with stable BMD. During bisphosphonate therapy for prevention or treatment, men 50 to 70 years of age should consume 1000 mg/d of calcium and women aged 51 years and older and men aged 71 years and older consume 1200 mg/d of calcium.

Alendronate has been approved by the FDA for prevention and treatment of osteoporosis. The prevention dose is a 5-mg tablet daily or a 35-mg tablet weekly. The treatment dose is a 10-mg tablet daily or a 70-mg tablet weekly. Alendronate is also approved for treatment of men with osteoporosis as well as treatment of both women and men with glucocorticoid-induced osteoporosis. Alendronate has been shown to reduce the incidence of spine and hip fractures by approximately 50% over 3 years in patients with previous fractures.

Ibandronate is FDA approved for the treatment and prevention of postmenopausal osteoporosis. The dosage is a 150-mg tablet monthly or 3 mg every 3 months by intravenous injection. There is FDA approval for the oral formulation for osteoporosis prevention only. Ibandronate primarily reduces risk of vertebral fractures by 50% in 3 years.

Risedronate is FDA approved for the prevention and treatment of osteoporosis. The treatment dose is a 5-mg tablet daily, a 35-mg tablet weekly, a 75-mg tablet on two consecutive days every month, or a 150-mg tablet monthly. Risedronate is also approved for treatment of osteoporosis in men and women with glucocorticoid-induced osteoporosis. Risedronate reduces the incidence of vertebral fracture by approximately 45% and nonvertebral fractures by one-third over 3 years.

Zoledronic acid has been FDA approved for the prevention and treatment of postmenopausal osteoporosis in women, for improvement of bone mass in men with osteoporosis, and for the prevention and treatment of glucocorticoid-induced osteoporosis in men and women. Recently zoledronic acid has been approved for secondary prevention of fractures in patients who have had recent low-trauma hip fracture. The treatment dose of zoledronic acid is 5 mg intravenously annually or once every 2 years for prevention.

Calcitonin

Calcitonin is FDA approved for the treatment of osteoporosis in women who are 5 or more years postmenopausal. Calcitonin (200 U) is delivered in a single daily intranasal spray. Subcutaneous administration is also available but is used less frequently. Calcitonin should be used with caution with patients who have an allergy to salmon, allergic rhinitis, or epistaxis. Very rarely, patients can also have an anaphylactic response that requires emergency attention and discontinuation of the medication.

Estrogen Agonists and Antagonists

The use of estrogen to maintain bone health in postmenopausal women has fallen out of favor because of data indicating that estrogen increases the risk of cardiovascular disease and breast cancer. Therefore, estrogen use for osteoporosis prevention should be limited to younger women with premature ovarian failure and postmenopausal women who also require its beneficial effects for hot flushes or vaginal dryness.

Raloxifine has been approved for the treatment of postmenopausal osteoporosis. The treatment dose is a 60-mg tablet to be taken with or without food.

Parathyroid Hormone

Teriparatide (recombinant human PTH [1-34]) has been FDA approved for the treatment of osteoporosis in postmenopausal women and men who are at high risk for fracture. "High risk" is defined as patients with a T-score of -3.0 or less or patients who have either had a fracture or decreased BMD while on bisphosphonate therapy. It is also approved for men and women at high risk of fracture due to long-time glucocorticoid use. Teriparatide has bone-building properties in addition to the antiresorptive properties of the other agents. It is the only bone-building treatment option for osteoporosis.

Teriparatide is an anabolic steroid that is administered by a 20-μg daily subcutaneous injection; it is approved for up to 24 months over a patient's lifetime. After the 24-month duration, an antiresorptive agent (such as bisphosphonates or denosumab) can be administered to maintain BMD gains achieved with teriparatide.

Receptor Activator of Nuclear Factor κB (RANK) Ligand Inhibitors

Denosumab is a receptor activator of nuclear factor κB (RANK) ligand inhibitors that is FDA approved for the treatment of osteoporosis in postmenopausal women who are at high risk of fracture. It is an antiresorptive agent, like the bisphosphonates with much the same effect and outcomes. It is also approved for treatment of osteoporosis in men and those undergoing treatment of certain cancers, such as prostate cancer, who are at high risk for fractures. Denosumab is given by subcutaneous injection (60 mg every 6 months).

Annual Reassessment of Patients with Low Bone Mass

Once an initial DEXA scan has been obtained, every effort should be made to have subsequent scans done on the same machine. Once a repeat scan has been done, change in BMD, not T-score, from year to year is the appropriate way to interpret whether there has been a significant change in BMD. Most reports will not show a statistically significant change in the BMD from the previous test. If not noted on the report, a calculated change of about 4% likely represents a statistically significant change. Annually, a complete clinical evaluation of the patient, determination of risk factors for bone loss, and evaluation for development of secondary causes of bone loss should be performed, starting with a history and physical examination.

Vitamin D Deficiency

In promoting absorption from the gut, vitamin D enables proper bone mineralization by maintenance of calcium and phosphorus levels. Vitamin D also modulates the actions of osteoblasts and osteoclasts to ensure proper bone growth and remodeling. Chronically low levels of vitamin D can lead to rickets in children and osteomalacia in adults (see MKSAP 17 Nephrology).

In addition to bone health, vitamin D plays a role in inflammation reduction, growth regulation of various cell types, immune function, and neuromuscular signaling.

In assessing serum levels of vitamin D, concentrations of 25-hydroxyvitamin D are the best indicator of vitamin D status. It reflects vitamin D produced cutaneously and that obtained from food and supplements and has a circulating half-life of 15 days.

There are three levels of vitamin D status: sufficient (25-hydroxyvitamin D ≥30 ng/mL [75 nmol/L]), insufficient (25-hydroxyvitamin D 21-29 ng/mL [52.4-72.4 nmol/L]), and deficient (25-hydroxyvitamin D ≤20 ng/mL [50 nmol/L]). Because vitamin D levels can be affected by sun exposure, fall through winter months are ideal times to measure vitamin D levels. It is best to measure vitamin D levels at the same time each year unless treatment is being followed. In general, the optimal levels of vitamin D are those that prevent PTH levels from increasing to above normal levels. Increased PTH levels will lead to increased calcium withdrawal from the bones. In an attempt to find the optimal vitamin D level, several studies have looked at vitamin D levels related to cancer incidence, muscle stability and falls, immune status, and mood, in addition to bone health. Among most experts, a level between 30 and 40 ng/mL (75-100 nmol/L) is deemed sufficient for preventive health. Based on these levels, about 30% to 60% of Americans have low vitamin D levels, therefore most expert groups recommend screening all patients at least once. Those with darker skin, decreased sun exposure, or increased demands (pregnancy) often have low levels.

Special populations will have lower levels of vitamin D owing to medical conditions or medication side effects. In addition, obesity has been correlated with lower vitamin D levels possibly related to fat sequestration. Certain antiseizure medications (phenobarbital and phenytoin) may increase the metabolism of vitamin D to inactive forms. Glucocorticoids can decrease vitamin D metabolism. Agents that decrease absorption such as orlistat and cholesterol lowering agents can decrease vitamin D absorption. Similarly, patients with malabsorption disorders, including those with celiac disease and those who had bariatric surgery, can have decreased levels of vitamin D. In these special patient populations, not only does screening for deficiency need to be more frequent, but repletion may be more challenging. It is recommended that these populations be given at least two to three times more vitamin D to maintain adequate levels.

Recommendations

The current National Osteoporosis Foundation and Endocrine Society recommendation for adults 19 to 70 years of age is at least 600 U/d of vitamin D to maximize bone health; however, to raise blood levels consistently above 30 ng/dL (75 nmol/L) may require 1500 to 2000 U/d. In adults older than 70 years of age, 800 U of supplemental vitamin D per day is recommended to maximize bone health; however, 1500 to 2000 U/d may be required to keep levels consistently above 30 ng/dL (75 nmol/L). In treating the deficient patient, 50,000 U of either ergocalciferol or cholecalciferol is recommended, once weekly for 8 weeks. Once sufficiency is attained, maintenance therapy of 1500 to 2000 U/d is recommended.

Vitamin D toxicity is a very rare entity but one to be aware of. The effects of vitamin D levels greater than 90 ng/mL (225 nmol/L) include hypercalcemia. As a fat-soluble vitamin, decreasing vitamin D levels that are once elevated can be a slow process requiring continued monitoring.

KEY POINTS

- The U.S. Preventive Services Task Force recommends screening for osteoporosis in women aged 65 years and older and in younger women whose fracture risk is equal to or greater than that of a 65-year old white women who has no additional risk factors.

- The presence of a vertebral compression fracture makes the clinical diagnosis of osteoporosis, regardless of T-score on dual-energy x-ray absorptiometry (DEXA) scan, and treatment is recommended.

- Fracture Risk Assessment Tool (FRAX) score can help identify which patients are most likely to benefit from osteoporosis treatment; bisphosphonate therapy is first-line therapy for postmenopausal osteoporosis treatment and prevention.

- A 25-hydroxyvitamin D level between 30 and 40 ng/mL **HVC** (75-100 nmol/L) is deemed sufficient for bone health; most expert groups recommend screening all groups at least once for evidence of deficiency since U.S. incidence is 30% to 60% of the population, however, it should not be a serial, recurring screening test.

Paget Disease of Bone

Paget disease of bone is characterized by rapid and chaotic bone remodeling leading to disorganized bone microarchitecture. This disease more commonly affects persons of European descent during the sixth decade, with a prevalence of 3% to 10% in the elderly. Paramyxovirus infection of osteoclastic precursors is thought to be one possible cause, although about 15% of people with Paget disease have a family member with the disease. Paget disease appears to be inherited in an autosomal dominant manner with incomplete penetrance.

Clinical Presentation

The most common clinical manifestation is asymptomatic elevated serum alkaline phosphatase levels; only 30% of patients have symptoms at diagnosis. In some patients, the dysfunctional bone structure creates expansion in the bone leading to pain, swelling, and warmth. Bones of the axial skeleton are most frequently affected, namely the pelvis (70%), femur (55%), lumbar spine (53%), skull (42%), and tibia (30%). As a result, patients tend to have headache, sensorineural hearing loss, and bowing of the long bones (**Figure 16**). The abnormal bone growth may also lead to nerve impingement causing pain or neurologic deficits. Rarely, patients can develop increased vascular shunting to bones with resultant right-sided heart failure, cellular transformation to osteosarcoma, and hypercalcemia of immobilization.

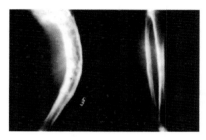

FIGURE 16. Radiograph showing Paget disease of bone in the left lateral tibia of a 71-year-old woman. Note the anterior bone, cortical thickening, and bone enlargement as compared with the normal radiograph on the right. The long-standing Paget disease resulted in a left leg that was 2.5 cm (1 in) shorter than the right.

Diagnosis

The diagnosis of Paget disease should be suspected in asymptomatic patients with an isolated elevation of alkaline phosphatase without evidence of liver disease. In these patients the most sensitive test is a nuclear bone scan which will detect areas of increased metabolic activity. Plain films of these areas should be obtained to identify pathognomonic pagetic lesions such as focal osteolysis with coarsening of the trabecular pattern and cortical thickening. In symptomatic patients with bone pain, plain films of painful areas may be the initial imaging test, although many experts recommend a baseline bone scan once the diagnosis is confirmed prior to initiating treatment.

Treatment

The main therapies for Paget disease of bone are the nitrogen-containing bisphosphonate medications (alendronate, pamidronate, risedronate, and zoledronic acid). The main indications for antiresorptive therapy are (1) pain caused by the increased metabolic activity; (2) planned surgery at site of pagetic bone disease, and (3) hypercalcemia due to multiple affected sites. There is no evidence that antiresorptive therapy is beneficial in asymptomatic patients. These medications are ideal because they suppress the rapid bone turnover that is characteristic of Paget disease. Decreases in alkaline phosphatase can be noted within 10 to 14 days after the initiation of therapy with a nadir reached in 3 to 6 months. NSAIDs and antineuropathic medications can also be used for pain control in these patients. For patients with pseudofractures, orthopedic stabilization may be required.

KEY POINTS

- The most common clinical manifestation of Paget disease of bone is asymptomatic elevated alkaline phosphate levels.
- The main therapy for Paget disease of bone is the nitrogen-containing bisphosphonate medications (alendronate, pamidronate, risedronate, and zoledronic acid).

Bibliography

Disorders of Glucose Metabolism

Bergenstal RM, Klonoff DC, Garg SK, et al; ASPIRE In-HOME Study Group. Threshold-based insulin-pump interruption for reduction of hypoglycemia. N Engl J Med. 2013 Jul 18;369(3):224-32. [PMID: 23789889]

Bergenstal RM, Tamborlane WV, Ahmann A, et al; STAR 3 STUDY Group. Effectiveness of sensor-augmented insulin-pump therapy in type 1 diabetes. N Engl J Med. 2010 Jul 22;363(4):311-20. [PMID: 20587585]

Committee on Practice Bulletins-Obstetrics. Practice Bulletin No. 137: Gestational diabetes mellitus. Obstet Gynecol. 2013 Aug;122(2 Pt 1):406-16. [PMID: 23969827]

Cowie CC, Rust KF, Byrd-Holt DD, et al. Prevalence of diabetes and high risk for diabetes using A$_{1c}$ criteria in the U.S. population in 1988-2006. Diabetes Care. 2010 Mar;33(3):562-8. [PMID: 20067953]

Cryer PE, Axelrod L, Grossman AB, et al. Evaluation and management of adult hypoglycemic disorders: an Endocrine Society Clinical Practice Guideline. J Endocrinol Metab. 2009 Mar;94(3):709-28. [PMID: 19088155]

Gregg EW, Chen H, Wagenknecht LE, et al. Association of an intensive lifestyle intervention with remission of type 2 diabetes. JAMA. 2012 Dec 19;308(23):2489-96. [PMID: 23288372]

Malanda UL, Welschen LM, Riphagen II, et al. Self-monitoring of blood glucose in patients with type 2 diabetes mellitus who are not using insulin. Cochrane Database Syst Rev. 2012 Jan 18;1:CD005060. [PMID: 22258959]

Nathan DM; DCCT/EDIC Research Group. The Diabetes Control and Complications Trial/Epidemiology of Diabetes Interventions and Complications Study at 30 years: Overview. Diabetes Care. 2014 Jan;37(1):9-16. [PMID: 24356592]

Qaseem A, Humphrey LL, Sweet DE, et al. Oral pharmacologic treatment of type 2 diabetes mellitus: a clinical practice guideline from the American College of Physicians. Ann Intern Med. 2012 Feb 7;156(3):218-31. [PMID: 22312141]

Yeh HC, Brown TT, Maruthur N, et al. Comparative effectiveness and safety of methods on insulin delivery and glucose monitoring for diabetes mellitus. Ann Intern Med. 2012 Sep 4;157(5):336-47. [PMID: 22777524]

Disorders of the Pituitary Gland

Colao A, Bronstein MD, Freda P, et al. Pasireotide versus octreotide in acromegaly: A head-to-head superiority study. J Clin Endocrinol Metab. 2014 Mar;99(3):791-9. [PMID: 24423324]

Colao A, Petersenn S, Newell-Price J, et al. A 12-month phase 3 study of pasireotide in Cushing's disease. N Engl J Med. 2012 Mar 8;366(10):914-24. [PMID: 22397653]

Freda PU, Beckers AM, Katznelson L, et al. Pituitary incidentaloma: an endocrine society clinical practice guideline. J Clin Endocrinol Metab. 2011 Apr;96(4):894-904. [PMID: 21474686]

Katznelson L, Laws ER Jr, Melmed S, et al. Acromegaly: an endocrine society clinical practice guideline. J Clin Endocrinol Metab. 2014 Nov;99(11):3933-51. [PMID: 25356808]

Klibanski A. Clinical Practice. Prolactinomas. N Engl J Med. 2010 Apr 1;362(13):1219-26. [PMID: 20357284]

Korbonits M, Storr H, Kumart AV. Familial pituitary adenomas-who should be tested for AIP mutations? Clin Endocrinol (Oxf). 2012 Sep;77(3):351-6. [PMID: 22612670]

Malchiodi E, Profka E, Ferrante E, et al. Thyrotropin-secreting pituitary adenomas: Outcome of pituitary surgery and irradiation. J Clin Endocrinol Metab. 2014 Jun;99(6):2069-76. [PMID: 24552222]

Melmed S, Casanueva FF, Hoffman AR, et al. Diagnosis and treatment of hyperprolactinemia: An Endocrine Society clinical practice guideline. J Clin Endocrinol Metab. 2011 Feb;96(2):273-88. [PMID: 21296991]

Nieman LK, Biller BMK, Findling JW, et al. The diagnosis of Cushing's syndrome: an Endocrine Society clinical practice guideline. J Clin Endocrinol Metab. 2008 May;93(5):1526-40. [PMID: 18334580]

Rajasekaran S, Vanderpump M, Baldeweq S, et al. UK guidelines for the management of pituitary apoplexy. Clin Endocrinol (Oxf). 2011 Jan;74(1):9-20. [PMID: 21044119]

Vasilev V, Daily AF, Petrossians P, et al. Familial pituitary tumor syndromes. Endocrine Practice. 2011 Jul-Aug;17 Suppl 3:41-6. [PMID: 21613050]

Disorders of the Adrenal Glands

Cordera F, Grant C, van Heerden J, et al. Androgen-secreting adrenal tumors. Surgery. 2003 Dec;134(6):874-80. [PMID: 14668717]

Eisenhofer G, Goldstein D, Walther M, et al. Biochemical diagnosis of pheochromocytoma: How to distinguish true- from false-positive test results. J Clin Endocrinol Metab. 2003 Jun;88(6):2656-66. [PMID: 12788870]

Fishbein L, Orlowski R, Cohen D. Pheochromocytoma/Paraganglioma: Review of perioperative management of blood pressure and update on genetic mutations associated with pheochromocytoma. J Clin Hypertens (Greenwich). 2013 Jun;15(6):428-34. [PMID: 23730992]

Funder JW, Carey RM, Fardella C, et al. Case detection, diagnosis, and treatment of patients with primary aldosteronism: an endocrine society clinical practice guideline. J Clin Endocrinol Metab. 2008 Sep;93(9):3266-81. [PMID: 18552288]

Lenders JW, Duh QY, Eisenhofer G, et al. Pheochromocytoma and paraganglioma: An endocrine society clinical practice guideline. J Clin Endocrinol Metab. 2014 Jun;99:1915-1942. [PMID: 24893135]

Morelli V, Reimondo G, Giordano R, et al. Long-term follow-up in adrenal incidentalomas: an Italian multicenter study. J Clin Endocrinol Metab. 2014 Mar;99(3):827-34. [PMID: 24423350]

Neary N, Nieman L. Adrenal insufficiency: etiology, diagnosis and treatment. Curr Opin Endocrinol Diabetes Obesity. 2010 Jun;17(3):217-23. [PMID: 20375886]

Nieman LK, Biller BM, Findling JW, et al. The diagnosis of Cushing's syndrome: an Endocrine Society Clinical Practice Guideline. J Clin Endocrinol Metab. 2008 May;93(5):1526-40. [PMID: 18334580]

Sprung CL, Annane D, Keh D, et al. Hydrocortisone therapy for patients with septic shock. N Engl J Med. 2008 Jan 10;358(2):111-24. [PMID: 18184957]

Young WF, Jr. Clinical practice. The incidentally discovered adrenal mass. N Engl J Med. 2007 Feb 8;356(6):601-10. [PMID: 17287480]

Zeiger MA, Thompson GB, Duh QY, et al. The American Association of Clinical Endocrinologists and American Association of Endocrine Surgeons medical guidelines for the management of adrenal incidentalomas. Endocr Pract. 2009 Jul-Aug;15 Suppl 1:1-20. [PMID: 19632967]

Disorders of the Thyroid Gland

American Thyroid Association (ATA) Guidelines Taskforce on Thyroid Nodules and Differentiated Thyroid Cancer, Cooper DS, Doherty GM, Haugen BR, et al. Revised American Thyroid Association management guidelines for patients with thyroid nodules and differentiated thyroid cancer. Thyroid. 2009 Nov;19(11):1167-214. Erratum in: Thyroid. 2010 Aug;20(8):942. [PMID: 19860577]

Bartalena L. Diagnosis and management of Graves disease: a global overview. Nat Rev Endocrinol. 2013 Dec;9(12):724-34. [PMID: 24126481]

Biondi B. Natural history, diagnosis and management of subclinical thyroid dysfunction. Best Pract Res Clin Endocrinol Metab. 2012 Aug;26(4):431-46. [PMID: 22863386]

Bogazzi F, Bartalena L, Martino E. Approach to the patient with amiodarone-induced thyrotoxicosis. J Clin Endocrinol Metab. 2010 Jun;95(6):2529-35. [PMID: 20525904]

Cooper DS, Biondi B. Subclinical thyroid disease. Lancet. 2012 Mar 24;379(9821):1142-54. [PMID: 22273398]

Demers LM, Spencer CA. Laboratory medicine practice guidelines: laboratory support for the diagnosis and monitoring of thyroid disease. Clin Endocrinol (Oxf). 2003 Feb;58(2):138-40. [PMID: 12580927]

Devdhar M, Ousman YH, Burman KD. Hypothyroidism. Endocrinol Metab Clin North Am. 2007 Sep;36(3):595-615, v. [PMID: 17673121]

Farwell AP. Nonthyroidal illness syndrome. Curr Opin Endocrinol Diabetes Obes. 2013 Oct;20(5):478-84. [PMID: 23974778]

Klubo-Gwiezdzinska J, Wartofsky L. Thyroid emergencies. Med Clin North Am. 2012 Mar;96(2):385-403. [PMID: 22443982]

Pearce EN, Farwell AP, Braverman LE. Thyroiditis. N Engl J Med. 2003 Jun 26;348(26):2646-55. Review. Erratum in: N Engl J Med. 2003 Aug 7;349(6):620. [PMID: 12826640]

Siegel RD, Lee SL. Toxic nodular goiter. Toxic adenoma and toxic multinodular goiter. Endocrinol Metab Clin North Am. 1998 Mar;27(1):151-68. [PMID: 9534034]

Stagnaro-Green A, Abalovich M, Alexander E, et al; American Thyroid Association Taskforce on Thyroid Disease During Pregnancy and Postpartum. Guidelines of the American Thyroid Association for the diagnosis and management of thyroid disease during pregnancy and postpartum. Thyroid. 2011 Oct;21(10):1081-125. [PMID: 21787128]

Reproductive Disorders

Bakalov VK, Vanderhoof VH, Bondy CA, Nelson LM. Adrenal antibodies detect asymptomatic auto-immune adrenal insufficiency in young women with spontaneous premature ovarian failure. Hum Reprod. 2002 Aug;17(8):2096-100. [PMID: 12151443]

Barbieri RL, Makris A, Randall RW, Daniels G, Kistner RW, Ryan KJ. Insulin stimulates androgen accumulation in incubations of ovarian stroma obtained from women with hyperandrogenism. J Clin Endocrinol Metab. 1986 May;62(5):904-10. [PMID: 3514651]

Belvisi L, Bombelli F, Sironi L, Doldi N. Organ-specific autoimmunity in patients with premature ovarian failure. J Endocrinol Invest. 1993 Dec;16(11):889-92. [PMID: 8144865]

de Moraes Ruehsen M, Blizzard RM, Garcia-Bunuel R, Jones GS. Autoimmunity and ovarian failure. Am J Obstet Gynecol. 1972 Mar;112(5):693-703. [PMID: 4551032]

Fernández-Balsells MM, Murad MH, Lane M, et al. Clinical review 1: Adverse effects of testosterone therapy in adult men: a systematic review and meta-analysis. J Clin Endocrinol Metab. 2010 Jun;95(6):2560-75. [PMID: 20525906]

Hoek A, Schoemaker J, Drexhage HA. Premature ovarian failure and ovarian autoimmunity. Endocr Rev. 1997 Feb;18(1):107-34. [PMID: 9034788]

Kauffman RP, Castracane VD. Premature ovarian failure associated with autoimmune polyglandular syndrome: pathophysiological mechanisms and future fertility. J Womens Health (Larchmt). 2003 Jun;12(5):513-20. [PMID: 12869299]

Kong MF, Jeffcoate W. Eighty-six cases of Addison's disease. Clin Endocrinol (Oxf). 1994 Dec;41(6):757-61. [PMID: 7889611]

Legro RS, Barnhart HX, Schlaff WD, et al; Cooperative Multicenter Reproductive Medicine Network. Clomiphene, metformin, or both for infertility in the polycystic ovary syndrome. N Engl J Med. 2007 Feb 8;356(6):551-66. [PMID: 17287476]

Mignot MH, Schoemaker J, Kleingeld M, Rao BR, Drexhage HA. Premature ovarian failure. I: The association with autoimmunity. Eur J Obstet Gynecol Reprod Biol. 1989 Jan;30(1):59-66. [PMID: 2647538]

Moncayo-Naveda H, Moncayo R, Benz R, Wolf A, Lauritzen C. Organ-specific antibodies against ovary in patients with systemic lupus erythematosus. Am J Obstet Gynecol. 1989 May;160(5 Pt 1):1227-9. [PMID: 2729399]

Plymate SR, Matej LA, Jones RE, Friedl KE. Inhibition of sex hormone-binding globulin production in the human hepatoma (Hep G2) cell line by insulin and prolactin. J Clin Endocrinol Metab. 1988 Sep;67(3):460-4. [PMID: 2842359]

Ryan MM, Jones HR Jr. Myasthenia gravis and premature ovarian failure. Muscle Nerve. 2004 Aug;30(2):231-3. [PMID: 15266640]

Vigen R, O'Donnell CI, Barón AE, et al. Association of testosterone therapy with mortality, myocardial infarction, and stroke in men with low testosterone levels. JAMA. 2013 Nov 6;310(17):1829-36. Erratum in: JAMA. 2014 Mar 5;311(9):967. [PMID: 24193080]

Calcium and Bone Disorders

Al-Azem H, Khan AA. Hypoparathyroidism. Best Pract Res Clin Endocrinol Metab 2012 Aug;26(4):517-22. [PMID: 22863393]

Bischoff-Ferrari H A, Willett WC, Orav E J, et al. A pooled analysis of vitamin D dose requirements for fracture prevention. N Engl J Med. 2012 Jul 5;367(1):40-9. [PMID: 22762317]

Holick MF. Vitamin D deficiency. N Engl J Med. 2007 Jul 19;357(3):266-81. [PMID: 17634462]

Holick MF, Binkley N, Bischoff-Ferrari HA, et al. Evaluation, treatment and prevention of vitamin D deficiency: an Endocrine Society clinical practice guideline. J Clin Endocrinol Metab. 2011 Jul;96(7):1911-30. [PMID: 21646368]

Marcocci C, Cetani F. Primary hyperparathyroidism. N Engl J Med. 2011 Dec 22;365(25):2389-97. [PMID: 22187986]

Institute of Medicine. Dietary Reference Intakes for Calcium and Vitamin D. Washington, DC: National Academy Press, 2010.

National Osteoporosis Foundation. Clinician's Guide to Prevention and Treatment of Osteoporosis. Washington, DC: National Osteoporosis Foundation, 2014.

Ralston SH. Paget's disease of the bone. N Engl J Med. 2013 Feb 14;368(7):644-50. [PMID: 23406029]

Sharma OP. Hypercalcemia in granulomatous disorders: a clinical review. Curr Opin Pulm Med. 2000 Sep;6(5):442-7. [PMID: 10958237]

Shoback D. Hypoparathyroidism. N Engl J Med. 2008 Jul 24;359(4):391-403. [PMID: 18650515]

Wolpowitz D, Gilchrest BA. The vitamin D questions: how much do you need and how should you get it? J Am Acad Dermatol. 2006 Feb;54(2):301-17. [PMID: 16443061]

Endocrinology and Metabolism Self-Assessment Test

This self-assessment test contains one-best-answer multiple-choice questions. Please read these directions carefully before answering the questions. Answers, critiques, and bibliographies immediately follow these multiple-choice questions. The American College of Physicians is accredited by the Accreditation Council for Continuing Medical Education (ACCME) to provide continuing medical education for physicians.

The American College of Physicians designates MKSAP 17 **Endocrinology and Metabolism** for a maximum of **14** *AMA PRA Category 1 Credits*™. Physicians should claim only the credit commensurate with the extent of their participation in the activity.

Earn "Instantaneous" CME Credits Online

Print subscribers can enter their answers online to earn CME credits instantaneously. You can submit your answers using online answer sheets that are provided at mksap.acponline.org, where a record of your MKSAP 17 credits will be available. To earn CME credits, you need to answer all of the questions in a test and earn a score of at least 50% correct (number of correct answers divided by the total number of questions). Take any of the following approaches:

➢ Use the printed answer sheet at the back of this book to record your answers. Go to mksap.acponline.org, access the appropriate online answer sheet, transcribe your answers, and submit your test for instantaneous CME credits. There is no additional fee for this service.

➢ Go to mksap.acponline.org, access the appropriate online answer sheet, directly enter your answers, and submit your test for instantaneous CME credits. There is no additional fee for this service.

➢ Pay a $15 processing fee per answer sheet and submit the printed answer sheet at the back of this book by mail or fax, as instructed on the answer sheet. Make sure you calculate your score and fax the answer sheet to 215-351-2799 or mail the answer sheet to Member and Customer Service, American College of Physicians, 190 N. Independence Mall West, Philadelphia, PA 19106-1572, using the courtesy envelope provided in your MKSAP 17 slipcase. You will need your 10-digit order number and 8-digit ACP ID number, which are printed on your packing slip. Please allow 4 to 6 weeks for your score report to be emailed back to you. Be sure to include your email address for a response.

If you do not have a 10-digit order number and 8-digit ACP ID number or if you need help creating a username and password to access the MKSAP 17 online answer sheets, go to mksap.acponline.org or email custserv@acponline.org.

CME credit is available from the publication date of December 31, 2015, until December 31, 2018. You may submit your answer sheets at any time during this period.

*Each of the numbered items is followed by lettered answers. Select the **ONE** lettered answer that is **BEST** in each case.*

Item 1

A 23-year-old woman is evaluated because of a 1-week history of palpitations. She also reports some heat intolerance and mild anxiety during the last several weeks, but she otherwise feels well. She is in the first trimester of an otherwise uncomplicated first pregnancy. Her only medication is a prenatal vitamin.

On physical examination, she is afebrile, blood pressure is 110/72 mm Hg, pulse rate is 105/min, and respiration rate is 13/min. BMI is 20. The skin is warm and moist. There is no proptosis or lid lag. Examination of the neck shows a diffusely enlarged thyroid with an audible bruit over both lobes. Cardiopulmonary and abdominal examinations are unremarkable. Neurologic examination reveals a fine resting tremor of the hands and brisk reflexes.

Laboratory studies:

Thyroid-stimulating hormone	<0.008 µU/mL (0.008 mU/L)
Free thyroxine (T_4)	5.5 ng/dL (70.9 pmol/L)
Total triiodothyronine (T_3)	400 ng/dL (6.2 nmol/L)
Thyroid-stimulating immunoglobulin index	4.5 (normal <1.3)

Which of the following is the most appropriate treatment?

(A) Methimazole
(B) Propylthiouracil
(C) Radioactive iodine
(D) Thyroidectomy

Grave's

Item 2

A 34-year-old man is evaluated for episodic palpitations of 8 months' duration. The palpitations last 5 to 10 minutes and then resolve spontaneously. They are usually associated with sweating and anxiety. Medical history is significant for thyroidectomy for medullary thyroid carcinoma diagnosed at 12 years of age. His father has also undergone thyroidectomy for medullary thyroid cancer. His only medication is levothyroxine.

On physical examination, blood pressure is 164/92 mm Hg, pulse rate is 106/min, and respiration rate is 12/min. Auscultation of the heart reveals a regular tachycardia without murmurs. The remainder of his examination is unremarkable.

Laboratory studies show a 24-hour urine excretion of catecholamines of 310 µg/m²/24 h (1832.1 nmol/m²/24 h) and metanephrines of 3400 µg/24 h (17,238 nmol/24 h).

In addition to the presenting diagnosis, which of the following disorders is this patient most likely to develop?

(A) Insulinoma
(B) Neurofibroma
(C) Primary hyperparathyroidism
(D) Prolactinoma

Item 3

A 31-year-old woman is evaluated following her recent discovery that she is pregnant at approximately 10 weeks' gestation. Medical history is significant for a prolactinoma diagnosed 2 years ago during an evaluation for amenorrhea. At the time of diagnosis, her serum prolactin level was 184 ng/mL (184 µg/L), and a 1.4-cm pituitary adenoma extending above the sella was detected on MRI without evidence of mass effect. She was treated with bromocriptine with return of regular menses. She discontinued the bromocriptine when she found that she was pregnant. She is currently without symptoms. She does not have new or severe headache. Medical history is otherwise unremarkable, and her only current medication is a prenatal multivitamin.

On physical examination, vital signs are normal. Visual fields are full to confrontation, and the remainder of her examination is normal.

Which of the following is the most appropriate next step in management?

(A) Check serum prolactin level
(B) Formal visual field testing
(C) Repeat pituitary MRI
(D) Restart bromocriptine

Item 4

A 48-year-old woman returns for a follow-up visit for management of type 1 diabetes mellitus. She reports doing well since the last visit. Overall, she believes that most of her blood glucose levels are at goal, but is concerned about occasional episodes of hyperglycemia occurring in the morning before breakfast. She eats a bedtime snack every night that is not covered with mealtime insulin. Review of her blood glucose log demonstrates morning fasting blood glucose values from 80 to 190 mg/dL (4.4-10.5 mmol/L). Her other premeal and bedtime values range from 100 to 120 mg/dL (5.5–6.7 mmol/L). She exercises two to three times per week in the evening. Medical history is significant for hypertension and hyperlipidemia.

Medications are insulin glargine, insulin lispro, ramipril, simvastatin, and aspirin.

On physical examination, blood pressure is 130/72 mm Hg and pulse rate is 67/min. BMI is 24. The remainder of the examination is unremarkable.

Results of laboratory studies show a hemoglobin A_{1c} level of 6.9% and serum creatinine level of 1.0 mg/dL (88.4 µmol/L). Serum electrolytes are normal.

Which of the following is the most appropriate management of this patient's occasional fasting hyperglycemia?

(A) Add insulin lispro at bedtime
(B) Add metformin
(C) Increase insulin glargine dose
(D) Measure 3 AM blood glucose level
(E) Continue current regimen

Item 5

A 70-year-old woman is seen for follow-up evaluation for possible Cushing syndrome. She presented with new-onset diabetes mellitus and a 9.1-kg (20-lb) weight gain over the last 6 months. Medical history is otherwise unremarkable, and she is currently taking no medications and has had no exposure to exogenous glucocorticoids in the past year.

On physical examination, blood pressure is 160/90 mm Hg, pulse rate is 80/min, and respiration rate is 12/min. BMI is 30. Facial plethora, central obesity, and bilateral supraclavicular fat pads are noted. There are violaceous abdominal striae measuring 1 cm wide and multiple ecchymoses on the extremities.

Initial laboratory studies show a serum cortisol level of 9 µg/dL (248.4 nmol/L) following a 1-mg dose of dexamethasone the night before, and a 24-hour urine free cortisol level that is greater than 3 times the upper limit of normal, which is confirmed on a second measurement. A plasma adrenocorticotropic hormone (ACTH) level is undetectable.

Which of the following is the most appropriate diagnostic test to perform next?

(A) CT scan of the adrenal glands
(B) Inferior petrosal sinus sampling
(C) Late night salivary cortisol measurement
(D) MRI of the pituitary gland

Item 6

A 44-year-old man is evaluated for management of type 2 diabetes mellitus. He was diagnosed with diabetes 6 months ago after being admitted to the hospital with diabetic ketoacidosis. He was discharged from the hospital on a basal and preprandial insulin regimen. Medications are regular insulin before meals and neutral protamine Hagedorn (NPH) insulin at bedtime. He completed diabetes education and nutrition classes and has been adherent with lifestyle modifications. His insulin doses have been decreased gradually over the last 4 to 5 months. His most recent hemoglobin A_{1c} level is 6.7%. Blood glucose values from his log book average 130 mg/dL (7.2 mmol/L).

On physical examination, temperature is 37.2 °C (99.0 °F), blood pressure is 128/68 mm Hg, and pulse rate is 72/min. BMI is 30. His physical examination is unremarkable.

Laboratory studies at the time of hospital admission:

Glucose, fasting	825 mg/dL (45.8 mmol/L)
Antibody to glutamic acid decarboxylase 65 (GAD-65)	Negative
Antibody to islet antigen 2 (IA-2)	Negative
C-peptide, fasting	0.5 ng/mL (0.16 nmol/L) Normal range: 0.8-3.1 ng/mL (0.26-1.03 nmol/L)

Which of the following is the most appropriate next step in his management?

(A) Discontinue current insulin regimen, initiate sliding-scale insulin
(B) Discontinue insulin, initiate metformin

(C) Repeat measurement of antibodies to glutamic acid decarboxylase 65 and islet antigen 2
(D) Repeat measurement of fasting C-peptide and glucose levels

Item 7

A 43-year-old man is evaluated in the emergency department for the "worst headache of my life." It occurred suddenly without warning. He has had mild headaches that come and go over the past 3 years, but nothing this severe. Soon after the headache began, he lost vision in his left eye, and the vision in his right eye became blurry. He vomited twice in the emergency department. His medical history is significant for progressive erectile dysfunction and loss of libido over the past 3 years.

On physical examination, temperature is 37.4 °C (99.3 °F), blood pressure is 156/92 mm Hg, pulse rate is 104/min, and respiration rate is 16/min. BMI is 28. He has loss of vision in his left eye and in the upper quadrants of his right eye. He also has left eye ptosis. Other cranial nerves are intact. Strength and sensation in all extremities are normal as are his speech and gait.

CT of the head shows acute pituitary hemorrhage. Pituitary MRI shows a 3.1 × 2.5 × 2.2-cm pituitary mass with central hemorrhage. The mass compresses the optic chiasm and the left cavernous sinus.

After administering high-dose glucocorticoids, which of the following is the most appropriate immediate management?

(A) Assess pituitary function
(B) Repeat imaging in 2 weeks
(C) Urgent transsphenoidal pituitary decompression
(D) Whole brain external beam radiation

Item 8

A 42-year-old woman is evaluated during an annual physical examination. She feels well. She has no pertinent personal or family medical history, and she takes no medications.

On physical examination, vital signs are normal. Palpation of the thyroid reveals a possible nodule in the right lobe that is not mobile with swallowing. The remainder of the gland is unremarkable, and there is no palpable cervical lymphadenopathy. Other physical examination findings are normal.

Laboratory studies reveal a serum thyroid-stimulating hormone level of 1.7 µU/mL (1.7 mU/L).

Ultrasound of the neck shows a right 1.5-cm hypoechoic nodule with internal microcalcifications.

Which of the following is the most appropriate next step in management?

(A) CT with contrast of the neck
(B) Fine-needle aspiration of the nodule
(C) Levothyroxine therapy
(D) Measurement of serum thyroglobulin level
(E) Thyroid scan with technetium

Item 9

An 18-year-old woman is evaluated for primary amenorrhea. Her cognitive function is normal, and she is not sexually active. Her personal and family medical history is unremarkable. She takes no medications.

On physical examination, temperature is 36.1 °C (97.0 °F), blood pressure is 110/70 mm Hg, pulse rate is 72/min, and respiration rate is 16/min; BMI is 20. Her height is 147 cm (58 in). Physical examination and secondary sex characteristics are normal, with Tanner stage IV breast and pubic hair development.

Pregnancy testing is negative. On subsequent laboratory studies estradiol level was undetectable, serum follicle-stimulating hormone level is 72 mU/mL (72 U/L), and serum luteinizing hormone level is 46 mU/mL (46 U/L).

Which of the following is the most appropriate management?

(A) Initiate estrogen and progestin therapy
(B) Measure serum prolactin
(C) Measure thyroid-stimulating hormone
(D) Perform pituitary MRI

Item 10

A 32-year-old man is evaluated for a 1-week history of severe neck pain. He also has heat intolerance, palpitations, and insomnia. Medical history is significant only for a viral upper respiratory tract infection 3 weeks ago. He takes no medications.

On physical examination, he appears anxious and is sweating. There is no proptosis or lid lag. Examination of the thyroid reveals a normal-sized gland that is very tender to palpation. There are no thyroid nodules. The heart rate is regular but tachycardic. The lungs are clear.

Laboratory studies:

Thyroid-stimulating hormone	<0.008 µU/mL (0.008 mU/L)
Free thyroxine (T_4)	3.2 ng/dL (41.3 pmol/L)
Total triiodothyronine (T_3)	310 ng/dL (4.8 nmol/L)
Thyroid-stimulating immunoglobulin index	<1.3 (normal, <1.3)
24-Hour radioactive iodine uptake	5% (low)

Which of the following is the most appropriate treatment?

(A) Methimazole
(B) Metoprolol
(C) Propylthiouracil
(D) Radioactive iodine

Item 11

A 30-year-old woman is evaluated for amenorrhea. She and her husband are interested in pregnancy in the next year, and they are concerned that they will not be able to conceive. Her menses became irregular about 2 years ago. In the past 12 months, she has had menses twice. Her last menstrual period was 4 months ago. She also notes low libido and dyspareunia. She has not had weight changes, constipation, hair loss or hirsutism, or skin changes.

Her medical history is significant for primary hypothyroidism and bipolar disorder. Medications are levothyroxine, lithium, and risperidone. She reports that she has been stable on these medications for a few years and feels well. She plans to discuss her medications with her psychiatrist prior to pregnancy.

On physical examination, blood pressure is 118/72 mm Hg and pulse rate is 82/min. BMI is 24. The thyroid is normal. Visual fields are intact.

Laboratory studies:

Follicle-stimulating hormone	1.3 mU/mL (1.3 U/L)
Luteinizing hormone	2.0 mU/mL (2.0 U/L)
Prolactin	102 ng/mL (102 µg/L)
Thyroid-stimulating hormone	1.1 µU/mL (1.1 mU/L)

Which of the following is the most likely cause of her hyperprolactinemia?

(A) Hypothyroidism
(B) Lithium
(C) Pituitary adenoma
(D) Risperidone

Item 12

A 55-year-old woman is evaluated for a new-patient visit. Medical history is significant for an eating disorder. Although she has maintained a normal weight for the past 20 years, she notes that prior to that time her weight would fluctuate in a range correlating with BMIs of 17 to 19. She has otherwise been healthy and currently feels well. She is postmenopausal and a never-smoker. Family history is significant for postmenopausal osteoporosis in her mother. Her medications are over-the-counter calcium and vitamin D supplements.

On physical examination, temperature is 36.3 °C (97.3 °F), blood pressure is 137/81 mm Hg, pulse rate is 76/min, and respiration rate is 11/min. BMI is 21. She has mild thoracic kyphosis but no skeletal tenderness. The remainder of the examination is unremarkable.

Results of laboratory studies are significant for a serum calcium level of 9.1 mg/dL (2.3 mmol/L) and 25-hydroxyvitamin D level of 40 ng/mL (99.8 nmol/L); thyroid function studies are normal.

Dual-energy x-ray absorptiometry (DEXA) scan shows T-scores of –1.8 in the femoral neck and –1.9 in the lumbar spine. Ten-year fracture risk using the Fracture Risk Assessment Tool (FRAX) is 6.9% for major osteoporotic fracture and 0.7% for hip fracture. Plain radiographs of the spine show no evidence of compression fracture.

Which of the following is the most appropriate management of this patient?

(A) Begin raloxifene
(B) Repeat DEXA scan in 2 years
(C) Replace calcium with cholecalciferol
(D) Start bisphosphonate therapy

Item 13

A 64-year-old man in the ICU is evaluated because of abnormal thyroid function tests. He was admitted 3 days ago for community-acquired pneumonia requiring intubation, mechanical ventilation, intravenous fluids, and dopamine support for his blood pressure.

On physical examination, temperature is 38.8 °C (101.8 °F), blood pressure is 95/60 mm Hg, and pulse rate is 130/min. The skin is warm and dry. There is no proptosis. Examination of the neck shows a normal-sized thyroid without nodules. Cardiovascular examination reveals regular tachycardia. On neurologic examination, reflexes are slightly delayed.

The serum thyroid-stimulating hormone (TSH) level is 0.1 µU/mL (0.1 mU/L), the serum free thyroxine level (T_4) is 0.9 ng/dL (11.6 pmol/L), and the serum total triiodothyronine (T_3) level is 50 ng/dL (0.8 nmol/L).

Which of the following is the most likely cause of this patient's abnormal thyroid function?

(A) Euthyroid sick syndrome
(B) Graves disease
(C) Hashimoto thyroiditis
(D) Subacute thyroiditis

Item 14

A 43-year-old man is evaluated during a follow-up visit for management of type 1 diabetes mellitus. He was diagnosed at 18 years of age and has multiple chronic complications from his diabetes, including end-stage kidney disease requiring hemodialysis, gastroparesis, frequent hypoglycemia with hypoglycemic unawareness, painful peripheral neuropathy, and proliferative retinopathy. The patient uses an insulin pump and a continuous glucose monitoring system to manage his diabetes. He is adherent with his regimen and performs multiple fingerstick blood glucose measurements with values ranging from 65 to 250 mg/dL (3.6-13.9 mmol/L). His most recent hemoglobin A_{1c} level is 7.5%.

Which of the following is the most appropriate next step in the management of this patient?

(A) Alter insulin pump settings to attain a hemoglobin A_{1c} goal of less than 7.0%
(B) Alter insulin pump settings to decrease the insulin doses
(C) Discontinue the insulin pump, start subcutaneous insulin injections
(D) Start gabapentin for treatment of painful peripheral neuropathy

Item 15

A 55-year-old woman is seen in follow-up for low bone mass and vitamin D deficiency. Cortical bone thinning was noted on radiographs of her right ankle following a fall 3 months ago. Subsequent evaluation included a dual-energy x-ray absorptiometry (DEXA) scan showing osteopenia. Her serum 25-hydroxyvitamin D level is 4 ng/mL (10 nmol/L). She was started on 50,000 U of vitamin D_2 (ergocalciferol)

weekly, 6 weeks ago. Medical history is significant for vitiligo and chronic fatigue. Medications are vitamin D_2 and calcium carbonate.

On physical examination, temperature is 36.1 °C (96.9 °F), blood pressure is 132/71 mm Hg, pulse rate is 83/min, and respiration rate is 12/min. BMI is 19. The remainder of her examination is unremarkable.

Laboratory studies:
Calcium	9.1 mg/dL (2.3 mmol/L)
Creatinine	0.9 mg/dL (79.6 µmol/L)
Parathyroid hormone	101 pg/mL (101 ng/L)
25-Hydroxyvitamin D, after 6 weeks	7 ng/mL (17.5 nmol/L)
24-Hour urine calcium	150 mg/24 h (3.7 mmol/24 h)

Which of the following is the most appropriate next step in management?

(A) Parathyroid sestamibi scan
(B) Refer for parathyroidectomy
(C) Switch to vitamin D_3 (cholecalciferol)
(D) Tissue transglutaminase antibody testing

Item 16

A 54-year-old woman is evaluated because of fatigue. Although she follows a daily 1400-kcal diet and exercises 3 to 4 nights per week for 30 minutes, she has gained 2.3 kg (5.0 lb) in the last month. She has hypercholesterolemia requiring statin therapy. Her mother was diagnosed with hypothyroidism shortly after the birth of her last child.

On physical examination, blood pressure is 145/90 mm Hg, pulse rate is 80/min, and BMI is 25. The skin is dry. The thyroid is mildly enlarged with a diffusely nodular texture. No discrete thyroid nodules are palpated. Reflexes are normal.

Laboratory studies:
Thyroid-stimulating hormone (TSH)	6.5 µU/mL (6.5 mU/L)
Free thyroxine (T_4)	0.9 ng/dL (11.6 pmol/L)
Thyroid peroxidase antibody	Positive

Similar results for TSH and T_4 were obtained 4 months ago.

Which of the following is the most appropriate next step in management?

(A) Initiate levothyroxine therapy
(B) Measure thyroid-stimulating immunoglobulins
(C) Repeat serum TSH measurement in 12 months
(D) Schedule thyroid radioactive iodine uptake and scan

Item 17

A 74-year-old woman is evaluated for a diagnosis of primary hyperparathyroidism made after an elevated serum calcium level was incidentally discovered on laboratory studies. She has no symptoms associated with hypercalcemia. Medical history is significant for hypertension and chronic kidney disease. Her only medication is amlodipine. She has never smoked.

On physical examination, temperature is 36.8 °C (98.3 °F), blood pressure is 134/87 mm Hg, pulse rate is 92/min, and respiration rate is 14/min. BMI is 27. The remainder of her examination is unremarkable.

Laboratory studies:

Calcium	11.3 mg/dL (2.8 mmol/L)
Creatinine	1.3 mg/dL (114.9 μmol/L)
Parathyroid hormone	76 pg/mL (76 ng/L)
Estimated glomerular filtration rate	40 mL/min/1.73 m²

Dual-energy x-ray absorptiometry (DEXA) scan shows a T-score of -1.3 in the right femoral neck. Her Fracture Risk Assessment Tool (FRAX) score indicates a 2.1% 10-year probability of hip fracture and 17% 10-year probability of any fracture.

Which of the following is the most appropriate therapy to recommend to this patient?

(A) Alendronate

(B) Cinacalcet

(C) Parathyroidectomy

(D) Clinical observation

Item 18

A 74-year-old woman is evaluated because of new-onset anxiety and insomnia. For the last 6 weeks, she has been waking up multiple times each night. She does not have heat intolerance, change in bowel habits, palpitations, or dyspnea on exertion. She takes no medications.

On physical examination, blood pressure is 125/68 mm Hg and pulse rate is 89/min. BMI is 18. There is no proptosis or lid lag. Examination of the thyroid reveals a 1.5-cm firm nodule in the left lobe that moves upward with swallowing. A fine resting hand tremor is present bilaterally.

Laboratory studies reveal a serum thyroid-stimulating hormone level of 0.05 μU/mL (0.05 mU/L), a serum free thyroxine (T_4) level of 2.9 ng/dL (37.4 pmol/L), and a serum total triiodothyronine (T_3) level of 250 ng/dL (3.8 nmol/L).

Ultrasound of the neck shows two thyroid nodules, a 1.5-cm nodule in the right lobe and a 2.0-cm nodule in the left lobe.

Which of the following is the most appropriate next step in management?

(A) Fine-needle aspiration of both thyroid nodules

(B) Initiation of methimazole

(C) Radioactive iodine (^{123}I) uptake and scan of the thyroid

(D) Total thyroidectomy

Item 19

A 34-year-old woman is evaluated for amenorrhea, headache, and fatigue. She reports that from the time of menarche until 2.5 years ago, her menses were regular and predictable. Two and a half years ago, her menses became irregular and then stopped completely 6 months ago. She has had a few

hot flushes and fatigue. She has noted galactorrhea. She began having headaches 2 years ago. In addition, she notes blurry peripheral vision.

The rest of her medical history is unremarkable. She takes no medications.

On physical examination, blood pressure is 112/72 mm Hg and pulse rate is 68/min. BMI is 21. White milky substance is expressed from her breasts bilaterally. Ocular movements and cranial nerves are intact. There are no stigmata of Cushing disease or acromegaly.

Laboratory studies:

Cortisol 8 AM after 1 mg of dexamethasone the night before	16 μg/dL (441.6 nmol/L)
Estradiol	<32 pg/mL (117.4 pmol/L)
Follicle-stimulating hormone	1.1 mU/mL (1.1 U/L)
Luteinizing hormone	0.8 mU/mL (0.8 U/L)
Prolactin	472 ng/mL (472 μg/L)
Thyroid-stimulating hormone	1.1 μU/mL (1.1 mU/L)

MRI shows a 2.4-cm pituitary tumor that elevates the optic chiasm and surrounds the left carotid artery.

Which of the following is the most appropriate treatment?

(A) Cabergoline

(B) Octreotide

(C) Radiation

(D) Surgery

Item 20

A 74-year-old woman is evaluated in the emergency department for several hours of altered mental status. She is from out-of-state and is visiting with relatives. One of her young relatives was recently ill with gastrointestinal symptoms. The patient developed anorexia 3 days ago and vomiting 2 days ago. She has been unable to tolerate any liquid or solid foods for the last 24 hours. Medical history is significant for type 2 diabetes mellitus, hypertension, hyperlipidemia, and hypothyroidism. Medications are aspirin, lisinopril, glimepiride, levothyroxine, and atorvastatin. Her last dose of medications was 48 hours ago.

On physical examination, her temperature is 37.5 °C (99.5 °F), blood pressure is 115/65 mm Hg, and pulse rate is 95/min. She is arousable but confused. Mucous membranes are dry. Her neck is supple. Cardiac examination reveals no murmurs. Her chest is clear to auscultation. Bowel sounds are present, and mild tenderness to palpation is noted throughout the abdomen. There is no rebound or guarding. There are no focal neurologic deficits.

Laboratory studies are pending.

Which of the following is the most likely cause of this patient's altered mental status?

(A) Cerebrovascular accident

(B) Hypoglycemia

(C) Hypothyroidism

(D) Statin toxicity

Item 21

A 38-year-old woman is evaluated because of a 3-week history of palpitations. She notes that her heart "races" at night and after minimal exertion. She also reports heat intolerance but has no change in bowel habits or menses.

On physical examination, the patient is restless and has pressured speech. Temperature is 36.8 °C (98.2 °F), blood pressure is 130/60 mm Hg, pulse rate in 110/min, and respiration rate is 12/min. Her skin is warm and moist, and a bilateral hand tremor is present. There is no proptosis or lid lag. The thyroid is enlarged without nodules or bruits.

Serum thyroid-stimulating hormone level is 0.08 µU/mL (0.08 mU/L), and the serum free thyroxine (T_4) level is 1.7 ng/dL (21.9 pmol/L).

Which of the following is the most appropriate next step in management?

(A) Measure serum triiodothyronine (T_3) level
(B) Measure serum thyroid peroxidase antibody titer
(C) Repeat thyroid function tests in 6 weeks
(D) Schedule ultrasound of the neck

Item 22

A 34-year-old woman is evaluated for a diagnosis of hypercalcemia after presenting to the emergency department 3 days ago for treatment of a kidney stone. She presented with severe right flank pain with nausea and vomiting. A 2-mm kidney stone was identified in the right ureter by ultrasonography that passed spontaneously; multiple additional intrarenal calcifications were noted to be present. Laboratory studies at that time showed normal kidney function and a serum calcium level of 11.5 mg/dL (2.9 mmol/L). Medical history is otherwise significant for hypertension and sarcoidosis. Her only medication is hydrochlorothiazide.

On physical examination, temperature is 36.8 °C (98.2 °F), blood pressure is 138/87 mm Hg, pulse rate is 89/min, and respiration rate is 12. BMI is 32. The remainder of the examination is unremarkable.

Laboratory studies are significant for a parathyroid hormone level of 4 pg/mL (4 ng/L).

Which of the following is most likely responsible for causing this patient's hypercalcemia?

(A) Calcium-sensing receptor mutation
(B) Elevated 1,25-dihydroxyvitamin D levels
(C) 25-Hydroxyvitamin D level
(D) Thiazide-induced renal calcium reabsorption

Item 23

A 40-year-old woman is evaluated for amenorrhea of 4 months' duration. She has had weight gain, facial hair, alopecia, and debilitating fatigue. Her medical history is significant for psoriasis. She seems to be gaining weight in her face, abdomen, and neck. She also bruises easily. Her only medication is clobetasol for psoriasis.

On physical examination, temperature is 37.6 °C (99.7 °F), blood pressure is 148/90 mm Hg, pulse rate is 88/min, and respiration rate is 12/min. BMI is 38. She is obese with a round face. She has terminal hairs on her chin, upper lip, chest, and back. Mild facial acne, central obesity, and a few wide purple striae on the back of her arms are also noted. She has supraclavicular fat. Her skin has psoriatic plaques. Muscle strength in the upper and lower extremities is 4/5.

Which of the following is the most likely diagnosis?

(A) Adrenocortical carcinoma
(B) Cushing disease
(C) Ectopic adrenocorticotropic hormone production
(D) Iatrogenic Cushing syndrome

Item 24

A 20-year-old woman is evaluated in the emergency department for polyuria, polydipsia, polyphagia, and an unintentional 5.4-kg (11.9-lb) weight loss over the past month. She has had increasing lethargy over the last 24 hours. Her medical history and family history are unremarkable. She takes no medications.

On physical examination, temperature is 37.5 °C (99.5 °F), blood pressure is 98/52 mm Hg, pulse rate is 120/min, and respiration rate is 30/min. BMI is 17. She is lethargic with dry mucous membranes, tachypnea, and tachycardia. Chest auscultation is clear. Abdominal examination shows diffuse mild tenderness and normal bowel sounds. There is no rebound tenderness or guarding with palpation.

Laboratory studies:

Hemoglobin	17 g/dL (170 g/L)
Leukocyte count	14,200/µL (14.2 × 10⁹/L)
Blood gases, arterial	
pH	7.25
PCO_2	21 mm Hg (2.8 kPa)
Creatinine	1.3 mg/dL (114.9 µmol/L)
Electrolytes	
Sodium	130 mEq/L (130 mmol/L)
Potassium	3.0 mEq/L (3.0 mmol/L)
Chloride	99 mEq/L (99 mmol/L)
Bicarbonate	9 mEq/L (9 mmol/L)
Glucose	620 mg/dL (34.4 mmol/L)
Lactic acid	8 mg/dL (0.89 mmol/L)

Intravenous 0.9% saline is initiated through a central venous catheter.

An electrocardiogram shows sinus tachycardia 120/min. Chest radiograph is normal.

Which of the following is the most appropriate next step in the management?

(A) Administer intravenous ceftriaxone
(B) Administer intravenous potassium chloride
(C) Administer intravenous sodium bicarbonate
(D) Initiate intravenous insulin therapy

Item 25

A 65-year-old woman is evaluated following a recent diagnosis of osteoporosis discovered on a screening dual-energy x-ray absorptiometry (DEXA) scan that showed T-scores of –2.5 at the femoral neck and –2.7 at the hip. Overall she feels well, although she notes a 5-cm (2-in) loss of height over the past 15 years and a 2.3-kg (5-lb) weight loss over the last year. She is postmenopausal. Medical history is unremarkable, and she is a never-smoker. Family history is negative for osteoporosis or nontraumatic fractures. She takes no medications.

On physical examination, temperature is 36.8 °C (98.2 °F), blood pressure is 144/68 mm Hg, pulse rate is 92/min, and respiration rate is 14/min. BMI is 22. The remainder of the examination is unremarkable.

Laboratory studies are significant for a normal basic metabolic profile and complete blood count. Serum calcium is 9.5 mg/dL (2.4 mmol/L) and serum phosphorus is 3.8 mg/dL (1.2 mmol/L). Serum 25-hydroxyvitamin D level is 32 ng/dL (79.9 nmol/L).

Which of the following tests is indicated prior to initiation of pharmacologic therapy?

(A) Serum and urine markers of bone turnover
(B) Serum estradiol level
(C) Serum parathyroid hormone level
(D) Serum thyroid-stimulating hormone level

Item 26

A 24-year-old woman is evaluated for excessive menstrual bleeding. She was recently diagnosed with polycystic ovary syndrome during an evaluation for hirsutism. Menarche occurred at age 11 years, and she has always had irregular menses occurring approximately every 60 days. However, her periods over the past year have been associated with heavy bleeding that is increasingly bothersome. Medical history is otherwise unremarkable, and she takes no medications. She currently does not desire fertility.

On physical examination, she is afebrile. Blood pressure is 110/70 mm Hg, pulse rate is 78/min, and respiration rate is 14/min. BMI is 32. Excess terminal hair growth is present on the upper lip, chin, and chest. The physical examination is otherwise normal.

A urine pregnancy test is negative.

Which of the following is the most appropriate therapy for this patient?

(A) Combined oral contraceptive pills
(B) Levonorgestrel intrauterine system
(C) Metformin
(D) Periodic progestin withdrawal

Item 27

A 55-year-old man is evaluated for abdominal fullness and nausea of 2 weeks' duration. He has no vomiting or fever. One month ago, he was diagnosed with type 2 diabetes mellitus. He reports an unintentional weight loss of 5 kg (11 lb) over the past month, generalized weakness, and poor appetite. Metformin is his only medication.

On physical examination, blood pressure is 158/90 mm Hg and pulse rate is 90/min. BMI is 29. His face is round and red. A dorsocervical fat pad is present. His abdomen is distended, but nontender. Violaceous

striae measuring 8 to 12 mm wide are noted on his upper arms and abdomen. There is 1+ bilateral lower extremity edema. Multiple ecchymoses and acanthosis nigricans are present.

Laboratory studies:

Adrenocorticotropic hormone	<5 pg/mL (1.1 pmol/L)
24-Hour urine cortisol excretion	
Initial measurement	280 μg/24 h (771.6 nmol/24 h)
Repeat measurement	300 μg/24 h (826.7 nmol/24 h)
Cortisol, serum	46 μg/dL (1269.6 nmol/L)
Urine	
Catecholamines	40 μg/m^2/24 h (236.4 nmol/m^2/24 h)
Metanephrines	1000 μg/24 h (5070 nmol/24 h)

CT scan of the abdomen with and without contrast reveals a 5.6-cm heterogeneous right adrenal mass with focal areas of calcifications and hemorrhage. The density of the mass is 50 Hounsfield units, and the contrast washout at 10 minutes is 20%.

Which of the following is the most appropriate next step in the management of this patient's adrenal mass?

(A) Chemotherapy
(B) Fine-needle biopsy
(C) Radiation therapy
(D) Surgical excision

Item 28

A 47-year-old man presents to the emergency department with weakness and shakiness. He has a long history of alcohol abuse but significantly decreased his usual daily alcohol intake over the past week because of gastrointestinal upset, nausea, and diarrhea. Medical history is otherwise unremarkable, and he takes no medications.

On physical examination, the patient is awake and oriented but tremulous. Mucous membranes are dry. Temperature is 37.3 °C (99.1 °F), blood pressure is 139/76 mm Hg, pulse rate is 101/min, and respiration rate is 15/min. BMI is 19. Cardiopulmonary examination is unremarkable. The abdomen is diffusely tender to palpation. Periodic spontaneous twitching is noted in the major muscle groups.

Laboratory studies are significant for a serum calcium level of 6.5 mg/dL (1.6 mmol/L), serum albumin level of 2.6 g/dL (26 g/L), serum potassium of 3.4 mEq/L (3.4 mmol/L), and normal kidney function studies. Serum parathyroid hormone and 25-hydroxyvitamin D levels are pending.

An electrocardiogram shows prolongation of the QT interval.

Which of the following is the most appropriate next diagnostic test to evaluate this patient's hypocalcemia?

(A) 1,25-Dihydroxyvitamin D level
(B) 24-Hour urine calcium excretion
(C) Ionized calcium level
(D) Magnesium level

Item 29

A 52-year-old woman presents for follow-up evaluation after being diagnosed with type 2 diabetes mellitus 6 weeks ago. Her initial hemoglobin A_{1c} level was 8.0%. Management at this time is with lifestyle modifications. She has worked closely with a diabetes educator and a nutritionist since her diagnosis. She has lost 3.2 kg (7 lb) by making changes to her diet and activity level. Review of her blood glucose log for the past 2 weeks shows preprandial blood glucose values in the 150 to 160 mg/dL (8.3-8.9 mmol/L) range and several 2-hour postprandial blood glucose values of 190 to 200 mg/dL (10.5-11.1 mmol/L). Her only other medical problem is hypertension for which she takes lisinopril.

On physical examination, blood pressure is 125/70 mm Hg and pulse rate is 74/min. BMI is 28. There is no evidence of diabetic retinopathy. She has normal monofilament and vibratory sensation in her extremities.

Except for her blood glucose parameters, basic laboratory studies obtained at the time of her initial diagnosis were normal.

In addition to continuing lifestyle modifications, which of the following is the most appropriate management for this patient's diabetes?

(A) Initiate dapagliflozin
(B) Initiate glipizide
(C) Initiate metformin
(D) Initiate sitagliptin

Item 30

A 28-year-old man is evaluated for fatigue and erectile dysfunction. His symptoms have been progressive over the past year. He notes decreased libido and reports loss of morning erections. He also feels tired, has difficulty concentrating, and notes diffuse joint aches. He believes he has less strength and has had to decrease his level of exercise.

Medical history is unremarkable. He had normal puberty and normal growth. He takes no medications.

On physical examination, temperature is 37.4 °C (99.3 °F), blood pressure is 108/72 mm Hg, pulse rate is 68/min, and respiration rate is 14/min. BMI is 23. The liver edge is palpable 4 cm below the costal margin. The penis is normal, and the testes are normal volume but soft and freely mobile without masses. Visual fields are intact.

Laboratory studies:

Follicle-stimulating hormone	3.0 mU/mL (3.0 U/L)
Luteinizing hormone	2.2 mU/mL (2.2 U/L)
Prolactin	12 ng/mL (12 µg/L)
Testosterone, total (8 AM)	178 ng/dL (6.2 nmol/L)
Testosterone, total (8 AM), repeated	162 ng/dL (5.6 nmol/L)
Thyroid-stimulating hormone	2.3 µU/mL (2.3 mU/L)

Pituitary MRI is normal.

Which of the following is the most appropriate next step in management?

(A) Begin testosterone replacement therapy
(B) Karyotyping

(C) Serum ferritin level and transferrin saturation
(D) Testicular ultrasound

Item 31

A 59-year-old man is evaluated for hypercalcemia. He was recently diagnosed with multiple myeloma. He does not have anorexia, nausea, constipation, polydipsia, polyuria, or confusion. Medical history is otherwise unremarkable, and he takes no medications.

On physical examination, temperature is 36.4 °C (97.5 °F), blood pressure is 134/80 mm Hg, pulse rate is 80/min, and respiration rate is 12/min. BMI is 30. The remainder of his physical examination is normal, and no weakness is noted on neurologic examination.

Serum calcium level is 10.8 mg/dL (2.7 mmol/L).

Which of the following is the most appropriate next laboratory test for evaluating this patient's hypercalcemia?

(A) 1,25-Dihydroxyvitamin D level
(B) Ionized calcium level
(C) Parathyroid hormone level
(D) Parathyroid hormone–related protein level

Item 32

A 37-year-old man is evaluated for a 2-year history of low libido, loss of morning erections, fatigue, and decreasing muscle mass. His medical history is otherwise unremarkable. He takes no medications.

On physical examination, vital signs are normal. BMI is 35. The remainder of the examination, including genital examination, is normal.

Laboratory studies:

Follicle-stimulating hormone	12 mU/mL (12 U/L)
Luteinizing hormone	10 mU/mL (10 U/L)
Prolactin	Normal
Morning testosterone (total)	148 ng/dL (5.1 nmol/L)
Confirmatory morning testosterone (total)	137 ng/dL (4.7 nmol/L)
Thyroid-stimulating hormone	Normal

A pituitary MRI is normal.

Before initiating therapy for this patient, which of the following should be determined?

(A) Bone mineral density
(B) Desire for fertility
(C) Fasting plasma glucose level
(D) Scrotal ultrasound

Item 33

A 55-year-old woman is evaluated in the emergency department because of a 1-week history of palpitations, chest pain, shortness of breath, diarrhea, and weight loss. Medical history is significant for an episode of chest pain 4 weeks ago; the chest pain was evaluated with an exercise stress test, which was positive. A subsequent cardiac catheterization was negative for epicardial coronary artery

CONT.

disease. She also has a history of Graves disease treated with daily methimazole; she stopped this medication on the day of her catheterization and has not restarted it since that time.

On physical examination, she is restless and confused. Temperature is 38.9 °C (102.0 °F), blood pressure is 175/94 mm Hg, pulse rate is 135/min and regular, and respiration rate is 20/min. The skin is warm and moist. There is mild proptosis with scleral injection. Examination of the thyroid reveals a diffusely enlarged gland that is nontender to palpation. A thyroid bruit is heard. Abdominal examination is unremarkable. There is edema of the lower extremities to the mid-lower leg. On neurologic examination, she is oriented to place but not to time, as she does not know the correct year.

Laboratory studies:

Leukocyte count	10,500/µL (10.5 × 10⁹/L)
Creatinine	1.3 mg/dL (115 µmol/L)
Thyroid-stimulating hormone	<0.008 µU/mL (0.008 mU/L)
Free thyroxine (T₄)	7.5 ng/dL (96.7 pmol/L)

Which of the following is the most likely diagnosis?

(A) Euthyroid sick syndrome
(B) Pheochromocytoma
(C) Subacute thyroiditis
(D) Thyroid storm

Item 34

A 39-year-old man is seen for a follow-up examination. Three months ago, he underwent an organ-sparing procedure for squamous cell carcinoma of the throat. As part of his surgery, his thyroid and all four parathyroid glands were removed. He was started on 1,25-dihydroxyvitamin D (calcitriol) and supplemental calcium carbonate following surgery. He subsequently completed a course of concurrent cisplatin-based chemotherapy and radiation therapy without significant complications and currently feels well with no new signs or symptoms. Medical history is otherwise unremarkable except for a 25-pack-year smoking history; he discontinued tobacco use at the time of diagnosis. Medications are calcitriol, calcium carbonate, and levothyroxine.

On physical examination, temperature is 37.0 °C (98.6 °F), blood pressure is 125/84 mm Hg, pulse rate is 85/min, and respiration rate is 12/min. BMI is 24. Well-healed surgical incisions are noted on the anterior neck. The remainder of the examination is unremarkable.

Laboratory studies:

Calcium	8.5 mg/dL (2.1 mmol/L)
Creatinine	0.8 mg/dL (70.7 µmol/L)
1,25-Dihydroxyvitamin D	Within therapeutic range
24-Hour urine calcium	375 mg/24 h (9.4 mmol/24 h)

Which of the following is the most appropriate management of this patient's postsurgical calcium therapy?

(A) Check 25-hydroxyvitamin D level
(B) Check parathyroid hormone level

(C) Continue current treatment regimen
(D) Decrease calcium supplementation

Item 35

A 40-year-old man with type 1 diabetes mellitus presents to the office. He seeks advice on his diabetes management as he intensifies his exercise routine in preparation for participation in a 10-K race. He reports prolonged hypoglycemia during intense exercise, despite eating a meal prior to the activity. His insulin regimen is insulin glargine and insulin glulisine. His most recent hemoglobin A₁c level was 7.0%.

Which of the following is the most appropriate management of this patient's hypoglycemia on the days that he exercises?

(A) Decrease meal-time insulin glulisine dose prior to exercise, continue insulin glargine dose
(B) Discontinue insulin glargine, continue insulin glulisine dose
(C) Increase meal-time protein prior to exercise, continue current insulin doses
(D) Switch insulin glulisine to a sliding-scale regimen, continue insulin glargine dose

Item 36

A 54-year-old man is evaluated because of fatigue. He also notes constipation and cold intolerance. Medical history is significant for tonsillar squamous cell carcinoma treated with radiation 3 years ago. There is no family history of thyroid disorders.

On physical examination, the skin is dry. Mild periorbital edema is present. The thyroid is of normal size and without nodules. Reflexes are delayed.

Laboratory studies show a hemoglobin level of 11 g/dL (110 g/L), a serum sodium level of 129 mEq/L (129 mmol/L), and a serum thyroid-stimulating hormone (TSH) level of 1.4 µU/mL (1.4 mU/L).

Which of the following is the most appropriate next step in management?

(A) Free thyroxine (T₄) measurement
(B) Repeat TSH measurement in 4 weeks
(C) Thyroid scintigraphy
(D) Thyroid ultrasound

Item 37

A 24-year-old woman is evaluated for hypercalcemia incidentally discovered on laboratory studies performed for another indication. She reports no hypercalcemia-related symptoms. Medical history is significant for gastroesophageal reflux disease and menstrual migraine. Family history is notable for a brother who has a "calcium" problem. Medications are omeprazole and sumatriptan as needed.

On physical examination, temperature is 36.2 °C (97.2 °F), blood pressure is 127/68 mm Hg, pulse rate is 73/min, and respiration rate is 12/min. BMI is 25. Chest, heart, and abdominal examinations are normal, as is the remainder of her examination.

Laboratory studies are significant for a serum calcium level of 11.2 mg/dL (2.8 mmol/L), parathyroid hormone level of 55 pg/mL (55 ng/L), and 25-hydroxyvitamin D level of 35 ng/mL (87.4 nmol/L). Kidney and thyroid function studies are normal.

Which of the following is the most appropriate next step in management?

(A) Bone densitometry
(B) Measurement of urine calcium and creatinine levels
(C) Parathyroid sestamibi scan
(D) Referral for parathyroidectomy

Item 38

A 25-year-old woman with type 1 diabetes mellitus is evaluated for recent-onset glycemic fluctuations without symptomatic hypoglycemia. She was diagnosed with diabetes 7 years ago. Her hemoglobin A_{1c} levels since diagnosis have ranged from 6.4% to 7.3%, with the most recent value at 7.3%. She reports eating a carbohydrate-consistent diet at each meal, with little variation in her selection of meals or snacks. She started a new job several months ago but continues her daily exercise routine and sleep schedule. She has no other medical problems or symptoms. Her diabetes treatment regimen is insulin glargine once daily and insulin lispro three times daily.

Physical examination findings and vital signs are normal.

Estimate glomerular filtration rate, serum creatinine level, and urine albumin-creatinine ratio are normal. Her blood glucose values from the previous week are shown below.

Blood glucose values:

Breakfast (mg/dL [mmol/L])	Lunch (mg/dL [mmol/L])	Dinner (mg/dL [mmol/L])	Bedtime (mg/dL [mmol/L])
124 (6.9)	190 (10.5)	109 (6.1)	210 (11.6)
110 (6.1)	92 (5.1)	112 (6.2)	126 (7.0)
115 (6.4)	118 (6.5)	112 (6.2)	126 (7.0)
117 (6.5)	127 (7.0)	204 (11.3)	110 (6.1)
108 (6.0)	101 (5.6)	122 (6.8)	114 (6.3)
101 (5.6)	111 (6.2)	106 (5.9)	72 (4.0)
126 (7.0)	187 (10.4)	102 (5.7)	196 (10.9)

Which of the following is the most likely cause of the fluctuating glycemic control?

(A) Antibodies to exogenous insulin
(B) Gastroparesis
(C) Inadequate insulin doses
(D) Inappropriate insulin timing

Item 39

A 20-year-old woman is admitted to the hospital for an elective adrenalectomy. Her history is significant for recent onset of hypertension, weight gain, generalized weakness, and easy bruising. Laboratory evaluation demonstrated an elevated urine free cortisol and lack of suppression of serum cortisol following a low-dose overnight dexamethasone suppression test. Subsequent testing revealed a suppressed adrenocorticotropic hormone level.

A contrast-enhanced adrenal CT scan revealed a well-circumscribed 3.7-cm right adrenal mass with a contrast washout of greater than 50% at 10 minutes.

Which of the following is the most appropriate perioperative management?

(A) Postoperative hydrocortisone
(B) Postoperative mitotane
(C) Postoperative norepinephrine
(D) Preoperative phenoxybenzamine

Item 40

A 62-year-old man is evaluated for right leg pain. The pain has developed progressively over the past 6 months and worsens with prolonged activity, such as playing golf. Medical history is unremarkable, and he takes no medications.

On physical examination, temperature is 36.3 °C (97.3 °F), blood pressure is 128/67 mm Hg, pulse rate is 73/min, and respiration rate is 10/min. BMI is 29. There is no pain to palpation over the femoral region, and he has normal range of motion.

Laboratory studies are significant for a serum alkaline phosphatase level of 200 U/L and serum calcium level of 9.0 mg/dL (2.3 mmol/L).

Plain radiograph of the right femur is shown.

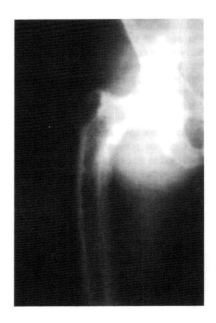

Which of the following is the most appropriate next step in management?

(A) Antiresorptive therapy
(B) Bone biopsy
(C) Evaluation for multiple myeloma
(D) Clinical observation

Item 41

A 29-year-old woman is evaluated during her first prenatal visit. She feels well. Medical history is significant only for hypothyroidism, for which she has taken levothyroxine, 100 μg/d, for the last 3 years. Her only other medication is a prenatal vitamin.

On physical examination, she is afebrile. Blood pressure is 98/72 mm Hg, pulse rate is 88/min, and respiration rate is 12/min. The thyroid is of normal size and without nodules. There is no cervical lymphadenopathy. Cardiovascular and pulmonary examinations are unremarkable. Abdominal examination reveals normal bowel sounds. The uterus is not palpable.

Laboratory studies show a serum thyroid-stimulating hormone level of 3.6 μU/mL (3.6 mU/L) and a serum total thyroxine (T_4) level of 4.5 μg/dL (58 nmol/L).

Which of the following is the most appropriate treatment of this patient's hypothyroidism?

(A) Continue levothyroxine dose
(B) Decrease levothyroxine dose
(C) Discontinue levothyroxine
(D) Increase levothyroxine dose

Item 42

A 62-year-old man is evaluated in the hospital for several hours of nausea, lightheadedness, and back and abdominal pain. He underwent uncomplicated mechanical aortic valve replacement 3 days ago. He had been doing well postoperatively until the development of his current symptoms. Medical history is significant only for hypothyroidism. Medications are therapeutic unfractionated heparin, levothyroxine, and as-needed oxycodone.

On physical examination, temperature is 37.2 °C (99.0 °F), blood pressure is 80/50 mm Hg, pulse rate is 110/min, and respiration rate is 18/min. BMI is 26. Examination of the chest shows a clean and dry sternal wound. Cardiac examination reveals regular tachycardia and mechanical S_2. There is no pain with palpation of the abdomen or lower back. His skin pigmentation is normal.

Laboratory studies:

Hemoglobin	7.3 g/dL (73 g/L)
	9.0 g/dL (90 g/L) postoperatively
Leukocyte count	11,000/μL (11 × 10⁹/L)
Activated partial thromboplastin time	70 s
Creatinine	1.0 mg/dL (88.4 μmol/L)
Sodium	130 mEq/L (130 mmol/L)
Potassium	6.0 mEq/L (6.0 mmol/L)
Cortisol, random	<2 μg/dL (55.2 nmol/L)

Which of the following is the most likely diagnosis?

(A) Autoimmune adrenalitis
(B) Bilateral adrenal hemorrhage
(C) Opiate-induced adrenal insufficiency
(D) Pituitary apoplexy

Item 43

A 44-year-old woman is evaluated for weight gain, muscle weakness, and metabolic syndrome. She has hirsutism but also notes hair loss on her head. She has been amenorrheic for 2 years.

Medical history is significant for hyperlipidemia, type 2 diabetes mellitus, hypertension, and obesity. Medications are atorvastatin, metformin, and lisinopril.

On physical examination, blood pressure is 156/92 mm Hg and pulse rate is 78/min. BMI is 42. She has a cushingoid appearance, acne, and moderate hirsutism affecting the chin, upper lip, breasts, back, and chest. There are several wide violaceous striae across the abdomen and the back of her arms.

Laboratory studies:

Adrenocorticotropic hormone (ACTH)	52 pg/mL (11.4 pmol/L)
Cortisol 8 AM after 1 mg of dexamethasone the night before	5.2 μg/dL (143.5 nmol/L)
24-Hour urine cortisol excretion	
Initial measurement	124 μg/24 h (341.7 nmol/24 h)
Repeat measurement	98 μg/24 h (270.0 nmol/24 h)

Intrapetrosal sinus sampling identifies a pituitary microadenoma as the source of the high ACTH level.

Which of the following is the most appropriate test to perform next?

(A) 8-mg dexamethasone suppression test
(B) 24-Hour urine free catecholamine and metanephrine measurement
(C) Dual-energy x-ray absorptiometry scan
(D) PET scan

Item 44

A 28-year-old woman is being discharged from the hospital with a diagnosis of autoimmune adrenalitis. Medical history is otherwise unremarkable, and she was on no medications prior to admission.

On physical examination, temperature is 37.0 °C (98.6 °F), blood pressure is 120/80 mm Hg, pulse rate is 80/min, and respiration rate is 12/min. BMI is 22. Increased skin pigmentation is noted over the extensor surfaces of the extremities bilaterally. The remainder of her examination is normal.

Which of the following is the most appropriate long-term medication regimen for this patient?

(A) Dexamethasone, 1 mg once daily
(B) Fludrocortisone, 0.05 mg once daily
(C) Hydrocortisone, 10 mg three times daily
(D) Prednisone, 5 mg once daily, and fludrocortisone, 0.05 mg once daily

Item 45

A 78-year-old woman is evaluated for a 2-week history of unintentional weight loss, night sweats, and neck swelling. She has more recently also had difficulty swallowing solid foods and positional shortness of breath. She does not have hoarseness, palpitations, or change in bowel habits. Prior to the development of these symptoms, she had been in her usual state of health with no illnesses. She has hypothyroidism and has been taking levothyroxine for 40 years, with a stable dose for the past 10 years.

On physical examination, temperature is 36.9 °C (98.4 °F), blood pressure is 140/88 mm Hg, pulse rate is 75/min, and respiration rate is 12/min. The thyroid is symmetrically enlarged, firm, and fixed. There is no thyroid bruit.

CT scan of the neck is shown.

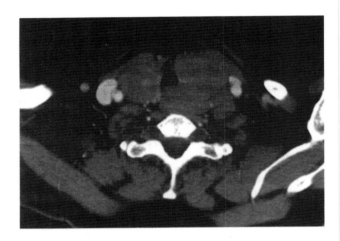

Which of the following is the most likely diagnosis?

(A) Graves disease
(B) Papillary thyroid cancer
(C) Primary thyroid lymphoma
(D) Subacute thyroiditis

Item 46

A 67-year-old man is evaluated for a recent diagnosis of primary hyperparathyroidism after an elevated serum calcium level was incidentally detected on laboratory testing. Medical history is significant only for hypertension, and his only medication is ramipril.

On physical examination, temperature is 35.8 °C (96.4 °F), blood pressure is 120/68 mm Hg, pulse rate is 62/min, and respiration rate is 14/min. BMI is 32. The remainder of his examination is unremarkable.

Laboratory studies:

Calcium	10.9 mg/dL (2.7 mmol/L)
Creatinine	0.9 mg/dL (79.6 µmol/L)
Parathyroid hormone	98 pg/mL (98 ng/L)
25-Hydroxyvitamin D	19 ng/mL (47.4 nmol/L)
Estimated glomerular filtration rate	>60 mL/min/1.73 m²

A dual-energy x-ray absorptiometry (DEXA) scan shows T-scores of –1.3 in the right femoral neck, –1.0 in the lumbar spine, and –1.4 in the non-dominant forearm. Fracture Risk Assessment Tool (FRAX) score indicates a 13% risk of major osteoporotic fracture and a 1.9% risk of hip fracture over the next 10 years.

Which of the following is the most appropriate management of this patient?

(A) Refer for parathyroidectomy
(B) Start alendronate
(C) Start calcitonin
(D) Start cinacalcet
(E) Start vitamin D₃ (cholecalciferol)

Item 47

A 57-year-old man is admitted to the hospital for evaluation of substernal chest pain. His medical history is significant for type 2 diabetes mellitus, coronary artery disease, hypertension, and hyperlipidemia. He manages his diabetes as an outpatient with diet, exercise, and metformin. His other medications are aspirin, metoprolol, atorvastatin, and sublingual nitroglycerin as needed. His inpatient plasma glucose values are 170 to 210 mg/dL (9.4-11.6 mmol/L). Results of all other laboratory studies are normal.

Which of the following is the most appropriate treatment for this patient's diabetes while hospitalized?

(A) Basal and prandial insulin
(B) Glipizide
(C) Metformin
(D) Sliding-scale insulin

Item 48

A 43-year-old woman is evaluated for progressive weight gain over the past 2 years. Her previous weight was 72.6 kg (160 lb) but has steadily risen to her current weight of 106.6 kg (235 lb). She notes a slight increase in her appetite but minimal change in her lifestyle or activity level. She has tried to lose weight with increased exercise and nutritional counseling but without significant results. More recently she reports having trouble sleeping and decreased exercise tolerance with activites such as walking up steps. Medical history is significant for impaired fasting glucose, hypertension, and hyperlipidemia. Medications are hydrochlorothiazide and atorvastatin. She has not been prescribed glucocorticoids or had glucocorticoid joint injections.

On physical examination, temperature is 37.2 °C (99.0 °F), blood pressure is 136/86 mm Hg, pulse rate is 88/min, and respiration rate is 12/min. BMI is 38. She has rounded facies, thin hair, mild hirsutism, and prominent fat deposition in the dorsocervical and supraclavicular areas. Her skin is thin, and she bruises easily, although striae are not present. Her examination is otherwise unremarkable.

Laboratory studies are significant for a fasting plasma glucose level of 120 mg/dL (6.7 mmol/L) and normal thyroid-stimulating hormone level.

Which of the following is the most appropriate next step in evaluation?

(A) Adrenocorticotropic hormone measurement
(B) 1-mg dexamethasone suppression test
(C) 8-mg dexamethasone suppression test
(D) Pituitary MRI
(E) Serum cortisol measurement

Item 49

A 50-year-old man undergoes follow-up evaluation for type 2 diabetes mellitus. His daily log demonstrates average blood glucose levels of 120 to 150 mg/dL (6.7–8.3 mmol/L), with hypoglycemia in the 50 mg/dL (2.8 mmol/L) range noted once or twice per week without a discernible pattern. He is unable to detect the hypoglycemia.

The patient has a medical history of diabetic retinopathy, chronic kidney disease, peripheral neuropathy, hypertension, hyperlipidemia, obstructive sleep apnea (on bilevel positive airway pressure), gastroesophageal reflux disease, and osteoarthritis in both knees. He reports intolerance to strenuous exercise due to knee pain. He is able to walk 15 minutes daily. He has worked closely with a nutritionist, resulting in a 5.0-kg (11-lb) weight loss over 1 year, which has plateaued recently.

Medications are insulin glargine, insulin aspart, lisinopril, carvedilol, pantoprazole, aspirin, and atorvastatin.

On physical examination, blood pressure is 140/90 mm Hg and pulse rate is 65/min. BMI is 37. Bilateral proliferative retinopathy is present. There are no carotid bruits or cardiac murmurs. Bilateral loss of monofilament and vibratory sensation on the feet and decreased ankle reflexes are noted. The remainder of the examination is normal.

Results of laboratory studies show hemoglobin A_{1c} level of 8.2% and serum creatinine level of 1.7 mg/dL (150.3 µmol/L).

Which of the following is the most appropriate treatment of this patient?

(A) Bariatric surgery
(B) Increase insulin
(C) Initiate metformin
(D) Initiate pramlintide

Item 50

A 47-year-old woman is evaluated for an incidentally discovered right adrenal mass.

On physical examination, blood pressure is 120/80 mm Hg in both arms and pulse rate is 84/min. The abdomen is nontender, and there are no palpable masses. The remainder of the examination is unremarkable.

Noncontrast CT of the abdomen demonstrates a 3.2-cm well-circumscribed, partially cystic right adrenal lesion with a density of 30 Hounsfield units. A low-dose dexamethasone suppression test is negative for evidence of cortisol hypersecretion.

Which of the following is the most appropriate next step in management?

(A) Adrenalectomy
(B) CT-guided transcutaneous biopsy
(C) Plasma aldosterone to plasma renin ratio
(D) Plasma free metanephrines
(E) No additional testing is indicated

Item 51

A 64-year-old man with type 2 diabetes mellitus and stage 4 chronic kidney disease is evaluated for continued glycemic management. He is followed closely by the nephrology service in preparation for impending hemodialysis, with initiation of erythropoietin therapy within the last 3 months. His average fasting and preprandial blood glucose values are in the 145 to 190 mg/dL (8.0-10.5 mmol/L) range. He does not have hypoglycemia. His insulin regimen consists of insulin detemir at bedtime and insulin glulisine before meals. His most recent hemoglobin A_{1c} value has decreased from 7.5% to 6.2%.

Which of the following is the most appropriate management for this patient's diabetes?

(A) Continue current therapy
(B) Decrease insulin detemir dose
(C) Discontinue preprandial insulin glulisine
(D) Measure postprandial glucose level

Item 52

A 34-year-old woman is evaluated for hirsutism and acne that began 4 months ago. She also reports that her voice has become deeper. Her menstrual periods have remained regular, occurring every 28 days.

She has one son 5 years of age. She reports that her pregnancy was uncomplicated and she had no difficulty conceiving. She had a tubal ligation following the birth of her child. She has a sister with polycystic ovary syndrome. She takes no medications.

On physical examination, blood pressure is 140/84 mm Hg, and pulse rate is 62/min. BMI is 21. She has hyperpigmented terminal hairs on the chin, neck, abdomen, and lower back and comedones and pustules on the face and upper back. There is frontotemporal hair loss. The remainder of the examination is unremarkable.

Laboratory studies:

Cortisol, free (urine)	26 µg/24 h (71.6 nmol/24 h)
Dehydroepiandrosterone sulfate	8.2 µg/mL (22.1 µmol/L)
Prolactin	8 ng/mL (8 µg/L)
Testosterone	96 ng/dL (3.3 nmol/L)

Which of the following is the most appropriate diagnostic test to perform next?

(A) Abdominal CT scan
(B) Low-dose dexamethasone suppression test
(C) Pelvic ultrasound
(D) Pituitary MRI

Item 53

A 27-year-old woman is evaluated for management of her type 1 diabetes mellitus. She was diagnosed 10 years ago. She has no known complications from her diabetes. She eats a healthy diet and exercises an average of 60 minutes per day in the evening. She takes insulin glargine and insulin aspart. She is adherent with her insulin regimen and checks her blood glucose level three to five times per day. Her average blood glucose value is 125 mg/dL (6.9 mmol/L), with fasting glucose values ranging from 80 to 150 mg/dL (4.4-8.3 mmol/L). She routinely measures her 2-hour postprandial glucose values, and they are consistently less than 150 mg/dL (8.3 mmol/L). She has several overnight blood glucose values ranging from 90 to 140 mg/dL (5.0-7.8 mmol/L). Her hemoglobin A_{1c} values over the last 6 months have been 7.3% to 7.5%. She is discouraged that her hemoglobin A_{1c} values remain above 7.0%.

Laboratory studies, including creatinine and complete blood count, are normal.

Which of the following is the most appropriate management of her elevated hemoglobin A_{1c} level?

(A) Begin continuous glucose monitoring

(B) Increase exercise

(C) Increase insulin aspart

(D) Increase insulin glargine

Item 54

A 25-year-old woman is evaluated after a recent diagnosis of polycystic ovary syndrome. She is concerned about hirsutism and irregular menses. She has no desire to be pregnant at this time. She takes no medications.

On physical examination, she is afebrile. Blood pressure is 110/60 mm Hg, pulse rate is 68/min, and respiration rate is 16/min; BMI is 37. Coarse hair is noted on the chin, jawline, and periumbilical area. The remainder of her physical examination, including pelvic examination, is normal.

Which of the following is the most appropriate treatment?

(A) Combined oral contraceptive pills

(B) Intermittent progestin withdrawal

(C) Levonorgestrel intrauterine system

(D) Spironolactone therapy

Item 55

A 46-year-old man is evaluated following a diagnosis of pheochromocytoma. He has no signs or symptoms at this time. Except for hypertension, his medical history is unremarkable. Medications are lisinopril and hydrochlorothiazide.

On physical examination, blood pressure is 170/90 mm Hg and pulse rate is 90/min. The remainder of the physical examination is unrevealing.

Which of the following is the most appropriate next step in management?

(A) Increase lisinopril dosage

(B) Perform contrast-enhanced adrenal CT scan

(C) Start phenoxybenzamine

(D) Start propranolol

Item 56

A 38-year-old man with panhypopituitarism is evaluated for worsening fatigue and weight gain over the past 3 months. He is sleeping 9 hours each night, but he feels tired during the day and has decreased his usual exercise level. He has morning

erections but reports low libido and occasional erectile dysfunction during intercourse. He wakes once during the night to urinate and drink water. He estimates that he urinates 5 to 8 times during the day, which is unchanged.

Medical history is significant for transsphenoidal resection of a craniopharyngioma at age 18 years. He has required anterior pituitary hormone replacement and desmopressin since that time. Medications are desmopressin, hydrocortisone, levothyroxine, somatropin, and testosterone enanthate.

On physical examination, temperature is 37.0 °C (98.6 °F), blood pressure is 118/64 mm Hg, pulse rate is 74/min, and respiration rate is 14/min. No orthostatic changes are noted. BMI is 24. There are no facial changes suggestive of acromegaly or Cushing syndrome. The thyroid is normal without goiter or nodules. Hair distribution and skin turgor are normal. There is no gynecomastia or striae. Normal penis and testicular volume are noted. Visual fields are intact on neurologic examination.

Laboratory studies:

Sodium	138 mEq/L (138 mmol/L)
Insulin-like growth factor 1	Normal
Prolactin	18 ng/mL (18 µg/L)
Thyroid-stimulating hormone	0.8 µU/mL (0.8 mU/L)
Thyroxine (T_4), free	0.7 ng/dL (9.0 pmol/L)
Testosterone (11 days after injection)	482 ng/dL (16.7 nmol/L)

Follow-up MRIs show no residual tumor.

Which of the following is the most appropriate management?

(A) Increase desmopressin

(B) Increase hydrocortisone

(C) Increase levothyroxine

(D) Increase testosterone enanthate

(E) Stop somatropin

Item 57

A 55-year-old man is evaluated following a screening for type 2 diabetes mellitus. He is asymptomatic. He has a history of hypertension and hyperlipidemia. There is no history of anemia, liver disease, or kidney disease. Medications are lisinopril and rosuvastatin.

On physical examination, blood pressure is 123/76 mm Hg and pulse rate is 72/min. BMI is 28. The remainder of the examination is unremarkable.

Laboratory studies:

Hematocrit	45.6%
Creatinine	1.0 mg/dL (88.4 µmol/L)
Glucose, fasting	128 mg/dL (7.1 mmol/L)
Hemoglobin A_{1c}	5.6%

Which of the following is the most appropriate diagnostic test to perform next?

(A) Fasting plasma glucose

(B) Hemoglobin A_{1c}

(C) Oral glucose tolerance test

(D) Random blood glucose

Item 58

A 34-year-old man is evaluated for a 2-year history of fatigue, low libido, and infertility. His family history is notable for a brother with infertility. His medical history is unremarkable, and he takes no medications.

On physical examination, vital signs are normal. His height is 195.6 cm (77 in), and his weight is 86.2 kg (190 lb). Genital examination reveals small, firm testes bilaterally.

Laboratory studies reveal a morning serum total testosterone level of 140 ng/dL (4.9 nmol/L) (which was confirmed on repeat testing), a serum follicle-stimulating hormone level of 24 mU/mL (24 U/L), and a serum luteinizing hormone level of 18 mU/mL (18 U/L). Repeated semen analyses reveal azoospermia.

Which of the following is the most appropriate diagnostic test to perform next?

(A) Karyotype
(B) MRI of the pituitary
(C) Scrotal ultrasound
(D) Serum prolactin measurement

Item 59

An 84-year-old man is evaluated for moderate fatigue. He otherwise feels well and does not have constipation, cold intolerance, weight gain or loss, anxiety, tremor, palpitations, or dyspnea. Medical history is significant for hypertension, and his only medication is felodipine.

On physical examination, he is alert and oriented. Blood pressure is 144/83 mm Hg; other vital signs are normal. The thyroid is not palpable. Cardiopulmonary examination is normal. There is no peripheral edema. Neurologic examination is nonfocal, and deep tendon reflexes are normal.

Laboratory studies:

Complete blood count	Normal
Comprehensive metabolic profile	Normal
Thyroid-stimulating hormone (TSH)	6.4 µU/mL (6.4 mU/L)
Free thyroxine (T_4)	1.3 ng/dL (16.8 pmol/L)

Which of the following is the most appropriate management?

(A) Levothyroxine therapy
(B) Measurement of serum total triiodothyronine (T_3) level
(C) Measurement of serum total T_4 level
(D) Repeat TSH and free T_4 measurement in 6 to 12 weeks

Item 60

A 62-year-old woman is evaluated for an incidentally discovered left adrenal mass. Two weeks ago, the patient was evaluated in the emergency department for diffuse abdominal pain and vomiting. A CT scan was obtained that was normal except for the adrenal mass. Three hours after presentation to the emergency department, the pain resolved spontaneously.

Her medical history is significant for diet-controlled type 2 diabetes mellitus diagnosed 1 year ago and osteoporosis diagnosed 4 years ago. Her only medication is alendronate.

On physical examination, temperature is 37.0 °C (98.6 °F), blood pressure is 120/80 mm Hg, and pulse rate is 70/min. BMI is 26. The remainder of the physical examination is normal.

Laboratory evaluation reveals a serum sodium level of 139 mEq/L (139 mmol/L) and serum potassium level of 4.1 mEq/L (4.1 mmol/L). The previously obtained CT scan shows a 2.0-cm well-circumscribed, left adrenal lesion with a density of 5 Hounsfield units.

In addition to screening tests for pheochromocytoma, which of the following is the most appropriate diagnostic test to perform next?

(A) Adrenal vein sampling
(B) Low-dose dexamethasone suppression test
(C) Plasma renin activity and aldosterone concentration measurement
(D) No further testing

Item 61

A 68-year-old man is seen in follow-up for a recent diagnosis of acromegaly. He presented with chronic fatigue, joint and back pain, and an increase in his shoe size over the past 2 years. Medical history is significant for hypertension and type 2 diabetes mellitus. Current medications are lisinopril, metformin, and as-needed acetaminophen.

On physical examination, blood pressure is 146/88 mm Hg and pulse rate is 90/min. BMI is 29. He has a prominent brow. Macroglossia is present. Lung and heart examinations are unremarkable. Musculoskeletal examination reveals large hands and knees with bone swelling and crepitus. Skin is thickened, and there is excessive perspiration. On neurologic examination, bitemporal hemianopsia is noted.

Laboratory studies are significant for an elevated serum insulin-like growth factor 1 level of 996 ng/mL (996 µg/L) and serum prolactin level of 42 ng/mL (42 µg/L).

MRI shows a 2.5 × 1.8-cm pituitary macroadenoma that elevates the optic chiasm and appears to envelop the left carotid artery and invade the left cavernous sinus. The optic chiasm is mildly atrophied.

Which of the following is the most appropriate next step in therapy for this patient?

(A) Dopamine agonist
(B) Growth hormone receptor blockade
(C) Somatostatin analogue
(D) Stereotactic radiation therapy
(E) Transsphenoidal pituitary surgery

Item 62

A 47-year-old man is evaluated postoperatively following thyroidectomy for papillary thyroid cancer. Preoperative evaluation showed no evidence of distant metastatic disease, and he underwent total thyroidectomy with central and left lateral neck dissections. The patient's medical history is otherwise unremarkable.

On physical examination, vital signs are normal. The neck surgical sites are clean and dry. The remainder of the examination is unremarkable.

The surgical pathology report reveals a 3.5-cm papillary thyroid cancer in the left lobe of the thyroid and six malignant lymph nodes out of 35 dissected. There is evidence of minor extrathyroidal extension and vascular invasion by the primary tumor.

Which of the following is the most appropriate postoperative treatment?

(A) Doxorubicin chemotherapy
(B) External-beam radiotherapy
(C) Radioactive iodine therapy
(D) No additional therapy

Item 63

A 66-year-old man is evaluated in the office after being treated in the emergency department for an exacerbation of chronic obstructive pulmonary disease. While in the emergency department, he was noted to have a random blood glucose level of 211 mg/dL (11.7 mmol/L). His hemoglobin A_{1c} was 7.8% at the time. A repeat random fingerstick blood glucose level in office is 204 mg/dL (11.3 mmol/L).

The patient reports recent polyuria and polydipsia. He has lost 6 kg (13.2 lb) over the last 3 months. He has chronic epigastric pain associated with loose, oily stools due to chronic pancreatitis.

He has a 20-pack-year history of tobacco use and prior alcohol use, however, he does not currently use alcohol. Current medications are enteric-coated pancreatic enzymes, vitamins, tiotropium inhaler, and an albuterol inhaler as needed.

On physical examination, temperature is 37.1 °C (98.8 °F), blood pressure is 130/75 mm Hg, and pulse rate is 90/min. BMI is 22. He has mild epigastric pain on palpation without rebound tenderness or guarding. The rest of his examination is unremarkable.

Which of the following is the most appropriate treatment for his diabetes?

(A) Exenatide
(B) Glipizide
(C) Insulin
(D) Metformin

Item 64

A 34-year-old woman is evaluated because she and her male partner have been trying to conceive for 13 months without success. Her medical history is notable for a 6-year history of irregular menses and a recent diagnosis of polycystic ovary syndrome. Her only medication is a prenatal vitamin.

On physical examination, vital signs are normal. BMI is 36. Terminal hair growth on the chin, upper lip, and sides of the face is noted. No evidence of abdominal or pelvic masses, clitoromegaly, or galactorrhea is detected.

Which of the following is the most appropriate treatment?

(A) Clomiphene citrate
(B) In vitro fertilization
(C) Injectable gonadotropin
(D) Metformin

Item 65

A 64-year-old woman is seen for follow-up evaluation. Two weeks ago, she was in a car accident, and an incidental pituitary adenoma was found on a cervical spine CT scan. She has no residual injuries from the car accident.

She is otherwise healthy and takes no medications. She went through menopause at age 51. She has night sweats two to three times per month and occasional hot flushes. These have improved over the past decade and are not bothersome. She is not sexually active. She has never taken hormone replacement therapy. She has had no change in vision, headaches, or galactorrhea.

On physical examination, temperature is 37.5 °C (99.5 °F), blood pressure is 110/63 mm Hg, pulse rate is 82/min, and respiration rate is 14/min. BMI is 26. There is axillary and pubic hair loss. Visual fields are intact. There are no findings suggestive of Cushing syndrome or acromegaly.

Laboratory studies:

Estradiol	<20 pg/mL (73.4 pmol/L)
Follicle-stimulating hormone	6.4 mU/mL (6.4 U/L)
Luteinizing hormone	3.2 mU/mL (3.2 U/L)
Prolactin	53 ng/mL (53 µg/L)
Thyroid-stimulating hormone	3.2 µU/mL (3.2 mU/L)
Thyroxine (T_4), free	1.1 ng/dL (14.2 pmol/L)

Pituitary MRI shows a 7-mm adenoma in the anterior sella. The tumor is not invasive. It does not approximate the optic chiasm. The pituitary stalk is mid-line.

Which of the following is the most appropriate management?

(A) Begin dopamine agonist
(B) Gamma knife stereotactic radiosurgery
(C) Repeat testing in 12 months
(D) Transphenoidal resection

Item 66

A 57-year-old man with a 15-year history of type 2 diabetes mellitus is evaluated for bilateral burning sensation in his feet for the last 6 to 12 months. The sensation worsens at night. His hemoglobin A_{1c} levels have remained less than 7.0% for the last 2 years but were between 8.0% and 9.0% before implementing significant lifestyle changes and transitioning to insulin therapy from metformin therapy 2 years ago.

His medical history includes coronary artery disease, first-degree atrioventricular block, nonproliferative diabetic retinopathy, hypertension, and hyperlipidemia.

Medications are regular insulin, neutral protamine Hagedorn (NPH) insulin, aspirin, metoprolol, atorvastatin, and lisinopril.

On physical examination, findings are compatible with distal polyneuropathy.

Which of the following is the most appropriate management of this patient's neuropathy?

(A) Amitriptyline

(B) Duloxetine

(C) Nerve conduction study

(D) Vitamin B$_{12}$ measurement

Item 67

A 72-year-old man presents to the emergency department overnight. His wife noted that he was diaphoretic and restless during the night, and his initial blood glucose level measured by emergency medical services was 41 mg/dL (2.3 mmol/L). He was given a single dose of intravenous glucose, which increased his blood glucose level to 85 mg/dL (4.7 mmol/L). His symptoms recurred en route to the hospital, and he responded to a second dose of intravenous glucose. While in the emergency department, he was provided food and his glucose level has remained above 80 mg/dL (4.4 mmol/L) without further treatment. The patient's wife reports several recent episodes of overnight diaphoresis over the last several weeks. His last meal prior to this episode was approximately 7 hours before symptom onset.

His medical history is significant for hypertension and osteoarthritis. Medications are lisinopril and as-needed ibuprofen.

On physical examination, the patient is alert and oriented. Blood pressure is 135/84 mm Hg, and pulse rate is 82/min. BMI is 23. The general physical and neurologic examinations are normal.

Laboratory studies are significant for a normal complete metabolic profile and blood count. An insulin secretagogue screen is obtained, and hypoglycemic studies consisting of measurement of insulin, C-peptide, proinsulin, and β-hydroxybutyrate levels are planned.

Which of the following is the most appropriate diagnostic strategy for this patient?

(A) Hypoglycemic studies now

(B) Mixed-meal testing with hypoglycemic studies at the time of symptomatic hypoglycemia

(C) Oral glucose tolerance testing with hypoglycemic studies at the time of symptomatic hypoglycemia

(D) 72-Hour fast with hypoglycemic studies at the time of symptomatic hypoglycemia

Item 68

A 24-year-old woman is evaluated for a 3-month history of amenorrhea accompanied by cyclic pelvic pain. Preceding the onset of amenorrhea, she had a recent dilatation and curettage to remove retained products of conception after a first-trimester spontaneous abortion. Her personal and family medical history is unremarkable. She takes no medications.

On physical examination, she is afebrile. Blood pressure is 110/60 mm Hg, pulse rate is 68/min, and respiration rate is 16/min. BMI is 24. Pelvic examination reveals a non-tender, mobile uterus.

Laboratory studies:

Estradiol	<80 pg/mL (293.6 pmol/L)
Follicle-stimulating hormone	6.2 mU/mL (6.2 U/L)
Luteinizing hormone	4.1 mU/mL (4.1 U/L)
Prolactin	Normal
Thyroid-stimulating hormone	Normal
Urine human chorionic gonadotropin	Negative

Which of the following is the most appropriate diagnostic test to perform next?

(A) MRI of the pituitary

(B) Peripheral karyotype

(C) Progestin withdrawal test

(D) Transvaginal ultrasound

Item 69

A 29-year-old woman comes to the office for a follow-up evaluation. She was diagnosed with type 2 diabetes mellitus 2 years ago. Her fasting and premeal blood glucose values range from 120 to 150 mg/dL (6.7-8.3 mmol/L). She has had no hypoglycemic events. She has been adherent with her insulin regimen along with diet and exercise modifications. Her hemoglobin A$_{1c}$ level has decreased from 9.0% to 7.5% over the last 12 months. She expresses frustration over the need for multiple medications to treat her diabetes. Medical history is otherwise unremarkable.

Medications are insulin glargine, insulin aspart, and metformin.

On physical examination, blood pressure is 120/72 mm Hg and pulse rate is 80/min. BMI is 27. The remainder of the examination is normal.

Hemoglobin A$_{1c}$ level is currently 7.4%. Results of all other laboratory studies are normal.

Which of the following is the most appropriate management of this patient's diabetes?

(A) Increase insulin glargine dose

(B) Measure 3 AM blood glucose level

(C) Measure postprandial blood glucose levels

(D) Switch metformin to sitagliptin

Item 70

A 32-year-old woman is evaluated for a 2-week history of foreign body sensation in her eyes. Despite flushing the eyes numerous times with saline, the sensation remains. She also feels pressure behind her eyes. She is not pregnant. Medical history is unremarkable.

On physical examination, scleral injection and periorbital edema are present bilaterally, right worse than left. Diplopia is noted on lateral gaze. There is no lid lag or proptosis. The thyroid is diffusely enlarged, and a bruit is noted. Neurologic examination discloses brisk reflexes and a bilateral hand tremor.

Laboratory studies reveal a serum thyroid-stimulating hormone level of less than 0.008 µU/mL (0.008 mU/L), a serum free thyroxine (T_4) level of 4.5 ng/dL (58.0 pmol/L), and a serum total triiodothyronine (T_3) level of 365 ng/dL (5.6 nmol/L).

Which of the following is the most appropriate next step in treatment?

(A) External-beam radiotherapy to the orbits

(B) Methimazole

(C) Radioactive iodine

(D) Total thyroidectomy

Item 71

A 42-year-old man is evaluated for resistant hypertension. He was diagnosed with hypertension at age 35 years and reports that his blood pressure has never been well controlled. He is taking his medications as prescribed. He does not have headaches, chest pain, palpitations, shortness of breath, or symptoms of panic attack. He has no history of cardiovascular disease, does not smoke, and does not drink alcohol. Medications are lisinopril, amlodipine, hydrochlorothiazide, metoprolol, and potassium chloride supplementation. He is not taking any over-the-counter medications.

On physical examination, blood pressure is 150/86 mm Hg and pulse rate is 65/min. BMI is 24. Examination of the heart is significant for an S_4 but no murmurs. The remainder of his examination is unremarkable.

Laboratory studies are significant for a serum creatinine level of 1.0 mg/dL (88.4 μmol/L), fasting plasma glucose level of 82 mg/dL (4.5 mmol/L), and serum potassium level of 3.2 mEq/L (3.2 mmol/L).

Which of the following is the most appropriate next diagnostic step?

(A) Dexamethasone suppression test

(B) Plasma aldosterone-plasma renin activity ratio

(C) Plasma metanephrines and catecholamines

(D) Renal artery Doppler flow study

Item 72

A 65-year-old man is evaluated because of painless neck swelling and difficulty swallowing that has progressively worsened over the last year. He does not have hoarseness, but he feels as though his voice is not as strong as it was in the past. Medical history is significant for multiple thyroid nodules. Fine-needle aspiration of three of the largest nodules 5 years ago showed that all nodules were benign on cytologic examination. Medical history is otherwise unremarkable, and he takes no medications.

On physical examination, vital signs are normal. The thyroid is diffusely enlarged and mobile with swallowing. He has facial flushing when raising his hands above his head as shown (see top of next column).

No cervical lymphadenopathy is noted. Cardiovascular and pulmonary examinations are normal. Reflexes are normal, and there is no visible tremor.

Laboratory studies show a serum thyroid-stimulating hormone (TSH) level of 4.0 μU/mL (4.0 mU/L).

Thyroid ultrasound shows innumerable coalescent nodules with no suspicious sonographic features.

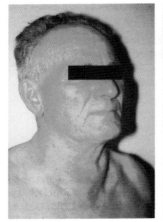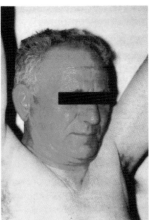

There is diffuse enlargement of the thyroid, and the inferior edge of the gland cannot be visualized. CT scan shows substernal extension of the goiter in the left lobe with mild tracheal narrowing and tracheal deviation to the right.

Which of the following is the most appropriate treatment?

(A) External-beam radiotherapy

(B) Levothyroxine

(C) Radioactive iodine

(D) Thyroidectomy

Item 73

A 26-year-old woman is evaluated because she and her husband have been trying to conceive for 14 months without success. Her husband fathered a child in a previous marriage. Her medical history is notable for pelvic inflammatory disease, which was diagnosed and successfully treated at age 18 years. Her only medication is a prenatal vitamin.

Physical examination findings are unremarkable.

Which of the following studies is most likely to be diagnostic?

(A) Diagnostic laparoscopy

(B) Hysterosalpingogram

(C) Peripheral karyotype of the patient

(D) Semen analysis of the patient's husband

(E) Transvaginal ultrasound assessment of follicle count

Item 74

A 46-year-old man is evaluated for a right lateral neck mass. He first noted the mass while shaving 2 weeks ago. He does not have hoarseness or difficulty swallowing. Medical history is significant only for hypertension. His only medication is hydrochlorothiazide.

On physical examination, blood pressure is 165/95 mm Hg, pulse rate is 88/min, and respiration rate is 12/min. There is a firm 2-cm mass in the right lateral neck and a mobile 1-cm right thyroid nodule.

Laboratory studies:

Calcium	10.5 mg/dL (2.6 mmol/L)
Creatinine	1.8 mg/dL (159.1 µmol/L)
Thyroid-stimulating hormone	4.8 µU/mL (4.8 mU/L)

Ultrasound of the neck reveals a hypoechoic thyroid nodule with microcalcifications measuring 1.6 cm. There is a 2.2-cm mass with internal calcifications in the area of the palpable abnormality.

Fine-needle aspiration of the thyroid nodule and the lateral neck mass reveals medullary thyroid cancer. *RET* testing is positive for a mutation in codon 634.

Which of the following is the most appropriate next step in management?

(A) 18-Fluoro-deoxyglucose positron emission tomography scan

(B) Plasma fractionated metanephrine levels

(C) Serum parathyroid hormone level

(D) Total thyroidectomy and lateral neck dissection

 Item 75

A 55-year-old woman is evaluated in the emergency department for altered mental status that has developed over the past week. Her family notes that she has become increasingly confused, and her oral intake has decreased significantly. Her medical history includes breast cancer that was diagnosed 5 years ago. Additional medical history is significant for hypertension. Her only medication is chlorthalidone.

On physical examination, the patient is minimally responsive. Mucous membranes are dry. Temperature is 36.2 °C (97.2 °F), blood pressure is 100/59 mm Hg, pulse rate is 110/min, and respiration rate is 12/min. BMI is 22. There is mild, diffuse abdominal tenderness to palpation. The remainder of the examination is unremarkable.

Laboratory studies are significant for a serum sodium level of 148 mEq/L (148 mmol/L), creatinine level of 4.0 mg/dL (353.6 µmol/L), baseline creatinine level is 1.6 mg/dL (141.4 µmol/L), and calcium level of 18.2 mg/dL (4.6 mmol/L).

Chlorthalidone is discontinued, and intravenous normal saline is started.

Which of the following is the most appropriate immediate next step in management?

(A) Calcitonin

(B) Cinacalcet

(C) Hemodialysis

(D) Zoledronic acid

Item 76

A 60-year-old man is evaluated during a routine follow-up examination. He has type 2 diabetes mellitus. Review of his blood glucose log demonstrates fasting blood glucose values ranging from 120 to 160 mg/dL (6.7-8.9 mmol/L) and variable 2-hour postprandial blood glucose values ranging from 50 to 190 mg/dL (2.8-10.5 mmol/L). His overnight blood glucose values range from 120 to 140 mg/dL (6.7-7.8 mmol/L). He is unable to detect hypoglycemia. The patient is concerned about hyperglycemia, and he desires to reach a hemoglobin A_{1c} level of less than 7%.

Medical history is significant for diabetic retinopathy, peripheral neuropathy, hypertension, and hyperlipidemia. Medications are neutral protamine Hagedorn (NPH) insulin, regular insulin, losartan, chlorthalidone, metformin, rosuvastatin, and aspirin.

On physical examination, blood pressure is 125/82 mm Hg and pulse rate is 80/min. BMI is 24. Retinal examination demonstrates nonproliferative retinopathy. His lower extremities have diminished sensation to a 10-g monofilament and vibration with a 128-Hz tuning fork.

Hemoglobin A_{1c} level is 7.2%, and the results of all other laboratory studies are normal.

Which of the following is the most appropriate treatment of this patient's diabetes?

(A) Continue current insulin and metformin doses

(B) Continue current insulin, increase metformin dose

(C) Decrease meal-time insulin, add pramlintide

(D) Decrease meal-time insulin, continue metformin

Item 77

A 28-year-old woman is evaluated for a 6-month history of infertility. In order to predict her fertile period, the patient has been using a home urinary luteinizing hormone (LH) kit. The kit can identify an LH surge and therefore predict ovulation and the optimal time for intercourse. Her urinary LH kit result has been consistently positive but her pregnancy test result consistently negative. She has been exercising recently in an attempt to lose weight. Her medical history is otherwise unremarkable, and she takes no medications.

On physical examination, vital signs are normal. BMI is 38. Coarse terminal hairs are noted on the chin, neck, and anterior chest. Pelvic examination is normal.

Pelvic ultrasound reveals a thickened endometrium and polycystic-appearing ovaries bilaterally.

Which of the following is the most likely diagnosis?

(A) Hypothyroidism

(B) Late-onset congenital adrenal hyperplasia

(C) Polycystic ovary syndrome

(D) Prolactinoma

Item 78

A 72-year-old woman is evaluated in follow-up for osteoporosis. Medical history is significant for a hip fracture 5 years ago sustained after a mild fall. Evaluation at that time included a dual-energy x-ray absorptiometry (DEXA) scan showing a left hip T-score of −2.8 and vertebral T-score of −2.7. She has been maintained on alendronate therapy since that time. Medical history is also significant for hypertension. Medications are alendronate, hydrochlorothiazide, calcium, and vitamin D. Family history

Answers and Critiques

Item 1   Answer: B

Educational Objective: Treat hyperthyroidism during pregnancy.

This patient has hyperthyroidism occurring during pregnancy and should be treated with propylthiouracil (PTU). Based on this patient's age and sex, the most likely cause of her hyperthyroidism is Graves disease. Clinical findings supporting this diagnosis are the diffuse thyromegaly, thyroid bruit, and elevated thyroid-stimulating immunoglobulin index. Treatment of hyperthyroidism during pregnancy is typically with medical management, and PTU, rather than methimazole, is the drug of choice during the first trimester. Although rare, methimazole has been associated with development of aplasia cutis (absence of a portion of skin on the scalp in a localized or widespread area) and choanal atresia (blockage of the posterior nasal passage due to failed recanalization of the nasal fossae during fetal development) when used in the first trimester. Once organogenesis is complete, methimazole can be substituted for PTU. Methimazole is typically the preferred agent in patients with hyperthyroidism because it has a longer intrathyroidal half-life than PTU and usually can be administered once daily.

Radioactive iodine is contraindicated during pregnancy because it can cause destruction of the fetal thyroid.

Thyroidectomy is generally avoided during pregnancy unless the hyperthyroidism cannot be controlled or the patient cannot tolerate either PTU or methimazole. When needed, surgery is typically performed during the second trimester, if possible.

KEY POINT

- In pregnant patients with hyperthyroidism, propylthiouracil, rather than methimazole, should be used in the first trimester because of the teratogenic effects of methimazole during this time.

Bibliography
Lazarus JH. Management of hyperthyroidism in pregnancy. Endocrine. 2014 Mar;45(2):190-4. [PMID: 24174179]

Item 2   Answer: C

Educational Objective: Diagnose the multiple endocrine neoplasia type 2 (MEN2) syndrome.

This patient is most likely to develop primary hyperparathyroidism. He has symptoms related to catecholamine excess from a pheochromocytoma and has a personal and family history of medullary thyroid cancer. This is typical of multiple endocrine neoplasia type 2A (MEN2A) resulting from a mutation in the *RET* proto-oncogene. Primary hyperparathy-

roidism due to multiple gland hyperplasia frequently occurs in patients with MEN2A. Patients with primary hyperparathyroidism may present with symptoms related to hypercalcemia (polydipsia, polyuria, and constipation), or the hyperparathyroidism may be found during an evaluation for osteoporosis or nephrolithiasis. Pheochromocytomas in MEN2A are usually benign and intra-adrenal in location, but can be multiple or bilateral.

Insulinoma and prolactinoma occur in multiple endocrine neoplasia type 1 (MEN1). In MEN1, one mutated allele of the *MEN1* gene is usually inherited, and a somatic mutation in the other allele is later acquired and results in the formation of neoplasia. The most common endocrine disorder in MEN1 is primary hyperparathyroidism resulting from one or more parathyroid adenomas.

Neurofibroma is not a clinical feature of MEN2A. Neurofibromas, café-au-lait spots, and pheochromocytoma are among the clinical features of the autosomal dominant disorder neurofibromatosis type 1.

KEY POINT

- Medullary thyroid cancer, pheochromocytoma, and primary hyperparathyroidism occur in patients with multiple endocrine neoplasia type 2A (MEN2A).

Bibliography
Krampitz GW, Norton JA. RET gene mutations (genotype and phenotype) of multiple endocrine neoplasia type 2 and familial medullary thyroid carcinoma. Cancer. 2014 Jul 1;120(13):1920-31. [PMID: 24699901]

Item 3   Answer: B

Educational Objective: Treat prolactinoma during pregnancy.

The patient should undergo formal visual field testing. During pregnancy, there is concern that prolactinomas can grow due to estrogenic stimulation. The risk of significant growth depends on the size of the prolactinoma prior to pregnancy. With microadenomas (<10 mm), the risk is considered to be low, whereas the risk is higher with macroprolactinomas (≥10 mm). Significant expansion may cause vision loss by compressing the optic chiasm. It is therefore appropriate to obtain visual field testing during pregnancy in women with macroadenomas even without symptoms to diagnose vision field loss (such as bitemporal hemianopsia) that may be due to an enlarging prolactinoma. Testing in these women is recommended every trimester of pregnancy. Because this patient is in her first trimester and has a history of a macroadenoma, visual field testing now is indicated.

It is not helpful to check the serum prolactin level. Prolactin is normally elevated in pregnancy and can be greater than 200 ng/mL (200 µg/L). Additionally, this patient has a known prolactinoma, so her prolactin will likely be elevated for both reasons. Elevated prolactin itself is not necessarily harmful. Prolactinomas cause concern when they cause hypogonadism or mass effect. In this patient, an elevated prolactin level will not change the treatment plan because it is expected to be elevated and does not help clarify whether the prolactinoma is causing harm.

Routine monitoring of women with prolactinomas with MRI during pregnancy is not indicated because the absolute risk of significant enlargement of pituitary adenomas is low. However, MRI is indicated in women with a pituitary macroadenoma and abnormalities on visual field testing or change in headache possibly attributable to expansion of the adenoma.

Bromocriptine is avoided in pregnancy when possible because its safety during gestation has not been established, although when a patient has symptoms of mass effect during pregnancy, bromocriptine may need to be restarted. However, it would not be appropriate to restart dopamine agonist therapy in this patient without a clear indication for treatment such as an enlarging pituitary adenoma.

KEY POINT

- Because prolactinomas may increase in size in pregnant women and lead to loss of vision, close clinical monitoring and formal visual field testing should be performed during each trimester.

Bibliography

Melmed S, Casanueva FF, Hoffman AR, et al. Diagnosis and treatment of hyperprolactinemia: an Endocrine Society clinical practice guideline. J Clin Endocrinol Metab. 2011 Feb;96(2):273-88. [PMID: 21296991]

Item 4   Answer: D

Educational Objective: Manage overnight hypoglycemia.

This patient should measure her blood glucose level at 3 AM. The etiology of fluctuating fasting glucose values in diabetes can be multifactorial, including overnight hypoglycemia, dawn phenomenon, or inadequate insulin doses. To maintain normal blood glucose levels upon rising, an early morning physiologic release of catecholamines, cortisol, and growth hormone occurs to stimulate endogenous glucose production from the liver. Overnight hypoglycemia caused by overtreatment of diabetes or prolonged effects of recent physical exertion can lead to low-normal fasting glucose values and amplify the release of catecholamines, cortisol, growth hormone, and glucagon to increase endogenous glucose production, which can lead to hyperglycemia (Somogyi effect). With the dawn phenomenon, fasting hyperglycemia occurs in the setting of inadequate basal insulin coverage to maintain the endogenous glucose value within a normal range. Food intake in the evening can also contribute to fasting hyperglycemia if it is inadequately covered with insulin. Overnight hypoglycemia and the dawn phenomenon can be distinguished by

measuring the glucose level at 3 AM. Medications that affect the overnight glucose level need to be decreased if the 3 AM glucose level is low. Medications that affect the overnight glucose should be increased or added if the 3 AM glucose level is elevated.

Fast-acting insulin such as insulin lispro at bedtime increases the risk of hypoglycemia.

Metformin will decrease gluconeogenesis from the liver and improve fasting hyperglycemia. However, for similar reasons, overnight hypoglycemia must be excluded before this treatment could be safely initiated.

Increasing the insulin glargine dose could also worsen overnight hypoglycemia if that is the cause of the fasting hyperglycemia.

Despite the hemoglobin A_{1c} level of less than 7%, the etiology of the patient's fasting hyperglycemia should be investigated. Detection of overnight hypoglycemia would necessitate immediate changes in her insulin regimen or food intake regardless of her hemoglobin A_{1c} value.

KEY POINT

- Overnight blood glucose monitoring can help detect hypoglycemia or dawn phenomenon.

Bibliography

Cryer PE, Axelrod L, Grossman AB, et al. Evaluation and management of adult hypoglycemic disorders: an Endocrine Society Clinical Practice Guideline. J Clin Endocrinol Metab. 2009 Mar;94(3):709-28. [PMID: 19088155]

Item 5   Answer: A

Educational Objective: Evaluate the cause of Cushing syndrome.

The most appropriate diagnostic test to perform next is a CT scan of the adrenal glands. This patient was suspected to have Cushing syndrome (CS) based on pathognomonic clinical findings and is not taking exogenous glucocorticoids. Two screening tests for CS are abnormal, which is adequate to establish the diagnosis. The next step in evaluation is measurement of the plasma adrenocorticotropic hormone (ACTH) level to differentiate between ACTH-dependent and ACTH-independent CS. With ACTH-dependent causes, the plasma ACTH is usually greater than 20 pg/mL (4.4 pmol/L). However, the low plasma ACTH reported in this patient is consistent with ACTH-independent CS. A CT scan of the abdomen to evaluate the adrenal glands is therefore indicated because the most common causes of ACTH-independent CS are adenomas and carcinomas of the adrenal cortex.

Inferior petrosal sinus sampling and MRI of the pituitary gland are used to confirm the presence of a corticotroph adenoma of the pituitary gland in ACTH-dependent CS, which is the most common cause of CS overall. However, neither is indicated in this patient because biochemical testing has not revealed ACTH-dependent CS.

The diagnosis of CS requires that at least two first-line screening tests be abnormal, including the low-dose dexamethasone suppression test (LDST) (both standard and overnight), 24-hour urine free cortisol (UFC), or late-night salivary cortisol. This patient failed to suppress cortisol levels following an overnight LDST and had an elevated 24-hour UFC level confirmed by a repeat collection. Therefore, measurement of late night salivary cortisol is unnecessary because the diagnosis of CS has already been established.

KEY POINT

- CT of the adrenal glands should be performed in patients with ACTH-independent Cushing syndrome because adenomas and carcinomas of the adrenal cortex are common causes.

Bibliography

Nieman LK, Biller BM, Findling JW, et al. The diagnosis of Cushing's syndrome: an Endocrine Society Clinical Practice Guideline. J Clin Endocrinol Metab. 2008 May;93(5):1526-40. [PMID: 18334580]

Item 6   Answer: D

Educational Objective: Manage ketosis-prone type 2 diabetes mellitus.

This patient should have a repeat measurement of fasting C-peptide and glucose levels. He has ketosis-prone type 2 diabetes mellitus. Patients with ketosis-prone type 2 diabetes do not fulfill the classic phenotype associated with autoimmune type 1 diabetes. These patients are often older, overweight or obese, and of black or Latino ethnicity. Patients with new-onset ketosis-prone diabetes require insulin therapy initially but might be able to be managed with oral agents in the future. Prior to switching from insulin to oral therapy, his pancreatic beta-cell function should be assessed with fasting C-peptide and glucose measurements. Ketosis-prone type 2 diabetes is heterogeneous condition in that the presence of autoantibodies is variable across the population, as is the degree of pancreatic beta cell function. His initial C-peptide level in the setting of hyperglycemia and diabetic ketoacidosis is not an accurate indication of his pancreatic function. Due to the toxic effects of prolonged hyperglycemia on the pancreatic beta cells, the fasting C-peptide and glucose or a glucagon-stimulated C-peptide should be measured 7 to 14 days after the correction of the acidosis in order to better assess function. If his repeat fasting C-peptide value is greater than or equal to 1.0 ng/mL (0.33 nmol/L) or his glucagon-stimulated C-peptide value is greater than or equal to 1.5 ng/mL (0.5 nmol/L), his beta cell function is preserved.

A sliding-scale insulin regimen that does not include basal insulin and does not begin insulin administration unless the blood glucose level is at or above a threshold level will cause wide swings from hyperglycemia to hypoglycemia, and this is inappropriate treatment.

Discontinuation of his insulin and switching to an oral agent such as metformin could be attempted with evidence of beta cell function preservation. Close follow-up would be necessary to monitor for worsening hyperglycemia or development of ketoacidosis, which would require restarting insulin therapy.

Determining autoimmunity, in conjunction with beta cell function, is helpful in assessing whether a patient has the potential to become insulin-independent in the future. His autoantibodies were negative at the time of his presentation, and it is unlikely that these would now be positive. It is not necessary to retest antibodies in this setting.

KEY POINT

- Prior to switching from insulin to oral therapy in patients with ketosis-prone diabetes, fasting C-peptide and glucose levels should be checked.

Bibliography

Maldonado MR, Otiniano ME, Cheema F, et al. Factors associated with insulin discontinuation in subjects with ketosis-prone diabetes but preserved β-cell function. Diabet Med. 2005 Dec;22(12):1744-50. [PMID: 16401322]

Item 7   Answer: C

Educational Objective: Treat pituitary apoplexy.

The patient has acute apoplexy caused by pituitary hemorrhage and requires urgent transsphenoidal decompression of the hemorrhage to preserve vision. Given his history of previous headache, loss of libido, and erectile dysfunction, he likely had a preexisting prolactinoma that acutely bled. Prolactinomas are almost always treated with dopamine agonists, but this patient requires urgent surgery to decrease pressure on the optic chiasm to save his vision. Transsphenoidal resection is the preferred method of pituitary surgery. He also requires urgent stress-dose glucocorticoids because of risk of secondary cortisol deficiency, which would be life-threatening.

The patient has appropriately received glucocorticoids for possible adrenocorticotropic hormone deficiency. There is no indication to assess other pituitary function. In the next 2 to 4 weeks, thyroid function will need to be assessed, but thyroxine (T_4) has a long half-life and does not need to be emergently measured or replaced. Treatment of hypogonadism or growth hormone deficiency is not urgent; surgical decompression is.

Waiting 2 weeks to repeat imaging could lead to permanent vision loss. He needs immediate intervention to preserve his vision. Similarly, whole brain external beam radiation is not appropriate for this patient who needs rapid surgical decompression.

KEY POINT

- Patients with pituitary apoplexy and vision loss should receive immediate stress-dose glucocorticoids in addition to undergoing urgent transsphenoidal pituitary decompression.

Bibliography

Rajasekaran S, Vanderpump M, Baldeweg S, et al. UK guidelines for the management of pituitary apoplexy. Clin Endocrinol. 2011 Jan;74(1):9-20. [PMID: 21044119]

Item 8   Answer: B

Educational Objective: Manage a solitary thyroid nodule.

Fine-needle aspiration (FNA) is the most appropriate next step in the evaluation to determine whether this patient's thyroid nodule is malignant or benign. She has already had an ultrasound examination. Ultrasonography is a sensitive means of identifying nodules and providing further characterization of the nodules, which is more predictive of malignancy than size alone. The ultrasonographic features that are considered more suspicious for malignancy include hypoechogenicity, microcalcifications, irregular margins, and increased intranodular Doppler flow. According to American Thyroid Association guidelines, this patient with a hypoechoic nodule that is 1.5 cm should have an FNA to rule out malignancy.

Nodular features are not readily identified on CT, and this study has a lower sensitivity than ultrasonography for identifying the presence of nodules. CT of the neck would therefore not provide any additional information about this patient, who has already had an ultrasound examination. In addition, CT would expose this patient to unnecessary radiation. If a patient has a substernal goiter, CT is beneficial for determining the extent of the goiter. However, this patient has no extension of the thyroid into the mediastinum.

Levothyroxine therapy to suppress growth of benign nodules is no longer recommended. Randomized clinical trials have failed to show a significant effect on nodule volume. Additionally, the required dose can induce thyrotoxicosis, which is associated with significant risk for cardiovascular complications.

Measurement of the serum thyroglobulin level is reserved for patients who have had a total thyroidectomy and is useful as a tumor marker for detection of residual or recurrent thyroid cancer. In a patient with an intact thyroid, serum thyroglobulin measurement is an insensitive and nonspecific means of testing for malignancy.

Thyroid scanning with technetium is unlikely to be helpful in this patient. Thyroid scanning is used to determine the functional status of the nodule. Isotope scanning is most useful in the setting of a nodule accompanied by a low serum thyroid-stimulating hormone level because toxic (or hyperfunctioning) nodules typically do not require FNA as the vast majority are benign. This patient has a normal serum thyroid-stimulating hormone level and is likely to have an indeterminate result ("cold" or "warm") on thyroid scanning.

KEY POINT

- Fine-needle aspiration is the most appropriate next step in the management of a patient with a solid thyroid nodule measuring greater than 1 cm on ultrasonography.

Bibliography

American Thyroid Association (ATA) Guidelines Taskforce on Thyroid Nodules and Differentiated Thyroid Cancer, Cooper DS, Doherty GM, Haugen BR, et al. Revised American Thyroid Association management guidelines for patients with thyroid nodules and differentiated thyroid cancer. Thyroid. 2009 Nov;19(11):1167-214. Erratum in: Thyroid. 2010 Aug;20(8):942. [PMID: 19860577]

Item 9   Answer: A

Educational Objective: Manage primary amenorrhea.

The most appropriate management is to initiate estrogen and progestin therapy in this patient with primary amenorrhea. Primary amenorrhea is defined as the lack of menses by age 16 years accompanied by a normal body hair pattern and normal breast development. Pregnancy must be ruled out in all patients with primary amenorrhea. Approximately 50% of patients with primary amenorrhea have a chromosomal abnormality. Primary ovarian insufficiency due to Turner syndrome, a syndrome characterized by short stature and the loss of a portion or all of one X chromosome, is one of the most common causes of primary amenorrhea. The diagnosis of Turner syndrome can be made on the basis of a karyotype, and this should be the next diagnostic test for this patient. Such a patient may also have fragile X premutation; however, no cognitive impairment is typically seen in this patient population. Diagnosing Turner syndrome is critical because affected patients have a higher incidence of cardiovascular disease, metabolic syndrome, and thyroid dysfunction. Patients with Turner syndrome may have either primary or secondary amenorrhea and commonly have normal secondary sexual characteristics. The mechanism involved appears to be early follicular depletion, such that ovaries are devoid of follicles and oocytes. Serum evaluations in these patients will reveal low estradiol levels (typically below the detectable level in the assay) and markedly elevated gonadotropin levels. This constellation of findings is consistent with hypergonadotropic hypogonadism. Such patients should receive hormone replacement therapy with estrogen and cyclic progestin to prevent endometrial hyperplasia, osteoporosis, and other sequelae of hypoestrogenism.

A pituitary prolactinoma causes secondary amenorrhea through direct inhibition of gonadotropin-releasing hormone secretion by prolactin. Because this patient has elevated levels of gonadotropins, neither a pituitary MRI nor a prolactin measurement is necessary.

Both hypothyroidism and hyperthyroidism also cause secondary amenorrhea. Hypothyroidism results in increased levels of thyrotropin-releasing hormone through negative feedback, and this hormone, in turn, stimulates prolactin secretion and suppresses gonadotropin secretion. Hyperthyroidism can cause rapid weight loss, which is known to cause functional hypothalamic amenorrhea. Since this patient has elevated gonadotropin levels and no signs of hyperthyroidism, thyroid-stimulating hormone measurement is not needed.

KEY POINT

- Patients with primary amenorrhea associated with hypergonadotropic hypogonadism should receive hormone therapy with estrogen to prevent endometrial hyperplasia and osteoporosis and cyclic progestin to prevent endometrial hyperplasia.

Bibliography

Cordts EB, Christofolini DM, Dos Santos AA, Bianco B, Barbosa CP. Genetic aspects of premature ovarian failure: a literature review. Arch Gynecol Obstet. 2011 Mar;283(3):635-43. [PMID: 21188402]

Item 10   Answer: B

Educational Objective: Treat subacute thyroiditis.

A β-blocker, such as metoprolol, is the most appropriate treatment for this patient with thyrotoxicosis who has subacute granulomatous (de Quervain) thyroiditis based on the low radioactive iodine uptake (RAIU) and the painful thyroid on examination. An antecedent event, in this case a viral illness, destroys the thyroid follicles and triggers the release of preformed thyroid hormones into the bloodstream, creating the thyrotoxic phase. During this phase, further release of thyroid hormones ceases, resulting in a low RAIU as seen in this patient. β-Blockers are beneficial in the thyrotoxic phase to block the adrenergic effects of the high circulating thyroid hormone levels. Treatment of subacute thyroiditis is otherwise typically supportive, with NSAIDs for pain as needed. In patients with severe pain, glucocorticoids may occasionally be used.

Blocking further release of thyroid hormones with a thionamide (either methimazole or propylthiouracil) is ineffective because the thyroid has already released preformed thyroid hormone into the bloodstream and is currently not producing or secreting additional thyroxine.

Administration of radioactive iodine for treatment of the hyperthyroidism is also ineffective because this patient's thyroid is not currently taking in iodine, as evidenced by the low uptake on his thyroid scan. More importantly, radioactive iodine will not treat this patient's underlying problem of damaged thyroid follicles and release of preformed thyroid hormone into the bloodstream.

KEY POINT

- Treatment of subacute granulomatous (de Quervain) thyroiditis typically is supportive, with NSAIDs and occasionally glucocorticoids for severe pain; β-blockers are beneficial in the thyrotoxic phase to block the adrenergic effects of the high circulating thyroid hormone levels.

Bibliography

Sweeney LB, Stewart C, Gaitonde DY. Thyroiditis: an integrated approach. Am Fam Physician. 2014 Sep 15;90(6):389-96. [PMID: 25251231]

Item 11   Answer: D

Educational Objective: Diagnose hyperprolactinemia caused by an antipsychotic agent.

Hyperprolactinemia is a known side effect of antipsychotic agents, and this patient's hyperprolactinemia is likely due to risperidone. Antipsychotics block dopamine and decrease inhibition of prolactin release at the pituitary, causing hyperprolactinemia. Stopping the medication can reverse the hyperprolactinemia but should only be done under the supervision of a psychiatrist. The patient's risperidone should not be discontinued unless her psychiatrist is consulted.

Hypothyroidism can cause hyperprolactinemia when uncontrolled, but her hypothyroidism is well treated. She has no symptoms of hypothyroidism, and her thyroid function tests are normal, so uncontrolled hypothyroidism is not the cause of her hyperprolactinemia.

Antipsychotic agents cause hyperprolactinemia by blocking dopamine, but lithium does not cause hyperprolactinemia.

Although the patient has a likely explanation for her hyperprolactinemia, a prolactinoma is still possible. Risperidone can cause prolactin levels above 200 ng/mL (200 μg/L), so her level of 102 ng/mL (102 μg/L) is not unreasonable. Remeasuring the prolactin level following discontinuation of the drug is recommended before further evaluation for a pituitary adenoma; the patient's psychiatrist should be consulted before withholding the risperidone for testing. A patient with hyperprolactinemia without a clear secondary or drug-induced cause should be assessed by an imaging study (preferably, MRI of the pituitary gland) to a exclude pituitary lesion.

KEY POINT

- Antipsychotic agents block dopamine and decrease inhibition of prolactin release at the pituitary, causing hyperprolactinemia.

Bibliography

Melmed S, Casanueva FF, Hoffman AR, et al. Diagnosis and treatment of hyperprolactinemia: an Endocrine Society clinical practice guideline. J Clin Endocrinol Metab. 2011 Feb;96(2):273-88. [PMID: 21296991]

Item 12   Answer: B

Educational Objective: Manage low bone mass.

A repeat dual-energy x-ray absorptiometry (DEXA) scan should be repeated in 2 years in this patient with low bone mass and relatively low 10-year fracture risk. The Fracture Risk Assessment Tool (FRAX) calculator defines the 10-year fracture risk for patients with T-scores in the -1.0 to -2.5 ranges. The FRAX calculator (www.shef.ac.uk/FRAX) incorporates multiple risk factors including sex, fracture history, femoral neck bone mineral density, glucocorticoid use, smoking, BMI, age, and alcohol intake to determine projected fracture risk. If the risk of major osteoporotic fracture is greater than or equal to 20% or the risk of hip fracture is greater than or equal to 3%, then the patient's benefit from therapy exceeds the risk, and she should be offered treatment. Because of her history of low body weight and limited nutritional intake during the time of development of peak bone mass, she is at increased risk for low bone mass or osteoporosis and is therefore an appropriate candidate for early screening. Her DEXA scan shows low bone mass. Spine film shows no evidence of fracture. Additionally, her calcium and vitamin D levels are normal. Continuing lifestyle activities (such as maximizing weight-bearing exercise and avoidance of tobacco or excessive alcohol) in addition to calcium and vitamin D supplementation is appropriate management of this patient.

Raloxifene is a selective estrogen receptor modulator (SERM) that is a treatment option for women with osteoporosis because it has been shown to increase bone mineral density and reduce the risk of vertebral (but not nonvertebral) fractures. However, raloxifene is also associated with an increased risk of thromboembolic events and vasomotor symptoms. There is limited data supporting use of raloxifene or other SERMs for treating patients with low bone mass, although some guidelines recommend considering treatment in patients with low bone mass and 10-year fracture risk determined by the FRAX calculator of greater than or equal to 20% for a major osteoporotic fracture or greater than or equal to 3% for hip fracture. Raloxifene would therefore not be appropriate therapy for this patient.

Cholecalciferol (D_3), a metabolite of vitamin D, is commonly used to supplement low serum vitamin D levels in patients with vitamin D deficiency. This patient has normal serum vitamin D levels; therefore, there is no indication for treatment with vitamin D metabolites.

Bisphosphonates are considered first-line therapy for osteoporosis, although they are not used routinely in women with low bone mass. Similar to the use of SERM therapy, guidelines recommend consideration of treatment with a bisphosphonate for low bone mass only if there is 10-year fracture risk determined by the FRAX calculator of greater than or equal to 20% for a major osteoporotic fracture or greater than or equal to 3% for hip fracture.

KEY POINT

- Treatment for low bone mass in postmenopausal women involves lifestyle modification (maximizing weight-bearing exercise and avoidance of tobacco or excessive alcohol) and vitamin D and calcium supplementation; the need for pharmacologic therapy is based on the 10-year estimated fracture risk (≥20% for a major osteoporotic fracture or ≥3% for hip fracture).

Bibliography
Kling JM, Clarke BL, Sandhu NP. Osteoporosis prevention, screening, and treatment: a review. J Womens Health. 2014 Jul;23(7):563-72. [PMID: 24766381]

Item 13   Answer: A

Educational Objective: Diagnose euthyroid sick syndrome.

This patient's clinical picture is consistent with euthyroid sick syndrome (also called nonthyroidal illness syndrome). Unless there is a strong suspicion of an underlying thyroid disorder that may be contributing to a patient's clinical findings, thyroid function tests should not be performed during critical illness. In hospitalized patients, especially ones as ill as the patient described here, thyroid function test results are highly likely to be abnormal. The first deviation that may occur during an acute illness is lowering of the serum total triiodothyronine (T_3) level. The serum thyroid-stimulating hormone (TSH) and serum free thyroxine (T_4) levels may also decline as the illness increases in severity. The pattern of these test results is often indistinguishable from that seen with central hypothyroidism. In fact, some controversy exists about whether the clinical picture of a low serum TSH level and low serum T_4 and T_3 levels is an adaptive response to the critical illness in order to alter the body's metabolism and thereby aid in recovery from the acute illness.

This patient does not have any definite findings of underlying Graves disease. The tachycardia and fever are likely the result of his severe infection. If he was also experiencing thyroid storm, high serum T_4 and T_3 levels would most likely be associated with the low serum TSH concentration.

The most common cause of hypothyroidism is Hashimoto thyroiditis. Physical examination findings can include a reduced basal temperature, diastolic hypertension, an enlarged thyroid gland, bradycardia, pallor, dry and cold skin, brittle hair, hoarseness, and a delayed recovery phase of deep tendon reflexes. Patients with Hashimoto thyroiditis have low T_4 and T_3 levels and elevated TSH. This patient's low TSH level is not compatible with Hashimoto thyroiditis.

This patient is unlikely to have subacute thyroiditis based on the timing of the illness. Although the infection could have triggered destruction of the thyroid, the subsequent release of preformed thyroid hormones into the serum should result in an elevation of serum T_4 and T_3 levels in the early phase of the disease, which is not consistent with the findings in this case.

KEY POINT

- Unless there is a strong suspicion of an underlying thyroid disorder that may be contributing to a patient's clinical findings, thyroid function tests should not be performed during critical illness because test results are highly likely to be abnormal.

Bibliography
Farwell AP. Nonthyroidal illness syndrome. Curr Opin Endocrinol Diabetes Obes. 2013 Oct;20(5):478-84. [PMID: 23974778]

Item 14   Answer: B

Educational Objective: Liberalize glycemic targets in a patient with multiple diabetic complications and advanced microvascular disease.

The most appropriate next step in management of this patient is to decrease the risk of hypoglycemia by decreasing the insulin doses delivered by the pump. This patient has had type 1 diabetes for 25 years with subsequent development of advanced microvascular disease. His frequent hypoglycemic events and hypoglycemic unawareness increase the risk of morbidity and mortality from recurrent hypoglycemia that may occur with stringent glycemic goals. Glycemic goals should be individualized to account for patient-specific factors, such as age and comorbidities. The American Diabetes Association suggests a hemoglobin A_{1c} goal of less than 8.0% in patients with a decreased life expectancy, history of severe hypoglycemia, multiple comorbidities, or advanced microvascular or macrovascular disease. The less stringent hemoglobin A_{1c} goal should be implemented to avoid recurrent hypoglycemia; however, the goal may need to be increased above 8.0% if it cannot be achieved safely.

Altering the pump settings to deliver more insulin to attain a hemoglobin A_{1c} goal of less than 7.0% will increase his risk of hypoglycemia. His hemoglobin A_{1c} goal should be liberalized to avoid hypoglycemia.

The risk of hypoglycemia can be reduced with lower insulin doses delivered by either an insulin pump or subcutaneous injections. Since the patient is already using an insulin pump, alteration of his insulin pump settings to deliver less insulin should occur next.

Gabapentin for treatment of his painful peripheral neuropathy is appropriate, but avoidance of recurrent hypoglycemia is the most serious issue that needs to be addressed next due to the associated increased risk of morbidity and mortality.

KEY POINT

- A less stringent hemoglobin A_{1c} goal is appropriate for persons with diabetes mellitus with a decreased life expectancy, history of severe hypoglycemia, multiple comorbidities, or advanced microvascular or macrovascular disease.

Bibliography

American Diabetes Association. (6) Glycemic targets. In: Standards of Medical Care in Diabetes-2015. Diabetes Care. 2015 Jan;38 Suppl 1:S33-40. [PMID: 25537705]

Item 15   Answer: D

Educational Objective: Determine causes of vitamin D deficiency.

This patient with refractory vitamin D deficiency, despite aggressive attempts at repletion, should be screened for celiac disease. The fact that supplementation with a therapeutic dose of vitamin D has failed to replete her body stores should raise concern for a malabsorption disorder. Based on her history of another autoimmune disorder (vitiligo), lower range BMI, and nonspecific signs and symptoms such as fatigue, subclinical celiac disease would be a reasonable cause of her malabsorption. Celiac disease may present with classic symptoms of diarrhea, overt malabsorption, and weight loss, but may also exist in a very mild form and may go largely undetected since patients have only nonspecific symptoms and subclinical malabsorption. If this patient tests positive for celiac disease, removing gluten from her diet will improve her intestinal lining and improve absorption of vitamin D. Even with therapy, patients with malabsorption will likely require increased doses of vitamin D supplementation.

Parathyroid imaging with a sestamibi scan is not indicated because the patient does not have primary hyperparathyroidism. Her parathyroid hormone level is elevated as an appropriate physiologic response to her markedly low vitamin D levels. Once her vitamin D levels are sufficient (>30 ng/dL [75 nmol/L]), her parathyroid hormone level should be remeasured to ensure that it has returned to the normal range. The parathyroid hormone level should be remeasured in approximately 4 weeks.

Referral for parathyroidectomy would also not be indicated in this patient without an established diagnosis of primary hyperparathyroidism.

A person her age with normal diet and minimal sun exposure should require about 1000 U daily of vitamin D to maintain adequate vitamin D stores. The choice to use cholecalciferol versus ergocalciferol is often based on the level of vitamin D deficit. Since the ergocalciferol is more readily available in the 50,000 U form and has a shorter half-life, it is recommended when a patient's vitamin D level is less than 10 ng/mL (25 nmol/L). Cholecalciferol is often used when the level is between 20 and 30 ng/mL (50-75 nmol/L) or for maintenance and therefore would not be ideal to replete this patient. Clinical discretion can be used for levels between 10 and 20 ng/mL (25-50 nmol/L).

Although vitamin D_3 (cholecalciferol) is a reasonable option for treatment of vitamin D deficiency, as mentioned above, cholecalciferol is best used for maintenance of vitamin D levels or repletion when the 25-hydroxyvitamin D level is between 20 ng/mL (50 nmol/L) and 30 ng/mL (75 nmol/L). Neither form of repletion, however, will be effective in the presence of significant malabsorption.

KEY POINT

- When vitamin D repletion efforts fail, secondary causes, such as malabsorption, should be considered.

Bibliography

Tavakkol A, DiGiacomo D, Green PH, Lebwohl B. Vitamin D status and concomitant autoimmunity in celiac disease. J Clin Gastroenterol. 2013 Jul;47(6):515-9. [PMID: 23328299]

Item 16   Answer: A

Educational Objective: Treat subclinical hypothyroidism.

The most appropriate next step in management is to initiate levothyroxine therapy. This patient has subclinical hypothyroidism with a mild elevation of the serum thyroid-stimulating hormone (TSH) level and normal serum free thyroxine (T_4) level. Her family history of hypothyroidism and her thyroid peroxidase antibody positivity increase the likelihood of progression to overt thyroid failure. In patients with a mild serum TSH elevation (between the upper limit of normal and 10 μU/mL [10 mU/L]), beginning levothyroxine therapy is reasonable if symptoms suggestive of hypothyroidism are present.

Thyroid-stimulating immunoglobulins (TSIs) are highly associated with Graves disease. When the diagnosis of

Graves disease cannot be made clinically in a patient with hyperthyroidism, measurement of the serum level of these antibodies is recommended, especially if radioactive iodine uptake studies are not available or if radioactive iodine exposure is contraindicated, as in pregnancy and breastfeeding. This patient does not have hyperthyroidism, and these tests are therefore not indicated.

Repeating a serum TSH measurement in this patient was reasonable, since up to 30% of patients with an initially abnormal serum TSH level will have a normalization of this value upon retesting. Since this patient has persistent elevation of TSH and symptoms that may be attributable to hypothyroidism, waiting 12 months before initiating therapy is not appropriate.

A radioactive iodine uptake (RAIU) scan is reserved for patients with hyperthyroidism. Patients with Graves disease typically have an elevated RAIU. Conversely, in patients with thyroiditis or exposure to exogenous thyroid hormone, the RAIU will be low (<5%) despite biochemical hyperthyroidism. Obtaining a thyroid RAIU in this patient is not indicated.

KEY POINT

- Levothyroxine therapy is reasonable in a patient with subclinical hypothyroidism and symptoms suggestive of hypothyroidism.

Bibliography

Garber JR, Cobin RH, Gharib H, et al; American Association of Clinical Endocrinologists and American Thyroid Association Taskforce on Hypothyroidism in Adults. Clinical practice guidelines for hypothyroidism in adults: cosponsored by the American Association of Clinical Endocrinologists and the American Thyroid Association. Endocr Pract. 2012 Nov-Dec;18(6):988-1028. Erratum in: Endocr Pract. 2013 Jan-Feb;19(1):175. [PMID: 23246686]

Item 17   Answer: C

Educational Objective: Define surgical indications for primary hyperparathyroidism.

The most appropriate treatment recommendation for this patient is parathyroidectomy. She has primary hyperparathyroidism as shown by her elevated serum calcium and parathyroid hormone levels. She also has evidence of kidney compromise with an elevated creatinine level and decreased estimated glomerular filtration rate (eGFR). Impaired kidney function (defined as eGFR <60 mL/min/1.73 m^2, 24-h urine calcium >400 mg/24 h [10 mmol/24 h], or the presence of nephrolithiasis or nephrocalcinosis by radiograph, ultrasound, or CT) is an indication for surgical treatment of hyperparathyroidism in otherwise asymptomatic patients. Other indications for surgery in asymptomatic patients include age younger than 50 years; a serum calcium level greater than or equal to 1 mg/dL (0.25 mmol/L) above upper limit of normal; a T-score of −2.5 or worse at the lumbar spine, total hip, femoral neck, or distal radius; or in those in whom medical surveillance is neither desired nor possible. Patients with these indications are considered to have the highest potential benefit from surgery.

A bisphosphonate, such as alendronate, would not be the treatment of choice for this patient as she does not have osteoporosis nor does she meet Fracture Risk Assessment Tool (FRAX) criteria for therapy. The FRAX calculator defines the 10-year fracture risk for patients with T-scores in the −1.0 to −2.5 range. The FRAX calculator (www.shef.ac.uk/FRAX) incorporates multiple risk factors including gender, fracture history, femoral neck bone mineral density, glucocorticoid usage, smoking, BMI, age, and alcohol intake to determine projected fracture risk. If the risk of major osteoporotic fracture is greater than or equal to 20% or the risk of hip fracture is greater than or equal to 3%, the patient's benefit from therapy exceeds the risk, and she should be offered treatment. Additionally, bisphosphonates should be used with caution in patients with compromised kidney function.

If the patient declines surgical intervention, a calcimimetic agent such as cinacalcet would be an appropriate therapy. Cinacalcet has recently been FDA approved as an alternative for patients unable or unwilling to undergo parathyroidectomy. Cinacalcet lowers calcium levels by stimulating the calcium-sensing receptors of the parathyroid glands and inhibiting parathyroid hormone secretion. However, it is expensive and has multiple drug interactions, which make it less desirable in this patient.

Because this patient is considered to be at increased risk of complications due to untreated hypercalcemia, clinical observation alone would not be appropriate.

KEY POINT

- Decreased estimated glomerular filtration rate (<60 mL/min/1.73 m^2) is an indication for surgical treatment of primary hyperparathyroidism in otherwise asymptomatic persons.

Bibliography

Bilezikian JP, Brandi ML, Eastell R, Silverberg SJ, Udelsman R, Marcocci C, et al. Guidelines for the Management of Asymptomatic Primary Hyperparathyroidism: Summary Statement from the Fourth International Workshop. J Clin Endocrinol Metab. 2014;99(10):3561-9. [PMID: 25162665]

Item 18   Answer: C

Educational Objective: Evaluate a toxic thyroid nodule.

Performing a radioactive iodine (^{123}I) uptake and scan is the most appropriate management for this patient, who most likely has a toxic nodule or nodules as the cause for her mild hyperthyroidism. Since multiple nodules were identified on ultrasound, it is important to ascertain which of the nodules are autonomous, as the likelihood of malignancy in such lesions is very low. Performing a thyroid scan will help identify whether one or more of the nodules is responsible for her thyroid function abnormalities.

A thyroid scan will also determine if fine-needle aspiration is indicated elsewhere in the gland. Nodules identified as autonomously functioning (or "hot") do not require fine-needle aspiration, whereas nodules that are either "cold" or "warm" (of similar uptake to the surrounding non-nodular thyroid tissue) may require cytologic evaluation.

This patient may ultimately benefit from methimazole therapy, but since her hyperthyroidism is mild, it is safe to wait to initiate medical therapy until after the thyroid scan is performed. In patients with a greater degree of thyrotoxicosis, beginning methimazole to lower the thyroid hormone levels prior to performing additional testing is reasonable. Once the hormone levels are nearing the normal range, the thionamide should be withheld for 5 days prior to the thyroid scan.

If the patient is found to have a toxic nodule or multiple toxic nodules, surgical removal is a reasonable treatment approach, particularly if there are compressive symptoms from the goiter. Since this is considered an elective procedure, administering low-dose methimazole to normalize of her thyroid hormone levels would be advisable prior to surgery.

KEY POINT

• Performing a radioactive iodine (^{123}I) thyroid uptake and scan is the most appropriate initial management for a patient who has mild hyperthyroidism most likely caused by a toxic nodule or nodules.

Bibliography
Jameson JL. Minimizing unnecessary surgery for thyroid nodules. N Engl J Med. 2012 Aug 23;367(8):765-7. [PMID: 22731671]

Item 19   Answer: A
Educational Objective: Treat a macroprolactinoma.

The patient has a macroprolactinoma, which is best treated with a dopamine agonist such as cabergoline. The most common cause of hyperprolactinemia is a prolactinoma, which is a benign adenoma. Microprolactinomas are less than 10 mm in diameter, and macroprolactinomas are 10 mm or greater in diameter. Prolactinomas are the most common type of secretory pituitary adenoma. The patient's tumor is causing significant mass effect, including compression of the optic chiasm, invasion into the cavernous sinus, secondary hypothyroidism, and likely growth hormone deficiency; however, even with these complications, the macroprolactinoma is best treated with medication instead of surgery. A dopamine agonist can cause a rapid decrease in the serum prolactin level and shrinkage of the prolactinoma. More specifically, in as many as 90% of patients, it can normalize prolactin levels, reverse hypogonadism, and shrink tumors by at least 50%. Because of these rapid decreases in tumor size, dopamine agonists can be used as first-line therapy, even in patients with mild visual field defects, as long as visual acuity is not threatened by rapid progression of the tumor or recent tumor hemorrhage.

Octreotide is used to treat acromegaly but has no role in the first-line treatment of prolactinoma.

Medical therapy is preferred over surgery and radiation for the treatment of prolactinomas. Stereotactic surgery (a specific kind of radiation therapy) would be considered in a patient with a tumor that is refractory to medical therapy and incompletely resectable.

Because this patient has a prolactinoma, the treatment of choice is a dopamine agonist, not surgery. There is an excellent chance that the prolactinoma will respond to cabergoline, and the patient can avoid surgery.

KEY POINT

• Dopamine agonists, such as cabergoline, are first-line therapy for symptomatic patients with prolactinomas.

Bibliography
Melmed S, Casanueva FF, Hoffman AR, et al. Diagnosis and treatment of hyperprolactinemia: An Endocrine Society clinical practice guideline. J Clin Endocrinol Metab. 2011 Feb;96(2):273-88. [PMID: 21296991]

Item 20   Answer: B
Educational Objective: Diagnose hypoglycemia in a patient with diabetes mellitus taking a sulfonylurea.

Hypoglycemia is the most likely cause of this patient's altered mental status. In patients taking a sulfonylurea for diabetes who develop dehydration, such as this patient with decreased oral intake in conjunction with nausea and vomiting, impaired kidney perfusion may lead to altered pharmacokinetics and an increased risk of hypoglycemia related to ongoing effects of the medication and minimal carbohydrate intake. Although sulfonylureas are very effective antihyperglycemic medications, most agents have relatively long half-lives, allowing convenient daily dosing. However, this slower clearance predisposes to hypoglycemia compared with other antiglycemic medications, particularly when kidney function is impaired. Glyburide, in particular, has a longer half-life than other sulfonylureas and its use is recommended against in older patients by the Beers Criteria, a list of medications that should be avoided or used with caution in older patients. Although she last took glimepiride more than 24 hours before her presentation with altered mental status, she was dehydrated, thus prolonging the glucose-lowering effects of this insulin secretagogue for several days.

Although patients with diabetes are at increased risk for atherosclerotic cardiovascular disease, this patient does not have focal abnormalities suggesting a cerebrovascular accident, and stroke itself is not a common cause of isolated altered mental status.

Levothyroxine also has a relatively long half-life allowing once daily dosing in most patients. Missing one or several doses of levothyroxine would therefore not likely lead to a degree of hypothyroidism causing acute mental status changes.

Statin toxicity is unusual, and the most common toxicity associated with statin use is musculoskeletal symptoms. Increased statin levels are not typically associated with mental status changes and would likely not be the cause of this patient's mental status changes.

Answers and Critiques

KEY POINT

- Sulfonylureas with long half-lives, such as glimepiride, may lead to acute kidney injury and hypoglycemia in older persons with diabetes mellitus.

Bibliography

American Diabetes Association. (7) Approaches to glycemic treatment. In: Standards of Medical Care in Diabetes-2015. Diabetes Care. 2015 Jan;38 Suppl 1:S41-8. [PMID: 25537707]

Item 21   Answer: A

Educational Objective: Evaluate triiodothyronine (T$_3$) hyperthyroidism.

The serum triiodothyronine (T$_3$) level should be measured next. This patient exhibits signs and symptoms of hyperthyroidism. Even though the available laboratory data are consistent with subclinical hyperthyroidism, the diagnostic evaluation is not complete until the T$_3$ level is checked. Although rare, an elevated T$_3$ level and a normal serum free thyroxine (T$_4$) level may be present in patients with hyperthyroidism. Measurement of the T$_3$ concentration should therefore be obtained in all patients suspected of having thyrotoxicosis. Measurement of the T$_3$ level is not indicated in patients with hypothyroidism because the T$_3$ concentration is conserved and may remain within the normal range, even in patients with significant hypothyroidism.

Measuring the thyroid peroxidase (TPO) antibody titer will not provide additional information about this patient. Determining TPO antibody status is helpful in patients with a mildly elevated serum thyroid-stimulating hormone (TSH) level and is associated with Hashimoto thyroiditis and future risk of developing permanent hypothyroidism. However, this patient demonstrates signs and symptoms consistent with hyperthyroidism.

Repeating the thyroid function tests (TFTs) in 6 weeks may be appropriate if the total or free T$_3$ level is found to be normal. If the T$_3$ is normal, the patient has subclinical hyperthyroidism, and repeating the TFTs may be indicated to determine if the abnormality is transient or permanent.

Ultrasound of the neck is appropriate for the evaluation of this patient if a nodule is suspected. However, this patient's diffusely enlarged thyroid gland is not suggestive of nodular disease. In addition, even if the physical examination were suggestive of nodular disease, the first step would be evaluation of the functional thyroid status.

KEY POINT

- Most patients with thyrotoxicosis will have elevations of both free thyroxine (T$_4$) and triiodothyronine (T$_3$), but isolated T$_3$ elevation is rare.

Bibliography

Vaidya B, Pearce SH. Diagnosis and management of thyrotoxicosis. BMJ. 2014 Aug 21;349:g5128. [PMID: 25146390]

Item 22   Answer: B

Educational Objective: Diagnose hypercalcemia in a patient with sarcoidosis.

This patient most likely has hypercalcemia due to increased 1,25-dihydroxyvitamin D levels. She has an elevated calcium level with a low parathyroid hormone level, indicating non-parathyroid hormone (PTH)–mediated hypercalcemia. The differential diagnosis of non–PTH-mediated hypercalcemia includes cancer-related hypercalcemia caused by osteolytic lesions of bone, humorally mediated by tumor-secreted parathyroid hormone-related protein (PTHrP), or granulomatous diseases, such as sarcoidosis. In granulomatous diseases, the hydroxylase in disease-associated macrophages actively converts 25-hydroxyvitamin D to the highly active 1,25-dihydroxyvitamin D metabolite. The increased levels of active vitamin D lead to increased absorption of calcium in the gut, promotion of increased bone resorption of calcium, and decreased calcium and phosphate excretion by the kidney.

Elevated serum calcium can be due to a mutation in the G-coupled protein calcium–sensing receptor (CASR) gene. These receptors are in the parathyroid glands and the kidneys. The sensor mutation results in a shift upward in the "normal" range of calcium that the receptor recognizes, resulting in a mildly elevated serum calcium level (usually <11.0 mg/dL [2.7 mmol/L]) and high normal or mildly elevated PTH level, unlike this patient whose PTH level was low.

25-Hydroxyvitamin D is the major circulating form of vitamin D and is minimally metabolically active relative to 1,25-dihydroxyvitamin D. Levels in this patient are likely to be low due to excessive conversion to the 1,25-dihydroxyvitamin D form, and would not identify the likely mechanism of hypercalcemia in this patient.

Hydrochlorothiazide, a thiazide diuretic, reduces blood volume by acting on the kidneys to reduce sodium (Na$^+$) reabsorption in the distal convoluted tubule. Thiazides increase the reabsorption of calcium in the distal convoluted tubule by their action on a Na$^+$-Cl$^-$ calcium co-transporter. However, any increase in calcium caused by thiazides is mild and rarely reduces the PTH level below the lower range of normal.

KEY POINT

- Granulomatous diseases, such as sarcoidosis, cause hypercalcemia through increased 1-α-hydroxylation activity that increases 1,25-dihydroxyvitamin D levels and calcium reabsorption.

Bibliography

Sharma OP. Hypercalcemia in granulomatous disorders: a clinical review. Curr Opin Pulm Med. 2000 Sep;6(5):442-7. [PMID: 10958237]

Item 23   Answer: D

Educational Objective: Diagnose Cushing syndrome from exogenous glucocorticoids.

The patient has iatrogenic Cushing syndrome caused by use of topical glucocorticoids in the treatment of psoriasis. Cushing syndrome presents similarly whether it is due to a pituitary adenoma (Cushing disease), adrenal tumor cortisol production, ectopic adrenocorticotropic hormone production, or excessive use of glucocorticoids. Her presentation would be consistent with any of these diagnoses; however, she is on high-potency topical glucocorticoids, so this alone explains her symptoms and presentation. Exogenous glucocorticoid use as a cause of Cushing syndrome is common, whereas the other causes are rare.

KEY POINT

- The most common cause of Cushing syndrome is an elevated level of cortisol resulting from both endogenous and exogenous exposure to glucocorticoids.

Bibliography

Nieman LK, Biller BMK, Findling JW, et al. The diagnosis of Cushing's syndrome: an Endocrine Society clinical practice guideline. J Clin Endocrinol Metab. 2008 May;93(5):1526-40. [PMID: 18334580]

Item 24 Answer: B

Educational Objective: Treat a patient with diabetic ketoacidosis.

This patient has diabetic ketoacidosis (DKA) and a low serum potassium level, so potassium chloride should be administered. The patient should be making adequate urine before administration of potassium replacement. Low potassium stores in the body will need correction prior to initiation of insulin therapy to avoid cardiac arrhythmias. Potassium chloride should be added to each liter of intravenous fluids to maintain the serum potassium level in the 4.0 to 5.0 mEq/L (4.0-5.0 mmol/L) range with the continued use of intravenous insulin therapy.

Antibiotic therapy is not warranted at this time. The mild leukocytosis upon presentation is most likely related to stress from DKA rather than an infectious process. In addition, the chest radiograph is normal.

Sodium bicarbonate provides no added benefit when the arterial blood pH is greater than 6.9 and may be associated with harm. A 2011 systematic review found that bicarbonate administration worsened ketonemia. Several studies found higher potassium requirements in patients receiving bicarbonate. Studies in children found a possible association between bicarbonate therapy and cerebral edema.

During the treatment of DKA, initiation of insulin therapy and correction of acidosis will shift the extracellular potassium back into the intracellular space. Significant worsening of the hypokalemia noted at presentation could occur if this is not corrected to a serum potassium level higher than 3.3 mEq/L (3.3 mmol/L) prior to initiation of insulin therapy, which could lead to the development of arrhythmias. Insulin therapy can be safely initiated once the serum potassium level is greater than 3.3 mEq/L (3.3 mmol/L).

KEY POINT

- During the initial management of diabetic ketoacidosis, hypokalemia should be corrected before initiation of intravenous insulin therapy to avoid significant worsening of the serum potassium levels that could cause cardiac arrhythmias.

Bibliography

Wilson JF. In the clinic. Diabetic ketoacidosis. Ann Intern Med. 2010 Jan 5;152(1):ITC1-15. [PMID: 20048266]

Item 25 Answer: D

Educational Objective: Identify secondary causes of bone loss prior to initiating bisphosphonate therapy.

Checking this patient's serum thyroid-stimulating hormone (TSH) level would be the most appropriate test to obtain prior to initiation of pharmacologic therapy. Although osteoporosis in postmenopausal women is most commonly associated with nonmodifiable risk factors such as age, sex, menopausal status, height, and build, it is always important to assess for possible secondary causes of bone loss that might be amenable to treatment, particularly if there is clinical suspicion in a specific patient. Appropriate laboratory testing for most patients with newly diagnosed osteoporosis includes complete blood count (for malignancy), complete metabolic profile (for calcium levels and kidney function), TSH, 25-hydroxyvitamin D, and urine calcium (screening for hypercalciuria), most of which were normal in this patient. However, this patient's history of unintentional weight loss over the past year may be her only symptom of hyperthyroidism, which could be contributing to her osteoporosis and would be important to treat in addition to therapy directed toward her osteoporosis. Therefore, measuring this patient's TSH level would be appropriate prior to starting therapy for osteoporosis.

Both serum and urine markers of bone turnover measure collagen breakdown products and other chemicals released from osteoclasts and osteoblasts as part of bone metabolism. However, they are not commonly used in most patients with osteoporosis primarily because there is significant variability in the different measures in an individual patient or between different patients, making standardization of results difficult. Therefore, their use is typically limited to research settings or in management of specific patients who have failed to respond to usual therapy for osteoporosis.

There is evidence that estrogen is effective for prevention and possibly treatment for osteoporosis, although the significant nonskeletal risks associated with this therapy have led to its not being used in favor of bisphosphonates. As this patient is postmenopausal and has no clinical suggestion of excess estradiol secretion, and bisphosphonate therapy would be considered preferable to estrogen despite serum levels, testing for estradiol would not be indicated in this patient.

Answers and Critiques

Hyperparathyroidism should always be considered as a possible secondary cause of bone loss. However, since this patient had normal calcium and 25-hydroxyvitamin D levels, hyperparathyroidism would be highly unlikely, and checking a parathyroid hormone level would not be indicated.

KEY POINT

- Testing for secondary causes of bone loss is appropriate before beginning pharmacologic therapy for newly diagnosed osteoporosis.

Bibliography

Hudec SM, Camacho PM. Secondary causes of osteoporosis. Endocr Pract. 2013;19:120-8. [PMID: 23186949]

Item 26   Answer: A

Educational Objective: Manage heavy menstrual bleeding caused by polycystic ovary syndrome.

This patient with polycystic ovary syndrome (PCOS) with heavy menstrual bleeding and hirsutism should be treated with combined estrogen-progestin oral contraceptive pills. Patients with PCOS remain in a stagnant follicular stage resulting in unopposed estradiol secretion from small ovarian follicles, causing proliferation of the endometrium in the absence of progesterone secretion from a corpus luteum. This predisposes patients to endometrial hyperplasia and heavy menstrual bleeding as a result of anovulatory bleeding. Intraovarian androgen production is also increased in PCOS, resulting in the hyperandrogenism and hirsutism associated with the disorder. Estrogen-progestin oral contraceptive pills are first-line therapy for the menstrual irregularities and hirsutism associated with PCOS. This therapy prevents unopposed estrogen-induced proliferation of the endometrium and suppresses the excess androgen production associated with PCOS. This would be appropriate therapy to treat both issues in this patient, who does not currently desire fertility.

Progestin therapy alone, either through periodic progestin withdrawal or use of a progesterone-eluting intrauterine device, will provide endometrial protection and treat this patient's menstrual irregularity. However, progestin therapy alone does not suppress androgen production and would not treat this patient's hirsutism.

Metformin has several favorable metabolic effects in patients with PCOS, including increased insulin sensitivity and reduced serum free testosterone. However, it has been shown to be less effective than oral contraceptives for improving the menstrual pattern and reducing serum androgens. It also does not provide endometrial protection and is considered a second-line therapy for patients with PCOS with significant menstrual irregularities and hirsutism who are unable to tolerate oral contraceptive pills.

KEY POINT

- In women with polycystic ovary syndrome, heavy menstrual bleeding, and hirsutism who do not desire fertility, estrogen-progestin oral contraceptive pills are first-line therapy to provide endometrial protection and suppress androgen production.

Bibliography

Legro RS, Arslanian SA, Ehrmann DA, et al; Endocrine Society. Diagnosis and treatment of polycystic ovary syndrome: an Endocrine Society clinical practice guideline. J Clin Endocrinol Metab. 2013 Dec;98(12):4565-92. [PMID: 24151290]

Item 27   Answer: D

Educational Objective: Treat adrenocortical carcinoma.

Adrenocortical carcinoma (ACC) is the most likely cause of this patient's Cushing syndrome, and surgical excision is the most appropriate management. The patient has classic clinical manifestations of Cushing syndrome (CS), and the 24-hour urine cortisol is markedly elevated on repeated measurements. Plasma adrenocorticotropic hormone (ACTH) is suppressed consistent with an ACTH-independent cause. The imaging characteristics of ACC include a large mass with irregular borders or shape, calcification, high attenuation (high Hounsfield units) on CT, and delay in contrast medium washout (less than 50% at 10 minutes), findings all present in this patient.

The treatment of ACC depends on the extent of disease at presentation. Surgical removal after appropriate biochemical assessment remains the best option, especially in patients with early disease. Even after apparent complete resection, adjuvant therapy with mitotane, a known adrenal cytotoxic drug, may be beneficial. Treatment with mitotane is recommended for patients with persistent disease and others with known metastases and is associated with objective remissions in approximately 25% of patients. The main factors limiting the use of mitotane include nausea, vomiting, lethargy, and neurologic side effects. Experience with other cytotoxic chemotherapy is limited, but has usually been ineffective. A poorer prognosis is associated with advanced stages of the disease, the presence of metastasis at diagnosis, an older age, and cortisol hypersecretion by the tumor. In patients without clinically evident disease after initial surgery, the median survival rate is 60% at 5 years.

Fine-needle biopsy cannot distinguish a benign adenoma from a carcinoma and is not used in the evaluation of ACC. It is sometimes used to distinguish ACC from metastatic disease. Its use in this patient is both unnecessary and inappropriate.

Radiation therapy is not used as the principal initial treatment in ACC; however, it may be used as adjuvant therapy after surgery to prevent tumor recurrence. Radiation therapy can also be used to treat areas of metastasis, such as to the bones or brain.

Answers and Critiques

KEY POINT

- Surgical removal after appropriate biochemical assessment is the most appropriate treatment for adrenocortical carcinoma, especially in patients with early disease.

Bibliography

Berruti A, Baudin E, Gelderblom H, et al. Adrenal cancer: ESMO Clinical Practice Guidelines for diagnosis, treatment and follow-up. Ann Oncol. 2012;23 Suppl 7:vii131-138. [PMID: 22997446]

Item 28   **Answer: D**

Educational Objective: Diagnose hypomagnesemia as a cause of hypocalcemia.

This patient's magnesium level should be checked. He has a very low calcium level that is likely contributing to his clinical findings of tremulousness, muscle irritability, and electrocardiogram changes. He struggles with alcohol abuse, and his low albumin level suggests malnutrition, likely due to his chronic alcohol intake as a primary source of calories. Magnesium deficiency is common in persons who abuse alcohol. Furthermore, he has had diarrhea for several days, which will also deplete his magnesium stores. This patient's low calcium level should promote parathyroid hormone (PTH) secretion to help correct the hypocalcemia. However, decreased levels of magnesium impair release of PTH; levels in patients with significant magnesium deficiency are either low or inappropriately in the normal range. Low magnesium levels are also associated with resistance to PTH activity at the level of bone, further contributing to hypocalcemia. Therefore, in patients with hypocalcemia and hypomagnesemia, it is crucial to correct the magnesium level (to at least 2 mg/dL [0.83 mmol/L]), as it is difficult to increase calcium levels until this is done.

1,25-Dihydroxyvitamin D has a short half-life, and its measurement only reflects the active levels of vitamin D. Since active levels tend to vacillate frequently based on immediate need, this level would not be diagnostically helpful. 25-Hydroxyvitamin D levels have a longer half-life and, therefore, more accurately reflect the total body stores of vitamin D.

Measuring 24-hour urine calcium excretion in this patient would not be diagnostically helpful as significant urinary loss of calcium is uncommon, and the urine calcium level in this patient would be expected to be low due to compensatory kidney retention of calcium.

Checking the ionized calcium level is indicated in settings where abnormal serum protein binding of calcium is possible. This test is not needed in this symptomatic patient who has no suggestion of excessive protein binding of calcium.

KEY POINT

- Low serum magnesium levels impair parathyroid hormone secretion and require repletion before serum calcium levels may be corrected.

Bibliography

Shoback, D. Hypoparathyroidism. N Engl J Med. 2008 Jul 24;359(4):391-403. [PMID: 18650515]

Item 29   Answer: C

Educational Objective: Manage early type 2 diabetes mellitus.

The most appropriate management for this patient is to initiate metformin. The patient is early in her diabetes disease course without evidence of microvascular disease. For otherwise healthy adults meeting these criteria, the American Diabetes Association recommends a hemoglobin A_{1c} level of less than 7.0%, preprandial glucose values of 70 to 130 mg/dL (3.9-7.2 mmol/L), and 1- to 2-hour postprandial glucose values of less than 180 mg/dL (10 mmol/L). Because the patient has not met these goals, a pharmacologic agent should be added at this time. Lifestyle recommendations consisting of increased physical activity, dietary modifications, and weight loss (if BMI is elevated) are the initial first step in treating diabetes. When lifestyle modifications fail to meet glycemic goals within 6 weeks, metformin is the recommended first-line therapy to be started in conjunction with continued lifestyle modifications. If glycemic goals are not met after 3 months of lifestyle modifications and metformin use, additional agents should be added to the regimen every 3 months until glucose goals are met.

Dapagliflozin, a sodium-glucose transporter-2 (SGLT-2) inhibitor, increases excretion of glucose through the kidney. It is a second-line agent that should be used after lifestyle modifications and metformin fail to reach glycemic goals.

The sulfonylurea glipizide stimulates insulin secretion from the pancreatic beta cells. This agent could improve the patient's postprandial hyperglycemia, but it may also induce weight gain in a patient actively working on weight loss. Glipizide is a second-line agent that should be used after lifestyle modifications and metformin fail to reach glycemic goals.

Sitagliptin, a dipeptidyl peptidase-4 (DPP-4) inhibitor, improves glycemic control by slowing gastric emptying and suppressing glucagon secretion. It is also considered a second-line agent that might be considered if lifestyle modifications and metformin fail to reach glycemic goals.

KEY POINT

- For most patients with type 2 diabetes mellitus, lifestyle modifications and metformin therapy are the most appropriate initial treatments.

Bibliography

American Diabetes Association. (7) Approaches to glycemic treatment. In: Standards of Medical Care in Diabetes-2015. Diabetes Care. 2015 Jan;38 Suppl 1:S41-8. [PMID: 25537707]

Answers and Critiques

Item 30   Answer: C

Educational Objective: Identify hemochromatosis as a cause of hypogonadotropic hypogonadism.

The patient has a clinical history suspicious for hemochromatosis and should be further evaluated by measuring serum transferrin saturation and ferritin levels. The patient has hypogonadism based on his clinical symptoms of decreased libido and erectile dysfunction, associated with a low morning serum testosterone level. A hypogonadotropic etiology is indicated by his low luteinizing and follicle-stimulating hormone levels. Causes of hypogonadotropic hypogonadism include infiltrative diseases such as hemochromatosis, sarcoidosis, cancer metastatic to the pituitary, and lymphoma. Pituitary tumors that impair gonadotropin function may also be a cause. This patient has several clinical findings suggestive of possible hemochromatosis, including a report of arthralgia and hepatomegaly on physical examination. Therefore, the next step in evaluation of this patient's hypogonadotropic hypogonadism is measurement of serum ferritin level and transferrin saturation to evaluate for possible hemochromatosis.

The cause of hypogonadism must be evaluated prior to the initiation of testosterone replacement. If testosterone therapy is started without testing for hemochromatosis, the diagnosis may be missed.

Although genetic disorders such as Klinefelter syndrome (47,XXY) may cause hypogonadism, patients with this syndrome have hypergonadotropic hypogonadism with elevated luteinizing and follicle-stimulating hormone values, unlike this patient. Therefore, karyotyping is not indicated.

A testicular ultrasound is used to evaluate the cause of primary testicular failure and is not indicated in the evaluation of hypogonadotropic hypogonadism. This patient's low gonadotropin levels indicate either a hypothalamic or pituitary disorder, instead of testicular disease. Although hemochromatosis may also directly affect testicular function in addition to its central hypogonadal effect, testicular ultrasound is not helpful in establishing the diagnosis of hemochromatosis as a cause of hypogonadism.

KEY POINT

- Patients with symptoms of hypogonadotropic hypogonadism should have serum transferrin saturation and ferritin concentration levels measured to identify hemochromatosis prior to initiating any therapy.

Bibliography

Bacon BR, Adam PC, Kowdley KV, et al. Diagnosis and management of hemochromatosis: 2011 Practice guidelines by the American Association for the Study of Liver Diseases. Hepatology. 2011:54(1):328-43. [PMID: 21452290]

Item 31   Answer: B

Educational Objective: Diagnose pseudohypercalcemia.

This patient's ionized calcium level should be checked. His total calcium level is elevated, but he is without clear symptoms associated with hypercalcemia. Approximately 40% to 45% of the calcium in serum is bound to protein, principally albumin, although the physiologically active form of calcium is in an ionized (or free) state. In most patients with relatively normal serum albumin levels, the total calcium usually accurately reflects the ionized calcium fraction. However, in clinical settings where increased protein binding of calcium may occur, the serum total calcium level may be elevated without a rise in the actual serum ionized calcium concentration. This may occur in patients with hyperalbuminuria (as may occur in those who are severely dehydrated), and in patients with a paraprotein capable of binding calcium (such as occasionally occurs in some patients with multiple myeloma). This phenomenon is sometimes termed pseudohypercalcemia (or factitious hypercalcemia). If present, a normal ionized calcium level may indicate that the elevated total calcium levels are due to excessive protein binding and potentially eliminate the need for further evaluation for hypercalcemia.

Measuring the 1,25-dihydroxyvitamin D level is useful in further assessing patients with non–parathyroid hormone (PTH)-mediated hypercalcemia to assess for excess vitamin D production. PTH testing is indicated in patients with hypercalcemia to differentiate between PTH-mediated and non–PTH-mediated hypercalcemia.

The hypercalcemia associated with multiple myeloma is caused primarily by tumor-induced, osteoclast-mediated bone resorption due to cytokines released by myeloma cells and is not PTH-mediated or due to excessive vitamin D levels. Measurement of PTH level and 1,25-dihydroxyvitamin levels may be indicated as part of this patient's evaluation only after true hypercalcemia has been established.

Parathyroid hormone–related protein (PTHrP) level measurement is useful in evaluating patients with non–PTH-mediated hypercalcemia but would not be indicated as a next study in this patient in whom pseudohypercalcemia has not been excluded.

KEY POINT

- In patients with conditions in which increased protein binding of calcium may occur, such as hyperalbuminemia or paraproteinemia, an artificially elevated total serum calcium level must be excluded.

Bibliography

Clines GA. Mechanisms and treatment of hypercalcemia of malignancy. Curr Opin Endocrinol Diabetes Obes. 2011 Dec;18(6):339-46. [PMID: 21897221]

Item 32   Answer: B

Educational Objective: Manage androgen therapy in the setting of hypogonadism.

Before initiating therapy for this patient with hypogonadism, his desire for fertility should be explored. Testosterone replacement therapy can be associated with decreased spermatogenesis and infertility. Exogenous testosterone suppresses both hypothalamic gonadotropin-releasing hormone and pituitary follicle-stimulating hormone and luteinizing hormone (LH) production, resulting in depletion of intratesticular testosterone. The effect is suppression of spermatogenesis so pronounced that testosterone replacement therapy has been studied as a male hormonal contraceptive. Based on Endocrine Society guidelines, men with hypogonadism should be treated with exogenous testosterone when they have consistent signs and symptoms of hypogonadism and low serum testosterone levels. Symptomatic men may report reduced libido, erectile dysfunction, mood changes, irritability, fatigue, or memory loss. Although this patient's symptoms would likely be improved with exogenous administration of androgen, replacement therapy may also result in infertility due to oligospermia. Patients with hypogonadism who desire fertility may require treatment with human chorionic gonadotropin (HCG). HCG has LH-like activity and stimulates the production of intratesticular testosterone, resulting in the high concentrations required for induction and maintenance of spermatogenesis.

Asymptomatic men with low serum testosterone levels may experience decreased bone mineral density and osteoporosis. Hormone replacement therapy will decrease the risk of osteoporosis. A bone mineral density measurement prior to the initiation of hormone replacement therapy is not needed.

Male hypogonadism is associated with increased visceral fat and insulin resistance, and hormone replacement therapy improves these metabolic parameters. There is no recommendation that hypogonadal patients initiating hormone replacement therapy be screened for diabetes mellitus with fasting plasma glucose measurement or other testing.

A 2010 systematic review of hypogonadal men receiving testosterone therapy found no evidence of increased risk of prostate cancer when compared with the placebo/nonintervention group. The Endocrine Society guideline on testosterone replacement therapy recommends a digital rectal examination and prostate-specific antigen (PSA) level determination at 3 and 6 months following the initiation of replacement therapy. Continued regular screening is recommended for men older than 40 years of age with a baseline PSA level greater than 6 ng/mL (6 µg/L). Scrotal ultrasound is unnecessary prior to initiation of testosterone therapy; a clinical testicular examination to rule out abnormalities or a testicular mass is sufficient.

KEY POINT

- Prior to initiation of testosterone therapy for hypogonadism, the desire for fertility should be ascertained because exogenous testosterone replacement therapy may result in oligospermia and infertility.

Bibliography

Samplaski MK, Loai Y, Wong K, Lo KC, Grober ED, Jarvi KA. Testosterone use in the male infertility population: prescribing patterns and effects on semen and hormonal parameters. Fertil Steril. 2014 Jan;101(1):64-9. [PMID: 24094422]

Item 33   Answer: D

Educational Objective: Diagnose thyroid storm.

This patient has thyroid storm, most likely precipitated by the iodine contained in the dye load from the cardiac catheterization in the context of undertreated Graves disease following her discontinuation of methimazole. Graves disease is the most common underlying condition associated with thyroid storm, and onset may be triggered by a number of factors in addition to iodine, including infection, surgery, myocardial infarction, trauma, or parturition. This patient has typical features of thyroid storm: fever, tachycardia, heart failure, gastrointestinal dysfunction, and mental status changes. Scoring systems exist that can be used to provide a more objective measurement of the severity of the thyrotoxicosis. Treatment of thyroid storm is directed toward supportive care, reduction of thyroid hormone production, decreasing peripheral conversion of thyroxine (T_4) to triiodothyronine (T_3), addressing adrenergic symptoms and thermoregulatory changes, and treating any identified precipitating factors. Thionamides and β-blockers are the mainstay of treatment to reduce thyroid hormone production and control adrenergic symptoms.

This patient's clinical presentation is not consistent with euthyroid sick syndrome. Although this patient's low level of serum thyroid-stimulating hormone (TSH) is consistent with euthyroid sick syndrome, her elevated serum thyroid hormone level is not. In euthyroid sick syndrome, serum thyroid hormone levels are typically low, creating a clinical picture similar to that seen in central hypothyroidism.

Pheochromocytoma typically presents with hypertension and tachycardia but thyromegaly is not a clinical feature of this disorder. Additionally, confusion and altered mental status are not presenting signs of the disease.

Subacute thyroiditis is typically precipitated by a recent viral illness. An iodine load, such as this patient had, is an unlikely cause. Although patients with subacute thyroiditis may present with significant thyrotoxicosis, the thyroid is typically painful to palpation, a clinical finding that was not present in this patient.

KEY POINT

- In patients with underlying Graves disease, thyroid storm may be precipitated by the iodine content found in contrast media.

Bibliography

Klubo-Gwiezdzinska J1, Wartofsky L. Thyroid emergencies. Med Clin North Am. 2012 Mar;96(2):385-403. [PMID: 22443982]

Item 34   Answer: D

Educational Objective: Manage postsurgical hypoparathyroidism.

This patient without parathyroid function should be advised to decrease his calcium supplementation intake. In patients without parathyroid function, stimulation of the kidney to convert 25-hydroxyvitamin D (from the liver) into the active form, 1,25- dihydroxyvitamin D (calcitriol), is lost, as is the signal to increase reabsorption of calcium in the kidney in the distal convoluted tubule and loop of Henle. As a result, both calcitriol and calcium supplementation must be provided, as was done in this patient. However, without reabsorption of calcium by the kidney, oral calcium will be absorbed and passed through the kidney, resulting in higher levels of urine calcium than in patients with normal parathyroid hormone levels. In monitoring calcium status in hypoparathyroid patients, the recommended goal should be a 24-hour urine calcium level of less than 300 mg/24 hours (7.5 mmol/24 h) with a concomitant serum calcium level in the low normal range (8.0-8.5 mg/dL [2.0-2.1 mmol/L]). If the urine calcium levels are surpassed, it is appropriate to decrease the calcium intake first; in patients with serum calcium levels greater than 8.5 mg/dL (2.1 mmol/L) and urine calcium greater than 300 mg/24 hours (7.5 mmol/24 h), concurrent decreases in both calcium supplementation and calcitriol are indicated.

Although 25-hydroxyvitamin D levels are the best indicator of total body vitamin D stores in patients with normal parathyroid function, it would not be helpful for therapeutic decision-making in this patient as the lack of PTH requires treatment with activated (1,25-dihydroxy) vitamin D. In this patient, 1,25-dihydroxyvitamin D levels measured concurrently with the serum and urine calcium levels are the most appropriate indicators of therapeutic effect.

Removal of the parathyroid glands does not allow the PTH level to be used to monitor appropriateness of therapy. It would be expected to be low or undetectable in this patient who has had resection of his parathyroid glands and chemotherapy and radiation.

It would be inappropriate to continue the current regimen given the elevated 24-hour urine calcium levels. Persistently elevated levels could lead to nephrolithiasis or nephrocalcinosis.

KEY POINT

- The urine and serum calcium goals are different in patients with hypoparathyroidism; the urine calcium goal is less than 300 mg/24 hours (7.5 mmol/24 h) and serum calcium goal is between 8.0 and 8.5 mg/dL (2-2.1 mmol/L) in these patients.

Bibliography
Khan MS, Waguespack SG, Hu M. Medical management of postsurgical hypoparathyroidism. Endocr Pract. 2011 Mar-Apr;17 Suppl 1:18-25. [PMID: 21134871]

Item 35   Answer: A

Educational Objective: Manage exercise-induced hypoglycemia.

This patient should decrease his meal-time insulin glulisine dose prior to exercise and continue his insulin glargine. Exercise can increase glucose utilization by the muscles, which can induce hypoglycemia in the setting of exogenous insulin. This patient consumes a meal and administers insulin glulisine, a

rapid-acting insulin, before intensive exercise. Since the duration of action of insulin glulisine can extend up to 4 hours, covering the meal consumption prior to exercise with a smaller dose of insulin glulisine can reduce the risk of hypoglycemia in the setting of intense or prolonged exercise.

Discontinuation of insulin glargine in a patient with type 1 diabetes will lead to hyperglycemia if the rapid-acting insulin isn't adjusted to provide basal insulin coverage. The hyperglycemia and insulin deficiency that develop in the absence of basal insulin coupled with the stress associated with exercise will lead to an increase in the release of counterregulatory hormones. In this scenario, there may not be sufficient insulin to decrease lipolysis and subsequent oxidation of free fatty acids. This could lead to diabetic ketoacidosis.

The meal-time insulin prior to exercise should be decreased; however, modification of the diet with increase in carbohydrates, rather than protein, can also help avoid exercise-induced hypoglycemia. Consumption of 15 to 30 grams of carbohydrates prior to exercise and/or a snack with complex carbohydrates after prolonged exercise can help mitigate the risk of hypoglycemia. Carbohydrates, especially simple ones, can rapidly provide glucose to the bloodstream and maximize glycogen stores in the liver that can be utilized for fuel during exercise. The digestion time for protein is prolonged compared with carbohydrates, thus providing a slower source of energy during exercise

A sliding-scale regimen of insulin glulisine is a reactive management plan for glucose control. In this scenario, it is possible that the patient could have an increased risk of hyperglycemia or hypoglycemia prior to, during, or after exercise secondary to insufficient or excessive doses of insulin from the sliding-scale regimen.

KEY POINT

- Because exercise can increase glucose utilization by the muscles, reducing the doses of mealtime insulin in a patient with diabetes mellitus will decrease the risk of hypoglycemia with intense or prolonged exercise.

Bibliography
American Diabetes Association. (4) Foundations of care: education, nutrition, physical activity, smoking cessation, psychosocial care, and immunization. In: Standards of Medical Care in Diabetes-2015. Diabetes Care. 2015 Jan;38 Suppl 1:S20-30. [PMID: 25537702]

Item 36   Answer: A

Educational Objective: Diagnose central hypothyroidism.

Measurement of the serum free thyroxine (T_4) level is the most appropriate next step in management for this patient who has clinical evidence of hypothyroidism (fatigue, constipation, cold intolerance, dry skin, delayed reflexes, anemia, and mild hyponatremia) but has had radiation to the base of the skull, including the pituitary gland. Although measurement of thyroid-stimulating hormone (TSH) is the most accurate reflection of thyroid status in patients with an intact hypothalamic-pituitary-thyroid axis, it is not a reliable measure of thyroid function in patients in whom there is loss of hypothalamic-pituitary function, such as seen in this patient. His low-normal TSH in the context of clinical hypothyroidism suggests possible central hypothyroidism, and measurement of the circulating level of thyroid hormone, the free serum T_4, would therefore be a more accurate indication of his thyroid status.

Repeating the TSH measurement would not be appropriate in this patient with signs and symptoms of hypothyroidism, as untreated hypothyroidism leads to increased cardiovascular morbidity and mortality. In addition, because of likely central hypothyroidism, the TSH level would remain an inaccurate indicator of thyroid function.

Thyroid scintigraphy is unlikely to distinguish the source of the hypothyroidism, as patients with primary or secondary hypothyroidism have decreased radioactive uptake. Thyroid scanning is most helpful in elucidating the cause of hyperthyroidism.

Ultrasound of the neck is normal in patients with central hyperthyroidism and would be unlikely to provide any additional information about this patient's thyroid status.

KEY POINT

- When central hypothyroidism is suspected, measurement of the serum free thyroxine (T_4) level is essential.

Bibliography

Persani L. Clinical review: Central hypothyroidism: pathogenic, diagnostic, and therapeutic challenges. J Clin Endocrinol Metab. 2012 Sep;97(9):3068-78. [PMID: 22851492]

Item 37   Answer: B

Educational Objective: Diagnose familial hypocalciuric hypercalcemia.

This patient's urine calcium and creatinine levels should be measured. Her laboratory values are consistent with hypercalcemia, and her parathyroid hormone level is toward the upper end of the normal range. In her age group and with a family member with a suspicious history, it is important to distinguish between primary hyperparathyroidism and familial hypocalciuric hypercalcemia (FHH). The distinction between primary hyperparathyroidism and FHH can be made by a 24-hour urine collection for calcium and creatinine, which will establish the amount of kidney calcium excretion and will allow evaluation of the calcium-creatinine ratio. Total urine calcium of less than 200 mg/24 h (5 mmol/24 h) and a calcium-creatinine ratio less than 0.01 are highly suggestive of familial hypocalciuric hypercalcemia. FHH results from a mutation in a specific calcium-sensing receptor in the parathyroids and kidneys, and results in an upward shift in the range of calcium and PTH leading to these clinical findings. Although a rare entity, making this diagnosis is crucial because it may prevent unnecessary parathyroidectomy for the patient. The course of FHH is

rarely associated with hypercalcemia and therefore does not require therapy to lower serum calcium levels. Screening other family members for the disorder is indicated.

Bone densitometry is not indicated in this age group in the absence of fragility fractures or other risk factors such as long-term high-dose glucocorticoid use or primary hyperparathyroidism.

A parathyroid sestamibi scan is a very useful nuclear imaging study for localization of adenomas in patients with primary hyperparathyroidism or parathyroid cancer. However, primary hyperparathyroidism has not been confirmed in this patient with suspicion for FHH, making this study premature.

The need for surgical treatment in this patient has also not been established. Therefore, surgical referral for parathyroidectomy would not be appropriate.

KEY POINT

- Measurement of 24-hour urine calcium and creatinine levels will distinguish between primary hyperparathyroidism and familial hypocalciuric hypercalcemia.

Bibliography

Shinall MC Jr, Dahir KM, Broome JT. Differentiating familial hypocalciuric hypercalcemia from primary hyperparathyroidism. Endocr Pract. 2013 Jul-Aug;19(4):697-702. [PMID: 23425644]

Item 38   Answer: D

Educational Objective: Evaluate timing of prandial insulin in a patient with diabetes mellitus.

The mismatch of timing of insulin administration to food intake with meals, possibly related to the time demands of her new job, is the most likely explanation for the erratic glycemic fluctuations noted on this patient's blood glucose log. The adequacy of her nocturnal long-acting insulin is reflected in her near-goal pre-breakfast blood glucose levels. However, the major fluctuations occurring around mealtimes are best explained by inconsistent use of her immediate-acting insulin relative to food intake. Meal coverage with insulin should mimic the physiologic pattern seen with endogenous insulin secreted from pancreatic beta cells. Administration of immediate-acting insulins should therefore ideally occur just prior to or at the time of the meal consumption. Because of the rapid onset of action with these agents, shifting the timing of administration away from this physiologic pattern may result in the blood glucose fluctuations seen in this patient. An important aspect of diabetes education is helping patients understand the actions of their prescribed insulin regimen and the importance of timing issues when using them.

Antibodies can develop in response to exposure to exogenous insulin; however, these antibodies are rarely clinically significant and would not adequately explain the blood glucose pattern seen in this patient.

Gastroparesis can cause erratic blood glucose values due to either rapid transit or delayed emptying of food within the digestive system. However, the lack of gastrointestinal symptoms, absence of clinical evidence of other diabetes-related complications, and her hemoglobin A_{1c} history suggesting good diabetic control make gastroparesis a less likely cause of her erratic blood glucose readings.

Inadequate insulin dosing can cause fluctuations in glycemic control. However, this patient reports little variability in her daily diet. She also has several days with evidence of adequate glycemic control on her current insulin regimen doses. Therefore, inadequate dosing is less likely to be the cause of her glycemic variability.

KEY POINT

- Because meal coverage with insulin should mimic the physiologic pattern seen with endogenous insulin secreted from the pancreatic beta cells as closely as possible, insulin administration in patients with diabetes mellitus should ideally occur prior to or at the time of the meal consumption.

Bibliography

DeWitt DE, Hirsch IB. Outpatient insulin therapy in type 1 and type 2 diabetes mellitus. JAMA. 2003 May 7;289(17):2254-64. [PMID: 12734137]

Item 39   Answer: A

Educational Objective: Manage a patient with Cushing syndrome following adrenalectomy.

The most appropriate management of this patient undergoing right adrenalectomy for Cushing syndrome (CS) is postoperative hydrocortisone. The patient has adrenocorticotropic hormone (ACTH)-independent CS, and a contrast-enhanced adrenal CT scan demonstrated a right adrenal mass with imaging characteristics consistent with a benign adenoma. Adrenocortical adenomas typically have low attenuation on unenhanced CT scan (density less than 10 Hounsfield units) and exhibit rapid washout of intravenous iodine contrast media (>50% at 10 minutes). Following adrenalectomy, patients with adrenal CS may develop acute adrenal failure because of hypothalamic-pituitary-adrenal (HPA) axis suppression and contralateral adrenal atrophy. All patients should be treated with stress-dose glucocorticoids and tapered to physiologic replacement until HPA axis recovery is confirmed. Most patients have adrenal insufficiency lasting as long as 12 months.

Postoperative administration of mitotane, an adrenolytic drug, is recommended as adjuvant therapy for patients with locally persistent or metastatic adrenocortical carcinoma (ACC). In these patients, mitotane is associated with objective remissions in approximately 25% of patients. This patient's CT scan findings are not consistent with ACC. Adrenal cancers are typically large (>4-6 cm) with irregular margins and areas of necrosis or calcification. Unenhanced CT will demonstrate high attenuation (density >10 Hounsfield units), and washout of intravenous iodine contrast media is less than 50% at 10 minutes.

Postoperative norepinephrine is not indicated. If the patient were to experience hypotension or shock postoperatively, treatment with vasopressors in addition to glucocorticoid replacement would be considered; however, this would not replace the administration of glucocorticoids in this population at risk for acute hypocortisolism.

Preoperative phenoxybenzamine is indicated in the management of patients with pheochromocytoma, not CS. The purpose of preoperative α-blockade is to provide blood pressure control and decrease the risk of cardiovascular complications related to excessive catecholamine release during intraoperative manipulation of the tumor.

KEY POINT

- Following adrenalectomy, patients with adrenal Cushing syndrome should be treated with stress-dose glucocorticoids during the postoperative period to avoid the risk of acute hypocortisolism.

Bibliography

Di Dalmazi G, Berr CM, Fassnacht M, et al. Adrenal function after adrenalectomy for subclinical hypercortisolism and Cushing's syndrome: A systematic review of the literature. JCEM. 2014;99:2637-2645. [PMID: 24878052]

Item 40   Answer: A

Educational Objective: Manage Paget disease of bone.

Initiating antiresorptive therapy in this patient with symptomatic Paget disease of bone is the most appropriate next step in management. Paget disease of bone is characterized by focal areas of accelerated bone remodeling that ultimately causes overgrowth of bone at one or more sites that may impair the integrity of affected bone. Areas commonly affected include the skull, spine, pelvis, and long bones of the lower extremities, such as in this patient who has thickened cortical bone and coarsening of the trabecular bone of the femur. The main indications for antiresorptive therapy in most patients include pain caused by increased bone metabolic activity (as in this patient) and hypercalcemia due to multiple affected sites. The most commonly used treatment agents are nitrogen-containing bisphosphonates (alendronate, pamidronate, risedronate, and zoledronic acid); these are the newer bisphosphonates and have been the most extensively studied for treatment of Paget disease of bone. Bisphosphonates stabilize bone turnover by suppressing bone resorption and new bone formation with a resulting reduction in serum alkaline phosphatase levels. There is no evidence that antiresorptive therapy is beneficial in asymptomatic patients.

Bone biopsy is rarely needed to establish the diagnosis of Paget disease of bone when there are characteristic radiographic findings of bone turnover (concurrent osteolytic and osteoblastic changes) and consistent laboratory studies (such as elevated serum alkaline phosphatase levels). Bone biopsy may be useful in certain situations in which bone lesions are primarily osteoblastic (suggesting possible metastatic disease) or osteolytic (possibly indicating multiple myeloma), neither of which are present in this patient.

The bone lesions of multiple myeloma are primarily osteolytic, in which case further evaluation for that diagnosis with a serum and urine protein electrophoresis would be appropriate. However, this patient's radiographic findings are not consistent with a diagnosis of multiple myeloma, and further evaluation for this disorder would therefore not be indicated.

Most patients with Paget disease of bone are asymptomatic and are identified only by elevated serum alkaline phosphatase levels detected on laboratory studies obtained for other reasons. In many patients with mild disease, clinical observation without initiation of therapy is appropriate. However, in this patient with symptomatic disease in a critical weight-bearing skeletal area, clinical observation without treatment would not be appropriate.

KEY POINT

- Treatment of Paget disease of bone with antiresorptive agents is indicated in symptomatic patients, those with elevated calcium levels, or patients with involvement of skeletal areas at high risk of complications, including fractures.

Bibliography

Ralston SH. Paget's disease of the bone. N Engl J Med. 2013 Feb 14;368(7):644-50. [PMID: 23406029]

Item 41   Answer: D

Educational Objective: Treat hypothyroidism in pregnancy.

This pregnant patient's levothyroxine dose should be increased to lower the serum thyroid-stimulating hormone. Maternal thyroid hormone production typically increases by 30% to 50% during pregnancy; therefore, in pregnant patients requiring levothyroxine supplementation, the replacement dose usually needs to be increased to provide adequate thyroxine (T_4) for the neurologic development of the fetus. The combination of this patient's elevated thyroid-stimulating hormone (TSH) level and low total T_4 level suggest that her levothyroxine dose should be increased. During pregnancy, the physiologic changes in thyroid hormone levels include a reduction in the serum TSH level and an increase in the serum total T_4 level. This change in the serum TSH level is partly due to the rise in the serum human chorionic gonadotropin (HCG) level; both hormones share sequence homology in their α subunit. As the serum HCG level rises with progression of pregnancy, the hormone can bind to the TSH receptors, resulting in a reduction in serum TSH levels. Consequently, the normal reference range for serum TSH during pregnancy shifts to a lower value, from 0.5 to 5.0 μU/mL (0.5-5.0 mU/L) pre-pregnancy to 0.03 to 2.5 μU/mL (0.03-2.5 mU/L) during the first trimester. Additionally, the serum total T_4 level rises 1.5-fold above the normal nonpregnant reference range. Part of this increase is due to the higher levels of estrogen associated with pregnancy, which cause an increase in serum total protein levels, including serum thyroid hormone-binding proteins. The increased thyroid hormone requirements of the fetus also contribute to this change in serum T_4 levels.

In this patient, with a serum TSH value above 2.5 μU/mL (2.5 mU/L) during the first trimester, the dose of levothyroxine needs to be increased rather than decreased or discontinued. The serum TSH level should be rechecked in 4 weeks to ensure that the dose adjustment continues to be adequate. Likewise, thyroid function tests should be repeated at least once during each trimester to ensure that additional adjustments in the levothyroxine dose are not needed.

KEY POINT

- On confirmation of pregnancy in a patient taking levothyroxine, serum thyroid-stimulating hormone should be checked to determine the need for levothyroxine dose adjustment.

Bibliography

Stagnaro-Green A, Abalovich M, Alexander E, et al; American Thyroid Association Taskforce on Thyroid Disease During Pregnancy and Postpartum. Guidelines of the American Thyroid Association for the diagnosis and management of thyroid disease during pregnancy and postpartum. Thyroid. 2011 Oct;21(10):1081-125. [PMID: 21787128]

Item 42   Answer: B

Educational Objective: Diagnose the cause of adrenal failure.

This patient most likely has primary adrenal failure due to bilateral adrenal hemorrhage. He has acute onset nausea, lightheadedness, back and abdominal pain, and hypotension. While nonspecific, these findings are consistent with adrenal failure. Additionally, laboratory studies show hyponatremia, hyperkalemia, and hypocortisolemia, which are also consistent with the diagnosis. A sudden drop in the hemoglobin and hematocrit, as seen in this patient, may be present without evidence of bleeding elsewhere. Risk factors for adrenal hemorrhage include anticoagulant therapy (and may occur with treatment levels within the therapeutic range), the postoperative state, abnormalities of hemostasis (such as heparin-induced thrombocytopenia or antiphospholipid antibody syndrome), and sepsis. Because adrenal hemorrhage is uncommon and the associated findings may be relatively nonspecific, an increased level of suspicion is required for the diagnosis in at-risk patients; failure to identify acute adrenal failure in a timely manner may lead to cardiovascular collapse. Adrenal hemorrhage can often be visualized on abdominal CT imaging. Treatment of acute adrenal failure is with stress-dose glucocorticoids (hydrocortisone, 50-100 mg intravenously every 6-8 hours) and supportive care with intravenous fluids and vasopressors as needed for hemodynamic compromise.

Although autoimmune adrenalitis may cause primary adrenal failure and is associated with the presence of other autoimmune diseases (such as hypothyroidism in this patient), the onset of symptoms related to hypocortisolism are usually more gradual, and skin hyperpigmentation is often seen on examination.

Chronic administration of long-acting opiate medications is a known cause of hypogonadotropic hypogonadism and a potential etiology of secondary adrenal insufficiency. The administration of relatively short-acting opiates (oxycodone) on an as-needed basis for postoperative pain is unlikely to cause clinically significant hypothalamic-pituitary-adrenal axis disturbance. Hypogonadotropic hypogonadism would also not present with hyperkalemia because mineralocorticoid secretion is preserved.

Pituitary apoplexy results from acute hemorrhage into the pituitary and may result in adrenal insufficiency. Although this patient might be at increased risk due to anticoagulation, he does not have headache or visual disturbances, which are common in pituitary apoplexy. Because pituitary apoplexy causes secondary adrenal insufficiency, it would not result in hyperkalemia.

KEY POINT

- Patients with bilateral adrenal hemorrhage typically present with clinical features of acute cortisol and aldosterone deficiency, including gastrointestinal disturbance, lethargy, weakness, hypotension, shock, hypoglycemia, and electrolyte imbalances, such as hyponatremia and hyperkalemia.

Bibliography

Rosenberger LH, Smith PW, Sawyer RG, et al. Bilateral adrenal hemorrhage: the unrecognized cause of hemodynamic collapse associated with heparin-induced thrombocytopenia. Crit Care Med. 2011 Apr;39(4):833-8 [PMID: 21242799]

Item 43   Answer: C

Educational Objective: Evaluate a patient with a new diagnosis of hypercortisolism for osteoporosis.

This patient with newly diagnosed hypercortisolism is at high risk for osteoporosis and fracture, and a screening dual-energy x-ray absorptiometry (DEXA) scan is indicated. The mechanism of osteoporosis in patients with Cushing syndrome is related to decreased intestinal calcium absorption, decreased bone formation, increased bone resorption, and decreased renal calcium reabsorption. Patients with low bone density should be considered for bisphosphonate treatment to reduce the risk of fracture.

An 8-mg dexamethasone suppression test can be used to help localize the source of adrenocorticotropic hormone (ACTH) in a patient with Cushing syndrome. Patients with pituitary Cushing disease respond to 8 mg of dexamethasone with a suppressed cortisol level. In comparison, patients with ectopic ACTH production do not respond to 8 mg of dexamethasone, and their cortisol levels remain elevated. However, this test is associated with a number of false-positive results. The 8-mg dexamethasone suppression test is not indicated for this patient because she has already had a more definitive test. Intrapetrosal sinus sampling has better sensitivity and specificity when completed by a skilled interventional radiologist.

Measuring 24-hour urine free catecholamine and metanephrine levels would be used to screen for pheochromocytoma. If this patient had an adrenal adenoma, she would certainly need to be screened for pheochromocytoma prior to surgery, but she does not have a known adrenal lesion. Her symptoms and comorbidities are explained by her diagnosis of Cushing disease, and she has no specific signs or symptoms that require an evaluation for pheochromocytoma.

A PET scan is not necessary or indicated in the evaluation of Cushing syndrome. Cushing disease is caused by a pituitary adenoma and is not malignant. Cushing syndrome due to ectopic ACTH production is often caused by a cancer. PET scan may be indicated to try to localize the source of ectopic ACTH, but the source of the excessive ACTH is already known to be from a pituitary adenoma.

KEY POINT

- Patients with hypercortisolism should have a screening dual-energy x-ray absorptiometry scan because they are at a high risk of osteoporosis and fracture.

Bibliography

Nieman LK, Biller BMK, Findling JW, et al. The diagnosis of Cushing's syndrome: an Endocrine Society clinical practice guideline. J Clin Endocrinol Metab. 2008 May;93(5):1526-40. [PMID: 18334580]

Item 44   Answer: D

Educational Objective: Manage primary adrenal failure.

The most appropriate regimen for the long-term treatment of this patient's primary adrenal failure would be prednisone, 5 mg once daily, and fludrocortisone, 0.05 mg once daily. In primary adrenal failure, there is a failure in the production of all the hormones of the adrenal cortex. Patients therefore require both glucocorticoid and mineralocorticoid replacement. Because she is no longer ill, physiologic replacement doses are appropriate. Prednisone primarily has glucocorticoid activity, with 5 mg being considered a physiologic replacement dose. It is also long-acting so may be administered once daily in combination with fludrocortisone, which has almost pure mineralocorticoid properties. Physiologic replacement doses of fludrocortisone are 0.05 to 2 mg per day.

Dexamethasone is primarily a glucocorticoid and could be used as the glucocorticoid portion of combination replacement therapy with a mineralocorticoid such as fludrocortisone. However, dexamethasone alone would not be appropriate therapy for primary adrenal failure due to its intrinsic lack of mineralocorticoid activity.

Fludrocortisone alone is also inappropriate because it would not provide glucocorticoid replacement.

Hydrocortisone has both glucocorticoid and mineralocorticoid properties, with primarily glucocorticoid activity at physiologic replacement doses of 12.5 to 25 mg in two to three divided doses daily. At total daily doses above 50 mg, hydrocortisone has adequate mineralocorticoid activity to allow for its use as monotherapy. However, treatment with hydrocortisone, 10 mg three times daily, does not provide

CONT.

adequate mineralocorticoid replacement, while it supplies a supraphysiologic amount of glucocorticoid that could lead to iatrogenic Cushing syndrome if administered on a long-term basis.

Patients with primary adrenal failure require additional glucocorticoid at times of physiologic stress. Treatment for minor stress (upper respiratory infection, fever, minor surgery under local anesthesia) is typically two to three times the basal dose of hydrocortisone (or equivalent), for moderate stress (minor or moderate surgery with general anesthesia) usually 45 to 75 mg/day, and major stress (major surgery, trauma, critical illness, or childbirth) up to 150 to 200 mg/day with a gradual taper following resolution of the stress.

KEY POINT

- Patients with primary adrenal failure require both glucocorticoid and mineralocorticoid replacement in physiologic doses.

Bibliography

Neary N, Nieman L. Adrenal insufficiency: etiology, diagnosis and treatment. Curr Opin Endocrinol Diabetes Obes. 2010 Jun;17(3):217-23.[PMID: 20375886]

Item 45   Answer: C

Educational Objective: Diagnose primary thyroid lymphoma.

The patient has primary thyroid lymphoma, which most often occurs in elderly women with a long-standing history of Hashimoto thyroiditis. The clinical presentation is typically one of rapid onset (weeks) of an enlarging goiter with weight loss and night sweats. The diagnosis is made by biopsy of the thyroid with flow cytometry. Treatment typically involves chemotherapy and/or radiation therapy. Thyroidectomy is usually not needed.

CT scan of the neck, rather than ultrasound, was ordered in this patient because of the compressive symptoms and positional breathing issues. CT scan allows visualization of the enlarged thyroid gland and assessment of the patency of the trachea. In this image, the "doughnut" sign can be seen, whereby the enlarged thyroid extends behind and completely encircles the trachea.

New-onset Graves disease is unlikely to occur in a patient of this age, particularly with her long-standing history of hypothyroidism. Furthermore, there is no bruit or other clinical sign of Graves disease, and the thyromegaly associated with Graves disease is not acute in onset.

This patient is unlikely to have papillary thyroid cancer, as these tumors typically grow very slowly, in contrast to the acute onset of her findings. Additionally, the thyroid is not typically diffusely enlarged, as seen on this CT scan. Rather, a distinct nodule and potentially concomitant cervical lymphadenopathy would be expected.

Subacute (de Quervain) thyroiditis is associated with acute onset of anterior neck pain. It is typically seen following a viral illness in the preceding months. The changes on

CT are typically a patchy infiltrate with minimal lymphadenopathy. This patient's image reveals marked diffuse enlargement of the thyroid, and she did not have a history of prior illness.

KEY POINT

- Primary thyroid lymphoma most often occurs in elderly women with underlying hypothyroidism; the typical presentation includes rapidly enlarging goiter, weight loss, and night sweats, and imaging reveals a diffusely enlarged thyroid.

Bibliography

Kim HC, Han MH, Kim KH, et al. Primary thyroid lymphoma: CT findings. Eur J Radiol. 2003 Jun;46(3):233-9. [PMID: 12758117]

Item 46   Answer: E

Educational Objective: Treat primary hyperparathyroidism and concomitant vitamin D deficiency.

The most appropriate treatment of this patient is to replete his vitamin D deficiency with a supplement such as vitamin D_3 (cholecalciferol). He has primary hyperparathyroidism as shown by his elevated serum calcium and parathyroid hormone levels. However, there is a high prevalence of concurrent vitamin D deficiency and insufficiency in patients with primary hyperparathyroidism, and low levels of 25-hydroxyvitamin D can stimulate parathyroid hormone secretion in non-adenomatous glands. Because of this, measurement of vitamin D levels should be ordered as part of the evaluation of primary hyperparathyroidism, and repletion should be provided if identified. In these patients, it is important to replace their vitamin D to a level of at least 30 ng/dL (75 nmol/L). After this level is reached, the patient should be placed on a vitamin D dosage to maintain that value. The choice to use cholecalciferol versus ergocalciferol is often based on the level of vitamin D deficiency. Since ergocalciferol is more readily available in the 50,000 U form and has a shorter half-life, it is recommended when a patient's vitamin D level is less than 10 ng/mL (25 nmol/L). Cholecalciferol is often used when the level is between 20 and 30 ng/mL (50-75 nmol/L) or for maintenance. Since this patient already has hypercalcemia and low-dose repletion is desired, the lower doses (400 U daily) of vitamin D_3 (over-the-counter cholecalciferol) should be used. This patient's serum calcium should be monitored at least monthly.

This patient does not meet the threshold for surgery. His serum total calcium level is less than 1 standard deviation from upper limit of normal, his bone density score is not in the osteoporotic or treatment range, he is older than 50 years of age, and his glomerular filtration rate is preserved.

Alendronate would be an excellent option for calcium reduction and simultaneous treatment of osteoporosis if his T-scores were lower or Fracture Risk Assessment Tool (FRAX) scores were higher. The FRAX calculator defines the 10-year fracture risk for patients with T-scores in the -1.0 to -2.5 range. The FRAX calculator (www.shef.ac.uk/FRAX)

incorporates multiple risk factors including sex, fracture history, femoral neck bone mineral density, steroid usage, smoking, BMI, age, and alcohol intake to determine projected fracture risk. If the risk of major osteoporotic fracture is greater than or equal to 20% or the risk of hip fracture is greater than or equal to 3%, the patient's benefit from therapy exceeds the risk and treatment should be offered.

Calcitonin is an option for reducing his calcium levels, but he is currently asymptomatic and does not warrant calcium lowering.

Cinacalcet, a calcimimetic agent, is another option for lowering calcium for symptomatic patients with kidney involvement. This patient has preserved kidney function and no symptoms. Due to the cost and potential side effects of cinacalcet, it would not be indicated at this time.

KEY POINT

- In patients with primary hyperparathyroidism and concomitant vitamin D deficiency, 25-hydroxyvitamin D levels should be repleted to at least 30 ng/dL (75 nmol/L) to prevent further parathyroid hormone stimulation.

Bibliography

Holick MF, Binkley N, Bischoff-Ferrari HA, Gordon C, Hanley D, Heaney R, Weaver C. Evaluation, treatment and prevention of vitamin D deficiency: an Endocrine Society clinical practice guideline. J Clin Endocrinol Metab. 2011 Jul;96(7):1911-30. [PMID: 21646368]

Item 47   Answer: A

Educational Objective: Manage diabetes mellitus in a hospitalized patient.

The most appropriate treatment for this patient's diabetes mellitus while hospitalized is a weight-based treatment plan that includes basal and prandial insulin. Hyperglycemia in the hospital is associated with poor outcomes. According to the American Diabetes Association and American Association of Clinical Endocrinologists, glucose goals in hospitalized patients in a non-ICU setting are premeal values less than 140 mg/dL (7.8 mmol/L) and random values less than 180 mg/dL (10 mmol/L). The American College of Physicians recommends avoiding values less than 140 mg/dL (7.8 mmol/L) to decrease the risk of hypoglycemic complications. The patient's plasma glucose values exceed the recommended guidelines and require treatment.

Oral agents do not have safety or efficacy data for use in the hospital. Glipizide is an insulin secretagogue that can potentially induce hypoglycemia in the hospital setting, particularly with unpredictable changes in oral intake.

With metformin use, hospitalized patients can develop poor organ perfusion, which can increase the risk of lactic acidosis. Intravenous contrast dye can also impair kidney function in the setting of metformin use in the hospital. Reinitiation of the patient's home regimen of metformin at or near the time of discharge is most appropriate after all procedures have been completed and organ function is stable and glucose levels have returned to baseline values.

Sliding-scale insulin is nonphysiologic and can result in large fluctuations in blood glucose levels. Sliding-scale insulin is not recommended as the sole insulin therapy in the hospital setting.

KEY POINT

- For non-critically ill hospitalized patients with diabetes mellitus and hyperglycemia, a weight-based treatment plan that includes basal and prandial insulin is recommended.

Bibliography

American Diabetes Association. (13) Diabetes care in the hospital, nursing home, and skilled nursing facility. In: Standards of Medical Care in Diabetes-2015. Diabetes Care. 2015 Jan;38 Suppl:S80-5. [PMID: 25537715]

Item 48   Answer: B

Educational Objective: Diagnose Cushing syndrome.

The most appropriate next diagnostic test for this patient is the 1-mg dexamethasone suppression test. She has the typical clinical features and findings of cortisol excess, or Cushing syndrome. The most common cause of Cushing syndrome is exogeneous glucocorticoid use; however, she has not received glucocorticoids. To evaluate for Cushing syndrome, biochemical evidence of hypercortisolism must be confirmed by use of several screening tests. Three screening tests are used for Cushing syndrome: the 1-mg dexamethasone suppression test (given late at night with assessment of cortisol suppression the next morning), 24-hour urine free cortisol excretion (to quantify total daily cortisol secretion), and measurement of evening salivary cortisol (which normally reaches a nadir at that time but remains elevated in patients with Cushing syndrome). At least two abnormal first-line screening tests are required for diagnosis. Only after establishing biochemical hypercortisolism should the source of excess cortisol production be sought.

Measurement of adrenocorticotropic hormone (ACTH) is not a screening test for Cushing syndrome. After documentation of excess cortisol production, ACTH levels may be useful in determining if hypercortisolism is ACTH-dependent or –independent; however, it is not an appropriate initial screening test.

An 8-mg dexamethasone suppression test is helpful in differentiating between Cushing disease (pituitary tumor-secreting ACTH) and ectopic ACTH production. However, it is not a screening test for Cushing syndrome and would be appropriate only in specific situations after Cushing syndrome is diagnosed.

A pituitary MRI should be ordered only after hypercortisolism and Cushing syndrome are diagnosed and a pituitary adenoma is suspected as a cause.

Measurement of serum cortisol levels lacks sensitivity and specificity for diagnosing Cushing syndrome, primarily due to the pulsatile nature of cortisol secretion, and is not used as a screening test.

KEY POINT

- To screen for Cushing syndrome, biochemical evidence of hypercortisolism must be confirmed by a 1-mg dexamethasone suppression test, 24-hour urine free cortisol testing, and/or measurement of evening salivary cortisol levels.

Bibliography

Nieman LK, Biller BMK, Findling JW, et al. The diagnosis of Cushing's syndrome: An Endocrine Society clinical practice guideline. J Clin Endocrinol Metab. 2008 May;93(5):1526-40. [PMID: 18334580]

Item 49   Answer: A

Educational Objective: Treat an obese patient with type 2 diabetes mellitus with bariatric surgery.

Patients with a BMI between 35 and 40 with one or more complications associated with obesity should be considered for bariatric surgery, with the goal of significant weight loss and improvement in metabolic abnormalities. This obese patient has type 2 diabetes mellitus with advanced microvascular disease along with other complications associated with obesity including hypertension, hyperlipidemia, obstructive sleep apnea, gastroesophageal acid reflux disease, and osteoarthritis. His attempts at lifestyle management with diet and exercise did not result in weight loss that substantially improved his metabolic abnormalities or obesity.

Increasing the insulin doses could potentially exacerbate the weekly hypoglycemic events occurring in a patient with hypoglycemic unawareness. This could also lead to more weight gain due to frequent treatments of hypoglycemia.

Metformin is contraindicated in men with a serum creatinine level above 1.5 mg/dL (132.6 µmol/L) due to the possibility of lactic acidosis and will not address the underlying problem of obesity.

Pramlintide slows gastric emptying, which can decrease appetite. The weight loss associated with the use of pramlintide is modest, and it may not be sufficient to improve the metabolic abnormalities and obesity-related complications in this patient. In addition, the patient's hypoglycemia may be exacerbated by pramlintide.

KEY POINT

- Obese persons (BMI between 35 and 40) with type 2 diabetes mellitus and associated complications should be considered for bariatric surgery.

Bibliography

Mechanick JI, Youdim A, Jones DB, et al. Clinical practice guidelines for the perioperative nutritional, metabolic, and nonsurgical support of the bariatric surgery patient-2013 update: cosponsored by American Association of Clinical Endocrinologists, The Obesity Society, and American Society for Metabolic & Bariatric Surgery. Endocr Pract. 2013 Mar-Apr;19(2):337-72. [PMID: 23529351]

Item 50   Answer: D

Educational Objective: Diagnose an incidentally noted adrenal mass.

The most appropriate next step in management is to evaluate for pheochromocytoma, preferably by measurement of plasma free metanephrines in this patient. Approximately 10% to 15% of incidentally discovered adrenal masses are functional, although most have no overt clinical manifestations. Therefore, all patients with an incidentally noted adrenal mass should be evaluated for the autonomous secretion of cortisol and catecholamines, and those with hypertension should also undergo testing for primary hyperaldosteronism. The low-dose dexamethasone suppression test should be performed to evaluate for subclinical Cushing syndrome given its superior sensitivity compared with other screening tests (24-hour urine free cortisol and late-night salivary cortisol); this test was negative in this patient. Measurement of 24-hour urine metanephrines and catecholamines is the usual first test in most asymptomatic patients to evaluate for catecholamine hypersecretion, although in those with imaging suggestive of pheochromocytoma, measurement of plasma free metanephrines is the preferred study because of its very high sensitivity and high negative predictive value for a normal study. Imaging in this patient reveals a well-circumscribed partially cystic lesion with high attenuation on noncontrast CT scan, which is in keeping with a pheochromocytoma and is not typical of an adrenocortical adenoma, which characteristically has low attenuation on CT scan (density <10 Hounsfield units) due to relatively high lipid content.

Management of an adrenal incidentaloma depends on its size, imaging characteristics (phenotype), and hormonal functioning. Almost all adrenal tumors that are overtly functional are larger than 6 cm in size or have unfavorable imaging characteristics should be considered for surgical removal. However, biopsy or surgical resection of any adrenal mass prior to ruling out a pheochromocytoma is not recommended, as any manipulation of a catecholamine-secreting tumor without appropriate preoperative management can precipitate a hypertensive crisis.

Measurement of the plasma aldosterone to plasma renin ratio is indicated as part of the evaluation of an incidentally discovered adrenal mass in a patient with hypertension, but not in this individual who has normal blood pressure.

Not performing additional testing may miss a subclinical pheochromocytoma and would therefore not be an appropriate next step in management.

KEY POINT

- A patient with an incidentally noted adrenal mass should undergo biochemical testing for subclinical Cushing syndrome and pheochromocytoma, and those with hypertension should also be evaluated for primary hyperaldosteronism.

Bibliography

Arnaldi G, Boscaro M. Adrenal incidentaloma. Best Pract Res Clin Endocrinol Metab. 2012; 26:405-419. [PMID: 22863384]

Answers and Critiques

Item 51   Answer: D

Educational Objective: Manage the limitations of hemoglobin A$_{1c}$ measurements in a patient with diabetes mellitus and chronic kidney disease.

This patient should measure his postprandial glucose level. The hemoglobin A$_{1c}$ measurement is not always reliable in the setting of chronic kidney disease; thus fingerstick blood glucose measurements should be closely evaluated to help guide therapy. This patient's slightly elevated fasting and premeal blood glucose values may be indicative of postprandial hyperglycemia that could be detected with postprandial glucose measurements and used to guide therapy. For patients trying to achieve hemoglobin A$_{1c}$ levels less than 7.0%, fasting and premeal glucose targets usually are set at approximately 80 to 130 mg/dL (4.4-7.2 mmol/L). This patient's slightly out of range fasting and premeal glucose measurements seem at odds with the recent drop in his hemoglobin A$_{1c}$ level to 6.2%. Specific scenarios unique to end-stage kidney disease can affect the accuracy of the hemoglobin A$_{1c}$ measurement. Hemoglobin A$_{1c}$ can be falsely elevated in the setting of chronic kidney disease due to carbamylated hemoglobin secondary to uremia interfering with some of the assays. Hemoglobin A$_{1c}$ can be falsely decreased in the setting of a reduced erythrocyte lifespan, iron deficiency, blood transfusions, and increased erythropoiesis with erythropoietin use. In this patient, the fingerstick blood glucose measurements do not correlate with the most recent hemoglobin A$_{1c}$ after initiation of erythropoietin. The hemoglobin A$_{1c}$ value is falsely decreased after erythropoietin therapy as a result of a change in the proportion of young and old erythrocytes and a change in the rate of glycation.

The patient's fingerstick blood glucose values are elevated, which further increases risk for microvascular and macrovascular damage. The current regimen should be adjusted to decrease hyperglycemia.

Decreasing the insulin detemir dose would increase hyperglycemia based on daily blood glucose data provided by the patient.

Discontinuation of the preprandial insulin glulisine based on the falsely decreased hemoglobin A$_{1c}$ level would increase the hyperglycemia noted in the fingerstick blood glucose values.

KEY POINT

- End-stage kidney disease in patients with diabetes mellitus can affect the accuracy of the hemoglobin A$_{1c}$ measurement, which should not be used to guide therapy.

Bibliography
Ng JM, Cooke M, Bhandari S, et al. The effect of iron and erythropoietin treatment on the A1c of patients with diabetes and chronic kidney disease. Diabetes Care. 2010 Nov;33(11):2310-3. [PMID: 20798337]

Item 52   Answer: A

Educational Objective: Diagnose an androgen-producing adrenal tumor.

The most appropriate diagnostic test to perform next is an abdominal CT scan to confirm the diagnosis of an androgen-producing adrenal tumor. Approximately 50% of androgen-producing adrenal tumors are benign adenomas, while the other half are malignant. Symptoms are usually minimal or absent in adult men. Women typically present with rapidly progressive signs and symptoms of androgen excess, including acne, hirsutism, and virilization (deepening of the voice, clitoromegaly, and male-pattern hair loss), and may also have irregular menses. In patients with clinical evidence of hyperandrogenism, biochemical testing is performed prior to imaging and should include measurement of serum testosterone and dehydroepiandrosterone sulfate (DHEAS), an adrenal androgen. This patient's biochemical evaluation has revealed marked elevation of DHEAS and mild elevation of testosterone, making an androgen-producing adrenal tumor the most likely diagnosis. DHEAS levels above 8 µg/mL (21.6 µmol/L) are diagnostic of an androgen-producing adrenal tumor. The elevated serum testosterone level seen in this patient is likely a consequence of the peripheral metabolism of adrenal androgens to testosterone. The serum testosterone level would be more than 150 to 200 ng/dL (5.2-6.9 nmol/L) in the setting of an androgen-producing ovarian tumor.

Performing a low-dose dexamethasone suppression test or pituitary MRI is not indicated because Cushing syndrome is unlikely with a normal 24-hour urine free cortisol level and in the absence of specific features of hypercortisolism (facial plethora, violaceous striae, and supraclavicular or dorsocervical fat pads).

Pelvic ultrasound is not an appropriate initial imaging test because the marked elevation of DHEAS makes an androgen-producing adrenal tumor much more likely than an ovarian neoplasm. Although the patient has a family history of polycystic ovary syndrome (PCOS), the tempo and severity of her clinical presentation are not in keeping with this disorder. Although adrenal androgen excess occurs in 30% to 40% of women with PCOS, only a mild elevation of DHEAS (3 µg/mL [8.1 µmol/L]) is expected.

KEY POINT

- In female patients, signs of androgen excess such as progressive hirsutism and virilization over a short period of time suggest the diagnosis of an androgen-producing adrenal or ovarian tumor.

Bibliography
Cavlan D, Bharwani N, Grossman A. Androgen- and estrogen-secreting adrenal cancers. Semin Oncol. 2010 Dec;37(6):638-48. [PMID: 21167382]

Item 53   Answer: A

Educational Objective: Manage diabetes mellitus with continuous glucose monitoring.

There is a discrepancy between this patient's fingerstick blood glucose values and her hemoglobin A$_{1c}$ values that can be quickly reconciled with a 72-hour continuous blood glucose monitoring system. Continuous blood glucose monitoring systems use an electrochemical enzymatic sensor to measure the glucose content of interstitial fluid via insertion of a subcutaneous needle. In some systems data recording can be made available in real time to the patient, whereas other models store the data for later access and analysis. Since she does not have kidney disease or anemia that could affect the accuracy of hemoglobin A_{1c} measurements, she likely has episodes of hyperglycemia not detected by her current monitoring efforts. Fingerstick blood glucose values only provide a small snapshot of the glucose variability that occurs throughout the day. Undetected hyperglycemia or hypoglycemia can lead to significant differences between the fingerstick blood glucose values and the expected hemoglobin A_{1c} level. Her wide range of fasting blood glucose values could be indicative of undetected overnight hypoglycemia. Intermittent continuous glucose monitoring is recommended when postprandial hyperglycemia, dawn phenomenon, or overnight hypoglycemia is suspected.

Lifestyle modifications are recommended for glycemic management; however, because this patient exercises in the evening, overnight hypoglycemia should be considered and evaluated with continuous glucose monitoring. Additional exercise may exacerbate the hypoglycemia.

This patient does not have evidence of postprandial hyperglycemia on her fingerstick blood glucose measurements, although it could be missed since she only measures after her meals periodically. Given the discrepancy in her blood glucose values and A_{1c} level, hypoglycemia should be ruled out first before increasing her insulin doses that may increase the risk of hypoglycemia.

KEY POINT

- Continuous glucose monitoring may be useful in persons with postprandial hyperglycemia, dawn phenomenon, or overnight hypoglycemia.

Bibliography

Klonoff DC, Buckingham B, Christiansen JS, et al. Continuous glucose monitoring: An Endocrine Society Clinical Practice Guideline. J Clin Endocrinol Metab. 2011; Oct;96(10):2968-2979. [PMID: 21976745]

Item 54   Answer: A

Educational Objective: Treat irregular menses and hirsutism in a patient with polycystic ovary syndrome.

The most appropriate treatment is combined oral contraceptive pills. Hirsutism is present in approximately 70% of women with polycystic ovary syndrome (PCOS). The combined oral contraceptive pill is the optimal treatment to address both this patient's concerns of menstrual irregularity and hirsutism. The estrogen component increases hepatic production of sex hormone–binding globulin, decreasing the patient's circulating free testosterone level. For women in whom hirsutism is a major concern, treatment is focused on reducing androgen production, decreasing the fraction of circulating free testosterone, and limiting androgen bioactivity to hair follicles. Coarse, thick hairs that are already noted on examination will need to be removed with a depilatory method; however,

terminal hair growth will be slowed with combined oral contraceptive use. Oral contraceptives that contain 30 to 35 µg of ethinyl estradiol appear to be more effective in managing hirsutism than formulations containing less ethinyl estradiol. Six months of treatment is considered the minimal interval in which to determine the level of response. Adherence to an oral contraceptive regimen will provide this patient with predictable menses as well as contraceptive benefit. In addition, the risk of endometrial hyperplasia is diminished.

Intermittent progesterone withdrawal, although effective for decreasing the risk of endometrial hyperplasia, would have no effect on this patient's concern regarding hirsutism.

The levonorgestrel intrauterine system is a long-acting, reversible contraceptive device that diminishes long-term risk of endometrial hyperplasia in patients with PCOS; however, it provides no benefit for hirsutism and has no effect on androgen production.

Spironolactone is a potent antiandrogen and is very effective against male-pattern hirsutism in patients with PCOS. However, it offers no benefit for control of the menstrual cycle. When spironolactone is prescribed, patients should be counseled regarding the potential teratogenicity in male fetuses, and a concurrent reliable contraceptive method should be established to prevent fetal exposure. Pregnancy can still occur in patients with oligo-ovulatory PCOS, and reliance on menstrual irregularity is not a substitute for a more proven contraceptive plan.

KEY POINT

- The combined oral contraceptive pill is the optimal treatment to address both irregular menses and hirsutism in patients with polycystic ovary syndrome.

Bibliography

Amsterdam ESHRE/ASRM-Sponsored 3rd PCOS Consensus Workshop Group. Consensus on women's health aspects of polycystic ovary syndrome (PCOS). Hum Reprod. 2012 Jan;27(1):14-24. [PMID: 22147920]

Item 55   Answer: C

Educational Objective: Manage a patient with pheochromocytoma.

The most appropriate next step in management is to begin treatment with an α-adrenoceptor antagonist, such as phenoxybenzamine. The purpose of preoperative α-blockade is to provide blood pressure control and decrease the risk of cardiovascular complications related to excessive catecholamine release during intraoperative manipulation of the tumor. Most patients are treated for 1 to 2 weeks before surgery with phenoxybenzamine with upward titration based on blood pressure. The target blood pressure is below 130/80 mm Hg seated and greater than 90 mm Hg (systolic) standing. Because of phenoxybenzamine's side effects including orthostasis, nasal stuffiness, fatigue, and retrograde ejaculation, some clinicians use short-acting specific α-antagonists, such as prazosin, doxazosin, or terazosin. In patients with tachycardia, β-blockers can be added after α-blockade is achieved. Labetalol, a combined α- and β-blocking agent, also can be used, especially in patients with tachyarrhythmias. A heart rate of 60 to 70/min seated and 70 to 80/min standing can be targeted in most patients. Patients with pheochromocytoma who are normotensive also should be treated with α-blockers because they often become hypertensive during surgical resection.

Increasing the dosage of lisinopril does not address the need for preoperative pharmacologic management of the patient's pheochromocytoma with α-blockade.

Although indicated for tumor localization following the biochemical diagnosis of pheochromocytoma, a contrast-enhanced adrenal CT scan should not be performed until after an α-adrenoceptor antagonist has been initiated. Administering iodine contrast media to a patient who has not received α-blockade could incite a hypertensive crisis.

Similarly, the β-adrenoceptor antagonist propranolol should not be given prior to α-blockade because unopposed α-adrenoceptor stimulation could also precipitate a hypertensive crisis.

KEY POINT

- In patients with a confirmed diagnosis of pheochromocytoma, α-blockade should be instituted before surgery to reduce the risk of cardiovascular complications and to control blood pressure.

Bibliography

Lenders JW, Duh QY, Eisenhofer G, et al. Pheochromocytoma and paraganglioma: an endocrine society clinical practice guideline. J Clin Endocrinol Metab. 2014 Jun;99(6):1915-42. [PMID: 24893135]

Item 56   Answer: C

Educational Objective: Manage hormone replacement therapy in a patient with panhypopituitarism.

The patient's hypothyroidism is inadequately treated, causing symptoms of fatigue and weight gain and a low free thyroxine (T_4) level. Therefore, his levothyroxine dose should be increased. Patients with secondary hypothyroidism from pituitary dysfunction have low or low-normal thyroid-stimulating hormone (TSH) values which cannot be used to assess the adequacy of thyroid hormone replacement. Because of this, the levothyroxine dose is adjusted based on free T_4 levels instead of TSH values. His free T_4 is low, suggesting inadequate treatment as the likely cause of his symptoms.

The patient's desmopressin dosing is adequate to treat his diabetes insipidus. His symptoms are well controlled without evidence of excessive urination, and his serum sodium level is normal. In addition, increasing the dose would risk potentially causing water retention and hyponatremia.

He is on a physiologic dose of hydrocortisone. Hydrocortisone dose is not adjusted based on laboratory test results because his endogenous adrenocorticotropic hormone (ACTH) and cortisol levels will remain low on adequate therapy and are therefore not used to alter therapy. Instead,

hydrocortisone is adjusted based on symptoms, such as orthostasis, weight loss, nausea, vomiting, and lightheadedness. He does not have these symptoms, so his cortisol deficiency is adequately treated. Increasing his hydrocortisone to higher than necessary doses increases the risk of iatrogenic Cushing syndrome and glucocorticoid-induced osteoporosis.

His testosterone value is normal, and he has normal morning erections. These are two signs that his hypogonadism is adequately treated. Possibly, his erectile dysfunction is a result of fatigue from hypothyroidism or is functional instead of physiologic.

There is no reason to stop somatropin. He has no evidence of residual tumor. Growth hormone (GH) replacement can improve lean mass distribution and quality of life in a patient with true GH deficiency, so it is reasonable to continue. Discontinuing GH will likely worsen his fatigue.

KEY POINT

- Patients with secondary hypothyroidism from pituitary dysfunction have low or low-normal thyroid-stimulating hormone values, so levothyroxine dose should be adjusted based on free thyroxine (T_4) level.

Bibliography

Schneider HJ, Aimaretti G, Kreitschmann-Andermahr, et al. Hypopituitarism. Lancet. 2007 Apr 28;369(9571):1461-70. [PMID: 17467517]

Item 57   Answer: A

Educational Objective: Diagnose type 2 diabetes mellitus.

A fasting plasma glucose measurement is the most appropriate diagnostic test for this patient. Diabetes mellitus can be diagnosed with an abnormal result of one screening test performed on two separate occasions. Although the hemoglobin A_{1c} is normal in this patient, the fasting plasma glucose is abnormally elevated within the diagnostic range for diabetes mellitus. When discrepant results occur among different screening tests for diabetes, the American Diabetes Association recommends repeating the abnormal screening test. If the repeat fasting plasma glucose measurement is abnormal, the diagnosis of diabetes is confirmed. Screening for type 2 diabetes should begin in all asymptomatic patients at age 45 years. In adult patients with a BMI greater than or equal to 25, screening should occur at any age if one or more additional risk factors for diabetes is present.

Use of the hemoglobin A_{1c} as an initial screening test in this patient is appropriate as there is no evidence for anemia or kidney or liver disease that could decrease the reliability of the test. The value was normal and does not warrant a repeat measurement as the next diagnostic test to perform in this scenario.

A 2-hour 75-g oral glucose tolerance test can be used as a screening tool for diagnosing diabetes. Since this test was not initially used for screening in this patient, it is most appropriate to repeat the abnormal screening test (fasting plasma glucose) that was already used for comparison.

A random blood glucose measurement would be useful in this patient if he presented with classic hyperglycemic symptoms in the setting of a blood glucose level of 200 mg/dL (11.1 mmol/L) or above, as that would be diagnostic of diabetes. This patient is not symptomatic.

KEY POINT

- When discrepant results occur among different screening tests for diabetes mellitus, the American Diabetes Association recommends repeating the abnormal screening test.

Bibliography
American Diabetes Association. (2) Classification and diagnosis of diabetes. In: Standards of Medical Care in Diabetes-2015. Diabetes Care. 2015;38 Suppl 1:S8-16. [PMID: 25537714]

Item 58   Answer: A

Educational Objective: Diagnose Klinefelter syndrome.

The most appropriate diagnostic test to perform next is a karyotype. This patient has evidence of hypergonadotropic hypogonadism based on elevated gonadotropin levels and low testosterone level. Klinefelter syndrome is a common cause of hypergonadotropic hypogonadism and azoospermia, resulting in infertility. A 47,XXY karyotype is diagnostic of Klinefelter syndrome. Mosaic variants of this condition exist but typically present with oligoasthenospermia, testicular failure, or hypogonadism. Concomitant symptoms often include sexual dysfunction and generalized fatigue. Tall stature is a common finding. Patients with Klinefelter syndrome may fail to achieve puberty or may present after sexual maturation with azoospermia. Fertility may be achieved from ejaculated sperm, if present, or extracted testicular sperm; however, advanced reproductive techniques such as in vitro fertilization and intracytoplasmic sperm injection are necessary to achieve pregnancy. Some couples may opt to include genetic testing by preimplantation genetic diagnosis and embryo biopsy to avoid transmission of the disorder to subsequent generations. Typically, gonadotropin levels are high in patients with Klinefelter syndrome, representing testicular hypofunction. After plans for conception are completed, supplementation with exogenous androgens may be considered to prevent osteoporosis. Conception with donor sperm is an alternative fertility treatment option.

MRI of the pituitary would be needed only to rule out a pituitary mass in the setting of hypogonadotropic hypogonadism. Because this patient's gonadotropin levels are high, a pituitary mass is unlikely.

Scrotal ultrasound would identify small testicles in a patient with suspected Klinefelter syndrome, but it would not identify the cause of this patient's elevated gonadotropin levels.

Serum prolactin level would likely be normal, as Klinefelter syndrome is characterized by primary hypogo-

nadism with normal prolactin levels. Therefore, measurement of serum prolactin is not the most useful test for this patient.

KEY POINT

- Klinefelter syndrome is a common cause of hypergonadotropic hypogonadism and azoospermia.

Bibliography
Krausz C, Chianese C. Genetic testing and counselling for male infertility. Curr Opin Endocrinol Diabetes Obes. 2014 Jun;21(3):244-50. [PMID: 24739313]

Item 59   Answer: D

Educational Objective: Interpret thyroid function test results in an elderly patient.

Clinical follow-up with repeat measurement of thyroid-stimulating hormone (TSH) and free thyroxine (T_4) is the most appropriate management for this patient. In persons over 80 years of age, the serum TSH level may be mildly elevated above the typical reference range for younger adults. The upper limit of the normal range in this elderly population without thyroid dysfunction may be as high as 8.0 µU/mL (8.0 mU/L). Since this patient's TSH level is 6.4 µU/mL (6.4 mU/L), his clinical symptoms are nonspecific, and his physical examination is normal, additional evaluation or treatment is not indicated at this time. However, his clinical symptoms should be monitored, and his serum TSH and free T_4 levels should be measured repeatedly several times over a period of months to ensure that the TSH value is not part of a trend to the development of overt thyroid dysfunction.

Because this patient's serum free T_4 level is normal and a diagnosis of hypothyroidism has not been established, he does not require levothyroxine therapy.

Measurement of the serum total triiodothyronine (T_3) level is not typically helpful in diagnosing hypothyroidism because total T_3 levels may remain within the normal range well into the evolution of hypothyroidism. However, total T_3 levels are useful in evaluating patients with possible hyperthyroidism because the value may be elevated out of proportion to the T_4 level, and failure to recognize an elevated T_3 value may underestimate the degree of hyperthyroidism present.

Total T_4 measures both the bound and unbound thyroid hormone fractions, whereas the free T_4 reflects the unbound portion of hormone, and may more accurately reflect available hormone levels in patients who may have an abnormality in protein metabolism (such as liver or kidney disease). However, measurement of total T_4 in addition to free T_4 would not provide additional diagnostic information in this patient.

KEY POINT

- In patients over 80 years of age, the serum thyroid-stimulating hormone level may be mildly elevated above the typical reference range.

Bibliography
Tabatabaie V, Surks MI. The aging thyroid. Curr Opin Endocrinol Diabetes Obes. 2013 Oct;20(5):455-9. [PMID: 23974775]

Item 60   Answer: B

Educational Objective: Evaluate an incidentally noted adrenal mass.

The most appropriate diagnostic test to perform next is the low-dose dexamethasone suppression test to screen for the autonomous secretion of cortisol. The increasing use of imaging studies for various medical indications has revealed otherwise unrecognized adrenal masses in less than 1% of the population younger than 30 years and up to 7% of those older than 70 years. Ten to 15% of adrenal incidentalomas are functional, although most have no overt clinical manifestations. Therefore, testing is usually necessary to identify functional tumors secreting catecholamines, cortisol, or aldosterone. Of the functional adenomas, most secrete excessive amounts of cortisol. In subclinical Cushing syndrome (CS), classic signs or symptoms of cortisol excess are not observed; however, complications of long-standing hypercortisolism may result. The patient has two disorders that can be seen in association with subclinical CS: type 2 diabetes mellitus and osteoporosis. Obesity and hypertension are also common. The low-dose overnight dexamethasone suppression test is recommended as the initial screening test for this condition due to its high sensitivity. Screening for pheochromocytoma, such as by measuring 24-hour urine fractionated metanephrines and catecholamines, is also indicated in all patients with an incidentally noted adrenal mass.

Adrenal vein sampling (AVS) is not needed. AVS is most often performed to evaluate for a bilateral versus unilateral adrenal cause of primary hyperaldosteronism.

Measurement of plasma renin activity and aldosterone concentration is not indicated in patients without hypertension.

No further testing is also inappropriate. Although the imaging characteristics of the mass are in keeping with a benign adrenal adenoma, further diagnostic evaluation is needed. This includes testing for autonomous hormonal secretion and subsequent radiographic surveillance (first at 3-6 months and then annually for 1-2 years).

KEY POINT

- Ten to 15% of adrenal incidentalomas are functional; biochemical testing is needed to identify functional tumors secreting catecholamines, cortisol, or aldosterone.

Bibliography

Zeiger MA, Thompson GB, Duh QY, et al. The American Association of Clinical Endocrinologists and American Association of Endocrine Surgeons medical guidelines for the management of adrenal incidentalomas. Endocr Pract. 2009 Jul-Aug;15 Suppl 1:1-20. [PMID: 19632967]

Item 61   Answer: E

Educational Objective: Treat acromegaly with transsphenoidal pituitary surgery.

Transsphenoidal resection of the pituitary adenoma is the initial treatment of choice in patients with acromegaly. It is also the only treatment that is potentially curative. Because this patient's tumor is invading the left cavernous sinus and compressing the optic chiasm, complete resection will likely not be possible; however, surgery can effectively debulk the tumor and preserve vision in addition to significantly decreasing growth hormone (GH) secretion as measured by insulin-like growth factor 1 (IGF-1) levels. In patients in whom complete resection is not possible, such as this patient, additional therapy may be required such as stereotactic radiation therapy or medical therapy to inhibit GH secretion or block its effect on the tissues. However, surgical resection remains an essential first step in the treatment of acromegaly.

A small number of GH-secreting pituitary adenomas co-secrete prolactin. Although dopamine agonist therapy with agents such as bromocriptine would treat the associated prolactin elevation, it is minimally effective in acromegaly and would not adequately treat GH secretion or address the mass effect of a GH-secreting adenoma.

A GH receptor blocker, pegvisomant, is available. Pegvisomant works in the peripheral tissues as an antagonist to GH but does not decrease its production by the tumor. This patient needs intervention to treat mass effect at this time because the tumor is damaging the optic chiasm and the patient's vision, and this treatment would not be expected to decrease the tumor size.

Somatostatin analogues, such as octreotide and lanreotide, inhibit GH secretion and are helpful in treating some patients with acromegaly. They are used primarily in patients with unresectable tumors without significant mass effect or those with a contraindication to surgery. They may also be used in patients with continued GH secretion following incomplete transsphenoidal resection. However, they would not be an appropriate treatment in this patient with a large, invasive, vision-threatening pituitary tumor.

Radiation therapy may be added to surgical or medical therapy to help increase the chance for remission or cure. Radiation to the pituitary carries a high risk of causing pituitary insufficiency and damage to surrounding tissues (particularly the optic nerves); therefore, it is not usually an initial treatment for acromegaly in most patients. In those in whom it is used, stereotactic surgery (gamma knife) is the preferred approach to minimize potential complications.

KEY POINT

- The primary therapy for acromegaly is transsphenoidal surgery to remove the causative growth hormone-secreting pituitary adenoma.

Bibliography

Melmed, S. Acromegaly pathogenesis and treatment. J Clin Invest. 2009 Nov;119:3189-202. [PMID: 19884662]

Item 62   Answer: C

Educational Objective: Treat high-risk thyroid cancer postoperatively.

Radioactive iodine (RAI) therapy is the most appropriate postoperative treatment in this patient who is at high risk of cancer recurrence based on his age, the size of the primary tumor, the presence of vascular invasion and extrathyroidal extension, and the number of involved lymph nodes. He therefore may benefit from adjuvant RAI therapy, which may decrease the likelihood of recurrent disease in patients with nodal metastases. This is given in conjunction with levothyroxine suppression therapy, which is indicated in all patients who have had a total thyroidectomy. Because of his high-risk disease, it would be appropriate to lower the thyroid-stimulating hormone level to less than 0.1 µU/mL (0.1 mU/L) in the absence of contraindications such as pre-existing cardiovascular disease or age greater than 65 years.

Traditional chemotherapeutic agents, such as doxorubicin, are generally ineffective in the management of differentiated thyroid cancer and would not be indicated for this patient. In patients with anaplastic carcinoma of the thyroid, however, some studies have demonstrated a possible benefit with concomitant use of paclitaxel-based chemotherapy and external-beam radiotherapy. This patient has classic papillary thyroid cancer histology and would not benefit from such treatment.

External-beam radiotherapy is rarely used in patients with differentiated thyroid cancer. An exception would be the management of patients with inoperable disease that threatens to cause local extension into vital structures in the neck such as the trachea, esophagus, or major blood vessels.

Because of the extent of disease found at surgery and this patient's high risk of recurrence, providing no additional therapy would not be an appropriate next step in management.

KEY POINT

- A patient who has undergone total thyroidectomy for thyroid cancer and is at high risk for disease recurrence should receive adjuvant radioactive iodine therapy.

Bibliography

Jonklaas J, Sarlis NJ, Litofsky D, et al. Outcomes of patients with differentiated thyroid carcinoma following initial therapy. Thyroid. 2006 Dec;16(12):1229-42. [PMID: 17199433]

Item 63   Answer: C

Educational Objective: Manage acquired type 1 diabetes mellitus.

This patient has an acquired form of type 1 diabetes mellitus caused by chronic pancreatitis (pancreoprivic diabetes), which necessitates the use of insulin for treatment of the hyperglycemia. Chronic pancreatitis results in permanent destruction of the pancreas and may impair both the endocrine and exocrine functions of the pancreas. The pancreatic exocrine abnormalities arise from loss of the pancreatic enzymes required for digestion and absorption of food. The pancreatic endocrine abnormalities can present in a similar manner as type 1 diabetes with hyperglycemia from insulin deficiency secondary to destruction of beta cells. Therefore

insulin is the recommended treatment. Unlike autoimmune type 1 diabetes, chronic pancreatitis also destroys the pancreatic alpha cells causing a glucagon deficiency that increases the risk of spontaneous hypoglycemia. Glucagon acts on the liver to increase glucose production through glycogenolysis and gluconeogenesis. The recovery from hypoglycemia is also impaired with alpha cell destruction. Early recognition of hypoglycemic symptoms and strategic hypoglycemic treatment plans should be emphasized with patients with pancreoprivic diabetes.

Exenatide, a glucagon-like protein-1 (GLP-1) mimetic, suppresses glucagon and promotes insulin secretion. The pancreatic beta cell and alpha cell destruction associated with chronic pancreatitis precludes this treatment option. Postmarketing reports of pancreatitis are also cause for concern for the use of this class of medication in patients with a history of pancreatitis.

The sulfonylurea glipizide increases insulin secretion. The effect would likely be minimal to nonexistent in this patient with hyperglycemia resulting from substantial beta cell destruction from chronic pancreatitis.

Metformin decreases hepatic glucose output by inhibiting gluconeogenesis and increases insulin-mediated glucose utilization in peripheral tissues. Metformin is a first-line agent for initial treatment of type 2 diabetes; however, this patient has an insulin deficiency from pancreatic beta cell destruction and should be treated as a patient with type 1 diabetes.

KEY POINT

- Hyperglycemia caused by chronic pancreatitis is an acquired form of type 1 diabetes mellitus and should be treated with insulin.

Bibliography

Mergener K, Baillie J. Chronic pancreatitis. Lancet. 1997 Nov 8;350(9088):1379-85. [PMID: 9365465]

Item 64   Answer: A

Educational Objective: Treat infertility related to polycystic ovary syndrome.

The most appropriate treatment is a selective estrogen receptor modulator (SERM) such as clomiphene citrate. SERMs are the established first-line treatment for ovulation induction in anovulatory patients with infertility from polycystic ovary syndrome (PCOS). Typically, therapy is started after menses and is given orally for 5 days. Common side effects include vasomotor symptoms and mood changes. Escalating doses of clomiphene are typically prescribed if a patient does not ovulate on lower doses. More recently, evidence suggests the effectiveness and possible superiority of aromatase inhibitor therapy (such as with letrozole) in women with PCOS for ovulation induction. However, this therapy is not currently FDA approved for this indication.

A small subset of patients with PCOS may require in vitro fertilization, but this therapy is typically explored only after several failed cycles of ovulation induction with clomiphene citrate.

In patients with clomiphene resistance, gonadotropin therapy would be an appropriate next step; however, caution is warranted because higher-order multiple gestation may result.

A 2012 Cochrane review of the effect of insulin-sensitizing drugs in women with infertility and PCOS included 44 trials, the majority of which involved metformin. Rates of pregnancy were improved with metformin compared with placebo and metformin plus clomiphene compared with clomiphene alone, but metformin did not change rates of live births compared with placebo or with clomiphene compared to clomiphene alone.

KEY POINT

- Selective estrogen receptor modulators such as clomiphene citrate are the established first-line treatment for ovulation induction in anovulatory patients with infertility from polycystic ovary syndrome.

Bibliography

Legro RS, Brzyski RG, Diamond MP, et al; NICHD Reproductive Medicine Network. Letrozole versus clomiphene for infertility in the polycystic ovary syndrome. N Engl J Med. 2014 Jul 10;371(2):119-29. Erratum in: N Engl J Med. 2014 Oct 9;317(15):1465. [PMID: 25006718]

Item 65   Answer: C

Educational Objective: Treat a microprolactinoma in a postmenopausal woman.

No therapy is necessary at this time, and the patient should be retested in 12 months. The patient has a microprolactinoma, but she is postmenopausal. Luteinizing hormone and follicle-stimulating hormone levels are normally high in postmenopausal women because of ovarian failure; however, her levels are lower than expected, likely because the elevated prolactin is providing negative feedback. This causes hypogonadism but is not clinically relevant because she is already hypogonadal from normal menopause. She has minimal symptoms from menopause and is tolerating it well.

The prolactinoma was found incidentally. On MRI, it has no concerning features, and her other pituitary hormone levels are normal. Although no treatment is necessary for this asymptomatic patient, it is advisable to retest in 6 to 12 months to make sure that the tumor does not grow.

Dopamine agonists, such as cabergoline, are used to treat symptomatic prolactinomas, but it is not necessary in this asymptomatic patient.

Radiosurgery is not necessary. It is an option to treat pituitary tumors that are not amenable to standard surgery or cannot be fully resected, but it is not indicated for this asymptomatic patient.

Transsphenoidal resection of the pituitary tumor is overly invasive and unnecessary because she is doing well. In addition, first-line therapy for symptomatic prolactinomas are dopamine agonists, not surgery.

KEY POINT

- Microprolactinomas in asymptomatic patients do not require treatment; however, surveillance is recommended.

Bibliography

Melmed S, Casanueva FF, Hoffman AR, et al. Diagnosis and treatment of hyperprolactinemia: an Endocrine Society clinical practice guideline. J Clin Endocrinol Metab. 2011 Feb;96(2):273-88. [PMID: 21296991]

Item 66   Answer: B

Educational Objective: Manage diabetic neuropathy.

Duloxetine is a reasonable initial option for this patient's painful peripheral neuropathy. The typical presentation for distal symmetric polyneuropathy is a bilateral "stocking-glove" distribution. Damage to the small nerve fibers can result in pain, numbness, burning, and tingling. It can also impair light touch and temperature sensation. Damage to the large nerve fibers leads to abnormal vibration sensation and proprioception. Diminished or loss of ankle reflexes is commonly seen early with diabetic polyneuropathy. Motor weakness can occur as the polyneuropathy progresses. Several classes of drugs are frequently used for symptomatic pain relief, including the tricyclic antidepressants (amitriptyline), other classes of antidepressants (duloxetine, venlafaxine), anticonvulsants (pregabalin, gabapentin, valproate), and capsaicin cream. There are few head-to-head comparison trials for these classes of drugs for distal symmetric polyneuropathy, thus selection must take into consideration the potential risks and benefits associated with each drug for an individual patient. Duloxetine has fewer risks than amitriptyline for this patient given his cardiac history.

Tricyclic antidepressants, such as amitriptyline, should be used cautiously in patients with known cardiac disease due to an association between this class of drugs and arrhythmias, heart block, and sudden death. The patient's history of cardiac disease and a first-degree atrioventricular block may increase his risk of side effects from amitriptyline.

A nerve conduction study is not routinely required for diagnosis or management in patients with diabetes with a typical presentation of symmetric distal polyneuropathy. Atypical clinical features should prompt additional work-up, including electrophysiologic testing.

Vitamin B_{12} deficiency has been associated with long-term use of metformin and can present with peripheral neuropathy. It is also commonly seen in the setting of megaloblastic anemia. It is unlikely that vitamin B_{12} deficiency is the cause of this patient's peripheral neuropathy as he has a classic presentation for symmetric distal polyneuropathy, discontinued metformin 2 years ago, and has a normal complete blood count.

KEY POINT

- Treatment options for diabetic polyneuropathy include the tricyclic antidepressants, other classes of antidepressants (duloxetine, venlafaxine), anticonvulsants (pregabalin, gabapentin, valproate), and capsaicin cream.

Bibliography

American Diabetes Association. (9) Microvascular complications and foot care. In: Standards of Medical Care in Diabetes-2015. Diabetes Care. 2015 Jan;38 Suppl 1:S58-66. [PMID: 25537710]

Item 67   Answer: D

Educational Objective: Evaluate hypoglycemia in a patient without diabetes mellitus.

This patient should undergo a 72-hour fast with hypoglycemic testing at the time of symptomatic hypoglycemia. He had symptomatic hypoglycemia with prolonged fasting (>5 hours) overnight that resolved with glucose administration. Since he is not currently hypoglycemic or symptomatic, fasting is necessary in an attempt to recreate the metabolic scenario that induced the hypoglycemia to allow definitive diagnosis. Glucose and hypoglycemic studies, including measurement of insulin, C-peptide, proinsulin, and β-hydroxybutyrate levels, should be obtained at the beginning of the fast and then repeated every 6 hours until the blood glucose level falls below 60 mg/dL (3.3 mmol/L), at which time they should be repeated every 1 to 2 hours until (1) symptomatic hypoglycemia (≤45 mg/dL [2.5 mmol/L]) occurs, (2) asymptomatic hypoglycemia (≤55 mg/dL [3.0 mmol/L]) occurs with previously documented Whipple triad, or (3) the 72-hour fast concludes. Whipple triad consists of three components: neuroglycopenia, concurrent hypoglycemia, and resolution of symptoms with correction of hypoglycemia.

Hypoglycemic studies are not adequately informative when the patient is not experiencing symptomatic hypoglycemia; therefore, testing now would not be appropriate.

Mixed-meal testing involves ingestion of a meal containing a mixture of protein, fat, and carbohydrates intended to raise the plasma blood glucose to assess the metabolic response to increased glucose. This test is appropriate when symptomatic hypoglycemia occurs within 5 hours after meal consumption (postprandial hypoglycemia). However, this patient's symptomatic hypoglycemia occurred 7 hours after his last meal; therefore, evaluation for postprandial hypoglycemia with a mixed-meal test would not be appropriate.

Oral glucose tolerance testing was previously used to evaluate postprandial hypoglycemia. However, it has not demonstrated effectiveness for this purpose and also would not be an appropriate study for evaluating fasting hypoglycemia.

KEY POINT

- Symptomatic fasting hypoglycemia is best evaluated with glucose and hypoglycemic studies preceding and during a 72-hour fast.

Bibliography

Cryer PE, Axelrod L, Grossman AB, et al. Evaluation and management of adult hypoglycemic disorders: an Endocrine Society Clinical Practice Guideline. J Endocrinol Metab. 2009 Mar;94(3):709-28. [PMID: 19088155]

Item 68   Answer: D

Educational Objective: Diagnose Asherman syndrome with transvaginal ultrasound.

The most appropriate diagnostic test to perform next is a transvaginal ultrasound. This patient has likely developed Asherman syndrome (AS). Because the hormonal evaluation in this patient supports an intact hypothalamic-pituitary-ovarian axis, a structural abnormality such as AS should be suspected. AS is an uncommon complication of dilatation and curettage, intrauterine device placement, or surgical procedures such as hysteroscopic myomectomy; it is caused by lack of basal endometrium proliferation and formation of adhesions (synechiae). Diagnosis should be considered in any woman with amenorrhea and previous exposure to uterine instrumentation. The typical presentation is with secondary amenorrhea, at times associated with cyclic pelvic pain, created by distention of the uterine cavity where pockets of functional endometrium persist but efflux of menstrual flow is blocked or slowed by adhesion formation. Although some patients with AS may be completely amenorrheic, others may demonstrate hypomenorrhea and report scant menses compared with the volume of their menstrual flow before the procedure. AS most commonly occurs in an inflammatory setting such as endometritis or septic abortion. AS may also occur as a result of an overly aggressive curettage. In a patient with AS, transvaginal ultrasound will show a thin endometrial stripe and may reveal small pockets of fluid where menstrual flow has been trapped by neighboring adhesions. A functional uterine examination, such as hysterosalpingogram or saline sonohysterogram, confirms the diagnosis. Treatment consists of hysteroscopic resection of lesions.

Given this patient's normal gonadotropin levels, a pituitary cause for her secondary amenorrhea is unlikely; therefore, imaging of the pituitary is not warranted at this time.

Premature ovarian insufficiency is not the most likely diagnosis given this patient's normal estradiol and gonadotropin levels; therefore, a peripheral karyotype would be expected to be normal and should not be performed.

Results of a progestin withdrawal test are used to delineate between an estrogen-deficient state (no bleeding) and an estrogen-sufficient state (withdrawal bleeding). If the patient is producing estrogen, she will have withdrawal bleeding within 1 week of completing a course of progesterone. If no withdrawal bleeding occurs after the progesterone challenge, then the patient has either a low-estrogen state and hypothalamic amenorrhea is the diagnosis, or there is uterine outflow blockage. This patient's history of a previous uterine procedure prior to the onset of amenorrhea and the possibility of denuded endometrium where synechiae are present will make a negative test (no withdrawal bleeding) uninterpretable.

KEY POINT

- The diagnosis of Asherman syndrome should be considered in any woman with amenorrhea and previous exposure to uterine instrumentation; the classic presentation is with secondary amenorrhea and sometimes cyclic pelvic pain.

Bibliography

Conforti A, Alviggi C, Mollo A, De Placido G, Magos A. The management of Asherman syndrome: a review of literature. Reprod Biol Endocrinol. 2013 Dec 27;11:118. [PMID: 24373209]

Item 69   Answer: C

Educational Objective: Identify postprandial hyperglycemia as a cause of elevated hemoglobin A_{1c} levels.

This patient should measure her postprandial blood glucose level. Given the patient's young age and lack of other major comorbidities, her hemoglobin A_{1c} goal is less than 6.5% to 7.0%. Postprandial hyperglycemia often remains undetected but still contributes to elevated hemoglobin A_{1c} values. The effect is more profound when the hemoglobin A_{1c} is close to 7.0%. Adequate meal-time coverage with insulin can be determined by measuring postprandial blood glucose levels. If her 1- to 2-hour postprandial blood glucose values are elevated above 180 mg/dL (10.0 mmol/L), her meal-time insulin should be increased or the composition of her meals should be altered to decrease her blood glucose. Changing her diet if it is causing postprandial hyperglycemia could eventually lead to lower insulin requirements.

Checking her postprandial blood glucose values first will help identify where the hyperglycemic issue arises that keeps her hemoglobin A_{1c} above goal.

Increasing her glargine dose will not adequately affect postprandial hyperglycemia and may lead to overnight or fasting hypoglycemia.

Overnight glucose abnormalities can be identified with the measurement of a 3 AM blood glucose level. Large fluctuations in fasting blood glucose values or consistent fasting hyperglycemia can be clues to overnight hypoglycemia with subsequent rebound hyperglycemia (Somogyi effect) or hyperglycemia as a result of rising catecholamines (dawn phenomenon). The patient reports stable fasting and preprandial glucose values throughout the day. The most likely timing for glucose abnormalities that would affect her hemoglobin A_{1c} value is in the postprandial state.

Sitagliptin is a dipeptidyl peptidase-4 (DPP-4) inhibitor that slows gastric emptying and suppresses glucagon secretion. Although it has a modest effect on hemoglobin A_{1c} lowering, metformin remains first-line therapy for type 2 diabetes and should be continued as part of her regimen.

KEY POINT

- Monitoring postprandial blood glucose levels can be useful to assess prandial insulin coverage in patients who have type 2 diabetes mellitus with at-goal preprandial readings but with hemoglobin A_{1c} values not at goal.

Bibliography

American Diabetes Association. (7) Approaches to glycemic treatment. In: Standards of Medical Care in Diabetes-2015. Diabetes Care. 2015 Jan;38 Suppl 1:S41-8. [PMID: 25537707]

Item 70   Answer: B

Educational Objective: Treat Graves ophthalmopathy.

Methimazole is most appropriate for this patient with Graves ophthalmopathy (GO). GO may be manifested by lateral gaze palsy, scleral injection, periorbital edema, and pressure sensation behind the eyes. Additional manifestations include proptosis, lid lag, and, if severe, decreased visual acuity. Excess deposition of glycosaminoglycans in the retro-orbital space results in increased pressure; the ensuing compression of the muscles and cranial nerves causes the ocular palsy. Most patients with GO have mild, nonprogressive symptoms that do not require specific treatment. The decision to treat depends upon the severity and activity of the disease. For patients who need treatment, initial therapy should target controlling the hyperthyroidism. Methimazole will rapidly lower circulating thyroid hormone levels, may reduce serum thyroid autoantibody titers, and may assist in controlling GO symptoms. Additional therapy to control symptoms includes use of ocular lubricants and taping of the eyelids at night (if the lids are unable to completely cover the eye). Because cigarette smoking increases the activity of GO and impairs the response to therapy, smoking cessation is of paramount importance.

External-beam radiotherapy is reserved for treatment of severe GO but typically is employed if symptoms persist or worsen in spite of return to the euthyroid state.

Because radioactive iodine (RAI) treatment has been associated with (at least transient) worsening of GO due to an initial increase in circulating antibody levels, its use is not recommended in patients with moderate to severe GO. When RAI is used, pretreatment with a glucocorticoid to mitigate the rise in antibody levels is recommended prior to RAI therapy.

Total thyroidectomy is typically recommended for long-term control of Graves disease in patients with active GO when medical therapy fails to induce a remission. However, returning the patient to a state of euthyroidism is advisable before surgery. Surgical decompression is also an option to control active GO, particularly if there is compression of the optic nerve.

KEY POINT

- Initial treatment of Graves ophthalmopathy is normalization of thyroid function.

Bibliography

Phelps PO, Williams K. Thyroid eye disease for the primary care physician. Dis Mon. 2014 Jun;60(6):292-8. [PMID: 24906675]

Item 71   Answer: B

Educational Objective: Diagnose primary hyperaldosteronism as a cause of secondary hypertension.

The most appropriate diagnostic test to perform next is to measure the plasma aldosterone-plasma renin activity ratio. This patient has resistant hypertension, defined as blood pressure that remains above goal despite concurrent use of three antihypertensive agents of different classes, one of which is a diuretic. Resistant hypertension may occur in as many as 10% of patients with hypertension. Although this patient is being treated with a diuretic, he has significant hypokalemia in the presence of treatment with an ACE inhibitor and potassium supplementation. This raises the possibility of primary hyperaldosteronism as a cause or contributing factor of his resistant hypertension. Appropriate initial evaluation for this diagnosis is measurement of the plasma aldosterone-plasma renin activity ratio. If positive, confirmatory testing is usually accomplished with intravenous salt loading, fludrocortisone suppression testing, or captopril testing. If confirmed, adrenal imaging is indicated to determine if hyperaldosteronism is due to a bilateral or unilateral cause. Mineralocorticoid receptor antagonists (such as spironolactone) are indicated for patients with a bilateral cause of primary hyperaldosteronism and those with a unilateral cause who refuse or are not candidates for surgery.

Dexamethasone suppression testing is used to evaluate for glucocorticoid excess. However, this patient is not taking exogenous glucocorticoids and has no physical examination findings (fat redistribution, striae) or laboratory studies (glucose metabolism abnormalities) suggesting Cushing syndrome. Therefore, testing for this possibility is not an appropriate next step in diagnosis.

Measurement of plasma metanephrines and catecholamines is used to evaluate for the possibility of pheochromocytoma, which classically presents with the triad of diaphoresis, headache, and tachycardia, none of which are present in this patient. In addition, pheochromocytoma would not explain the patient's hypokalemia.

Renal artery Doppler flow studies may be helpful in evaluating for renovascular hypertension. However, most cases of renovascular hypertension occur in patients over 50 years of age and are associated with atherosclerotic cardiovascular disease or evidence of functional impairment of the kidney, neither of which are apparent in this patient.

KEY POINT

- Patients with suspected primary hyperaldosteronism as a cause of resistant hypertension should be screened with a plasma aldosterone-plasma renin activity ratio.

Bibliography

Funder JW, Carey RM, Fardella C, et al. Case detection, diagnosis, and treatment of patients with primary aldosteronism: an endocrine society clinical practice guideline. J Clin Endocrinol Metab. 2008;93(9):3266-81. [PMID: 18552288]

Item 72   Answer: D

Educational Objective: Treat substernal goiter with compressive symptoms.

This patient should undergo thyroidectomy to treat his obstructive substernal goiter and prevent further airway compromise, which may be rapid and fatal. The thyroid nodule biopsy findings obtained 5 years ago most likely represent adenomatous hyperplasia, and the sonographic features of the gland and slow progression of the compressive symptoms support a diagnosis of a benign lesion. He has evidence of compressive symptoms on physical examination, with facial flushing when raising his arms (Pemberton sign). The flushing indicates venous outflow obstruction by the goiter as the vessels course through the thoracic inlet. Additionally, his symptoms of dysphagia and change in voice quality may suggest a compressive effect on the esophagus and recurrent laryngeal nerves, respectively. Surgical removal of the thyroid offers the best option for immediate relief of symptoms and identification of a possible underlying malignancy.

External-beam radiotherapy can result in eventual shrinkage of the thyroid but will not provide immediate relief of his obstructive symptoms, is unlikely to be curative, potentially increases the risk of secondary malignancy, and is associated with significant morbidity.

Levothyroxine therapy has been shown to reduce thyroid volume by up to 20%, but the clinical significance of this small change in volume with such a large goiter is unlikely to improve symptoms. Additionally, levothyroxine therapy may take many months to years to reduce the thyroid volume, and this patient needs immediate relief of his obstructive symptoms.

Radioactive iodine has been used to shrink multinodular goiters; the volume change is also gradual and optimal reduction averages 40%. However, radioactive iodine therapy may be risky in this patient because acute swelling of the thyroid after iodine uptake can lead to compromise of the vascular structures at the level of the thoracic inlet and further compression of the trachea.

KEY POINT

- In patients with multinodular goiter with compressive features, thyroidectomy is most likely to provide immediate relief of symptoms, decrease the risk of fatal airway compromise, and possibly identify underlying malignancy.

Bibliography

Aslam R1, Steward D. Surgical management of thyroid disease. Otolaryngol Clin North Am. 2010 Apr;43(2):273-83. [PMID: 20510714]

Item 73   Answer: B

Educational Objective: Evaluate primary infertility with a hysterosalpingogram.

The test most likely to be diagnostic is a hysterosalpingogram (HSG) to evaluate tubal patency. Primary infertility due to a tubal abnormality is common and is best evaluated with dynamic testing of the female reproductive tract under fluoroscopy with an HSG. This patient, owing to her history of pelvic inflammatory disease, is likely to have a distal tubal occlusion and resultant hydrosalpinx. Many women with hydrosalpinx have no symptoms; however, symptoms may include pelvic pain (both unilaterally and bilaterally) and chronic vaginal discharge. Confirmatory evaluation should

Answers and Critiques

include diagnostic laparoscopy, but this is not typically performed as first-line evaluation given the need for general anesthesia, intubation, and recovery. Repair of the fallopian tubes may be possible with microsurgical techniques; however, reocclusion is possible and the risk of subsequent ectopic pregnancy is high. Many women elect to proceed with in vitro fertilization in lieu of tubal surgery.

Ovarian reserve assessment and semen analysis are essential when evaluating a couple with infertility. Ovarian reserve assessment can be accomplished with early follicular phase testing of follicle-stimulating hormone (FSH) or anti-müllerian hormone (AMH). Transvaginal ultrasound in the early follicular phase allows for counting of antral follicles in each ovary, which if present at greater than eight bilaterally support normal ovarian reserve. However, given this patient's history of pelvic inflammatory disease and her husband's history of fathering a child in a previous marriage, HSG is the diagnostic test that is most likely to reveal an abnormality.

Semen analysis can be performed after a short window of abstinence on an ejaculated sperm specimen. However, it is unlikely to be helpful in this patient's husband.

Karyotyping is usually not indicated as part of the initial evaluation of unexplained female infertility because of the low incidence of discovered abnormalities.

Specialized laboratories with andrology services evaluate sperm concentration, sperm motility, and sperm morphology. Ovarian reserve may be evaluated by serum testing (day 3 follicle-stimulating hormone level, AMH level) or by transvaginal ultrasound assessment of antral follicle count.

> **KEY POINT**
>
> - Primary infertility due to a tubal abnormality is common, particularly in women with a history of pelvic inflammatory disease, and is best evaluated with a hysterosalpingogram.

Bibliography

Maheux-Lacroix S, Boutin A, Moore L, et al. Hysterosalpingosonography for diagnosing tubal occlusion in subfertile women: a systematic review with meta-analysis. Hum Reprod. 2014 May;29(5):953-63. [PMID: 24578476]

Item 74   Answer: B

Educational Objective: Evaluate newly diagnosed medullary thyroid cancer.

The next most appropriate step in the management of this patient with medullary thyroid cancer (MTC) and multiple endocrine neoplasia type 2A (MEN2A) is to evaluate for the presence of a pheochromocytoma by measurement of fractionated plasma metanephrines. All patients with a cytologic diagnosis of MTC should undergo testing of the tumor for genetic abnormalities as the initial step in their evaluation as 25% of patients with MTC will have the inherited form. Identification of a *RET* mutation in this patient means that the he has MEN2A, an inherited syndrome associated with hyperparathyroidism

and pheochromocytoma. Failure to identify and treat a pheochromocytoma prior to surgery can result in an intraoperative hypertensive crisis and, potentially, death.

While it is important to assess the risk of metastatic disease in this high-risk patient, 18-fluoro-deoxyglucose positron emission tomography scanning is not the ideal imaging modality in patients with MTC, as there is a high false-negative rate. CT of the lungs and liver is a more effective means of identification of distant metastases.

While evaluation for hyperparathyroidism by measuring the serum parathyroid hormone level is indicated in this patient with MEN2A, it is not the most appropriate next step in management. Testing for hyperparathyroidism is recommended prior to surgery because the parathyroid disease can be managed simultaneously with the thyroid cancer, but would not be an appropriate step before evaluating a patient with MEN2A for the presence of pheochromocytoma.

Total thyroidectomy and lateral neck dissection should not be performed until it is confirmed that this patient does not have a coexisting endocrine neoplasm owing to the high intraoperative risk associated with untreated pheochromocytoma. If identified, pheochromocytomas should be surgically removed prior to thyroidectomy.

Genetic counseling is a very important component of the treatment plan for all patients with newly diagnosed MEN2A as first-degree relatives are at high risk for also having the *RET* mutation. With a nearly 100% penetrance for development of MTC in carriers of *RET* mutations, referral to a team with experience in the management of these disorders is critical for timely diagnosis and treatment.

> **KEY POINT**
>
> - All patients with multiple endocrine neoplasia type 2A should undergo testing to exclude pheochromocytoma prior to thyroidectomy; an elevated level of plasma fractionated metanephrines should prompt treatment for pheochromocytoma before addressing the thyroid malignancy.

Bibliography

American Thyroid Association Guidelines Task Force,2015 Thyroid. [PMID: 25810047]

Item 75   Answer: C

Educational Objective: Treat severe hypercalcemia.

This patient has severe, malignancy-related (non–parathyroid hormone [PTH]-mediated) hypercalcemia with associated mental status changes and acute kidney injury. Hemodialysis is generally reserved for patients with extremely high serum calcium levels (>18 mg/dL [4.5 mmol/L]) associated with acute kidney injury that precludes other acute treatments because it is able to rapidly lower serum calcium and provide careful management of volume status and electrolytes. Both hemodialysis and peritoneal dialysis are options, although hemodialysis more rapidly lowers calcium levels.

CONT.

Calcitonin is a rapidly acting agent that interferes with osteoclast function and promotes kidney excretion of calcium. However, its calcium-lowering effect is relatively weak, and it is only able to lower serum calcium levels by 1 to 2 mg/dL (0.25-0.50 mmol/L) over 4 to 6 hours, which would not be optimal lowering of this patient's very high calcium level. Calcitonin will bring her calcium levels down, but not enough to alleviate her symptoms.

Cinacalcet, a calcimimetic agent, is an option for lowering calcium for symptomatic patients, but it is not indicated to acutely reduce life-threatening hypercalcemia.

Intravenous bisphosphonates are used for treatment of malignancy-induced hypercalcemia, with zoledronic acid or pamidronate the most common agents. However, onset of action is not rapid, and bisphosphonates are contraindicated in severe kidney injury. Therefore, zoledronic acid would not be an appropriate next step in treatment.

Once the serum calcium has been lowered by dialysis, calcitonin or an intravenous bisphosphonate may be used to keep the calcium levels at a manageable level. The use of dialysis in the patient is strictly for resolution of the acute mental status changes from the elevated calcium level, and longer-term management of hypercalcemia is required.

KEY POINT

- For patients with serum calcium levels greater than 18 mg/dL (4.5 mmol/L) with neurologic symptoms or acute kidney injury, hemodialysis is an appropriate choice to quickly reduce calcium levels.

Bibliography

Rosner MH, Dalkin AC. Onco-nephrology: the pathophysiology and treatment of malignancy-associated hypercalcemia. Clin J Am Soc Nephrol. 2012:7:1722-9. [PMID: 22879438]

Item 76   Answer: D

Educational Objective: Treat hypoglycemic unawareness.

This patient should decrease his meal-time insulin and continue metformin. He has hypoglycemic unawareness secondary to a diminished counterregulatory response that has developed in the setting of repeated episodes of hypoglycemia. His hypoglycemia occurs in the postprandial state, thus the meal-time insulin should be decreased to allow permissive hyperglycemia for 2 to 3 weeks. Permissive hyperglycemia is defined as allowing an increase in blood glucose values to the level at which no further episodes of hypoglycemia occur. Using less stringent glycemic goals during this period will provide the body an opportunity to reset the counterregulatory response to hypoglycemia to a more appropriate blood glucose range, if possible. Although developing mutual hemoglobin A_{1c} goals with the patient is important, hypoglycemia in this scenario precludes reaching his goal safely. Once he no longer has hypoglycemia, changes to the meal-time insulin doses or to meal content and volume can be evaluated to fine-tune his regimen while avoiding hypoglycemia.

Continuing the current regimen places the patient at increased risk for continued hypoglycemia in the setting of hypoglycemic unawareness.

Increasing the metformin dose may improve insulin sensitivity and decrease hepatic gluconeogenesis, which could improve the hyperglycemia and/or worsen the hypoglycemia. An increased metformin dose does not address the serious complication of hypoglycemic unawareness, which must be corrected first.

Pramlintide could decrease the hemoglobin A_{1c} to the patient's goal; however, hypoglycemia is a side effect of pramlintide in conjunction with insulin use. This may further increase the risk of hypoglycemia in this scenario. Pramlintide is an amylin mimetic that decreases glucagon secretion and increases satiety by decreasing gastric emptying. Pramlintide should be considered when the intended reduction in hemoglobin A_{1c} is modest and the desired effects are a reduction in both weight and postprandial hyperglycemia.

KEY POINT

- Treatment for hypoglycemic unawareness is to reduce the insulin dose and allow permissive hyperglycemia at all times for several weeks to provide the body an opportunity to reset the counterregulatory response to hypoglycemia to a more appropriate blood glucose range.

Bibliography

Cryer PE, Axelrod L, Grossman AB, et al. Evaluation and management of adult hypoglycemic disorders: an Endocrine Society Clinical Practice Guideline. J Endocrinol Metab. 2009 Mar;94(3):709-28. [PMID: 19088155]

Item 77   Answer: C

Educational Objective: Diagnose elevation of luteinizing hormone related to polycystic ovary syndrome.

The most likely cause of this patient's false-positive results using the urinary luteinizing hormone (LH) kit is polycystic ovary syndrome (PCOS). Women with PCOS typically have elevated resting LH levels, which may be mistaken on home urinary LH kits for ovulation. The primary clinical manifestations of PCOS are menstrual irregularity (oligomenorrhea or amenorrhea), ovulatory dysfunction with resultant infertility, insulin resistance, and hyperandrogenism. Oligo-ovulation or anovulation can result in endometrial hyperplasia and/or infertility. Hyperandrogenism presents as hirsutism, acne, or androgenic alopecia. Most patients with PCOS also have insulin resistance, and studies have shown an increased incidence of metabolic syndrome, obesity, impaired glucose tolerance, and frank type 2 diabetes mellitus. PCOS remains a diagnosis of exclusion that is made both clinically and with ancillary testing. A patient with PCOS with a positive urinary LH measurement result may interpret this as a true LH surge and expect ovulation to be imminent. Attempts at conception with intercourse or insemination may be focused on this reading and may therefore be ineffective. A more accurate assessment of LH surge and anticipated ovulation in patients with PCOS would be through transvaginal identification of ovarian folliculogenesis and confirmatory serum assessment of reproductive hormones.

Late-onset (nonclassic) congenital adrenal hyperplasia, although a common cause of hirsutism and oligo-ovulation, is typically associated with normal or low LH levels owing to the negative feedback of elevated androgens of adrenal origin on the anterior pituitary.

Functional hypothalamic amenorrhea affects 3% of women between the ages of 18 and 40 years and is a diagnosis of exclusion. Risk factors for this condition include a low body weight and fat percentage, rapid and substantial weight loss, eating disorders, excessive exercise, severe emotional stress, severe nutritional deficiencies, and chronic or acute illness. FSH and LH levels are inappropriately low or normal and cannot account for a positive urinary LH test.

Hypothyroidism and elevated serum prolactin levels suppress rather than elevate serum LH levels and would not account for this patient's increased urinary LH measurement.

KEY POINT

- Women with polycystic ovary syndrome typically have elevated resting luteinizing hormone (LH) levels, which may be mistaken on home urinary LH kits for ovulation.

Bibliography

Rotterdam ESHRE/ASRM-Sponsored PCOS Consensus Workshop Group. Revised 2003 consensus on diagnostic criteria and long-term health risks related to polycystic ovary syndrome. Fertil Steril. 2004 Jan;81(1):19-25. [PMID: 14711538]

Item 78   Answer: C

Educational Objective: Treat a high-risk patient with osteoporosis.

After counseling about smoking cessation, this patient should continue her current alendronate therapy. She has documented osteoporosis and is at high risk for subsequent fractures due to multiple risk factors, including current smoking and a previous fracture. Her bone mineral density (BMD) has been well maintained on an oral bisphosphonate for the last several years. The best way to evaluate a dual-energy x-ray absorptiometry (DEXA) scan from measurement to measurement is to compare the bone mineral density readings from year to year, not the T-score. A change in BMD that is less than about 4% (or the percentage noted by the DEXA machine manufacturer) is not considered a statistically significant change. This regimen should be considered successful therapy since the goal of bisphosphonates is not to build bone mass but to stabilize bone loss. Since this patient has had stable BMD while on alendronate, there is no indication to convert to a more invasive, expensive option at this time. It will be important, however, to continue to follow her for atypical fractures of the long bone due to her prolonged bisphosphonate treatment. If leg pain or an atypical fracture is noted, bisphosphonate therapy should be discontinued.

Denosumab is a receptor activator of nuclear factor κB (RANK) ligand inhibitor FDA approved for the treatment of osteoporosis in postmenopausal women who are at high risk of fracture. Since this patient has not failed bisphosphonate therapy (shown a significant decrease in BMD while on bisphosphonate therapy) nor is she intolerant of the current therapy, there is no reason to change her therapy.

Teriparatide is appropriate as first-line therapy for patients at high risk for fracture (T-score < -3.0) or who have experienced progressive osteoporotic disease while on bisphosphonate therapy. This change would be unnecessary since the patient's BMD has been maintained for the past 5 years.

A drug holiday is indicated for patients who have been on bisphosphonate therapy for 3 to 5 years, have had no progression of the disease, and have minimal risk factors for additional fractures. This patient has multiple risk factors for fractures; therefore, a drug holiday would not be appropriate.

KEY POINT

- In patients at high risk for osteoporosis, it is appropriate to continue bisphosphonate therapy alone if adequate bone stability has been achieved.

Bibliography

National Osteoporosis Foundation (www. my.nof.org/bone-source). Clinician's Guide to Prevention and Treatment of Osteoporosis. Washington, DC: National Osteoporosis Foundation; 2014.

Item 79   Answer: D

Educational Objective: Manage primary hyperaldosteronism.

The most appropriate treatment for this patient is spironolactone. He has primary hyperaldosteronism (PA) due to a bilateral adrenal source as evidenced by the lack of lateralization on adrenal vein sampling (AVS). Bilateral adrenal hyperplasia is the most common etiology of PA, accounting for approximately 60% of cases, and spironolactone is the treatment of choice. Spironolactone is a mineralocorticoid receptor (MR) antagonist that can improve blood pressure, normalize serum potassium concentration, and reduce excess cardiovascular risk related to hyperaldosteronism. Eplerenone is an alternative MR antagonist that is less likely to cause gynecomastia in men because of greater MR selectivity; however, use of eplerenone for this indication is off-label. Antagonists of the aldosterone-sensitive sodium channel (amiloride) can be used as second-line therapy.

Bilateral adrenalectomy is not appropriate for the routine management of PA, as this would risk primary adrenal failure, thus necessitating life-long glucocorticoid and mineralocorticoid therapy.

Dexamethasone, a long-acting synthetic glucocorticoid, has a role in treating only a small percentage of patients who have glucocorticoid-remedial hypertension, a very rare autosomal dominant condition resulting from ectopic expression of aldosterone synthase in the cortisol-producing zona fasciculata. Administration of dexamethasone will suppress pituitary adrenocorticotropic hormone (ACTH) secretion in these patients and therefore mineralocorticoid production. However, hyperaldosteronism in most patients is independent of ACTH secretion, and suppression with exogenous glucocorticoid is not an effective therapy.

Left adrenalectomy should not be performed because the patient has a bilateral cause of PA. The left adrenal adenoma detected by CT scan is an incidental finding and is likely not the cause of this patient's hyperaldosteronism. Because nonsecreting adrenal adenomas are common, AVS is needed in most patients with hyperaldosteronism to determine the source of aldosterone secretion when imaging studies show an adrenal adenoma to assess its contribution to excess mineralocorticoid production. AVS should be done at a high-volume referral center due to a high risk of complications when significant procedural experience is lacking.

KEY POINT

- For patients with primary hyperaldosteronism due to bilateral adrenal hyperplasia, medical therapy with a mineralocorticoid antagonist such as spironolactone is the treatment of choice because of its proven efficacy to lower blood pressure, normalize serum potassium concentration, and reduce cardiovascular risk.

Bibliography

Funder JW, Carey RM, Fardella C, et al. Case detection, diagnosis, and treatment of patients with primary aldosteronism: an endocrine society clinical practice guideline. J Clin Endocrinol Metab. 2008 Sep;93(9):3266-81. [PMID: 18552288]

Item 80   Answer: B
Educational Objective: Manage hyperprolactinemia caused by hypothyroidism.

The most appropriate treatment for this patient is to begin levothyroxine. She has primary hypothyroidism with an elevated thyroid-stimulating hormone level and a low free thyroxine (T_4) level. Her symptoms are consistent with hypothyroidism. Hypothyroidism is a cause of hyperprolactinemia. When patients present with hyperprolactinemia and hypothyroidism, the hypothyroidism should be treated and then the patient should be reevaluated to ensure that the hyperprolactinemia resolves. The patient's pituitary gland is normal. There is no tumor.

The hypothyroidism should be treated first, and then the patient's prolactin level should be retested. There is no indication for cabergoline, a dopamine agonist, at this point. Cabergoline is an appropriate therapy for a patient with hyperprolactinemia caused by a prolactinoma. This patient's hyperprolactinemia is explained by hypothyroidism.

Sertraline does not cause hyperprolactinemia or hypothyroidism. Antipsychotic agents are a common cause of hyperprolactinemia, but selective serotonin reuptake inhibitors such as sertraline are not.

There is no indication for pituitary MRI at this time because her hyperprolactinemia is explained by hypothyroidism. It is necessary to make sure that her hyperprolactinemia normalizes after treatment with levothyroxine.

KEY POINT

- In patients with hyperprolactinemia and hypothyroidism, the hypothyroidism should be treated first, then the patient should be reevaluated to ensure that the hyperprolactinemia resolves.

Bibliography

Melmed S, Casanueva FF, Hoffman AR, et al. Diagnosis and treatment of hyperprolactinemia: An Endocrine Society clinical practice guideline. J Clin Endocrinol Metab. 2011 Feb;96(2):273-88. [PMID: 21296991]

Item 81   Answer: B
Educational Objective: Diagnose cystic fibrosis as a cause of congenital bilateral absence of the vas deferens and azoospermia.

Congenital bilateral absence of the vas deferens is a common cause of obstructive azoospermia and is frequently associated with cystic fibrosis (CF). It may also present with unilateral absence of the vas deferens. Many patients are unaware that they have CF because they may have a mild form that causes only nonspecific symptoms such as chronic sinusitis. Partner testing for CF-carrier status should be encouraged to assess the likelihood of transmission to a subsequent generation. Sperm production is often normal in these patients; however, the absence of the vas deferens limits any observable sperm in the ejaculate. Therefore, testicular biopsy is necessary to retrieve sperm for use in advanced reproductive techniques (ART) such as in vitro fertilization and intracytoplasmic sperm injection. Utilization of donor sperm is an alternative for couples not interested in ART.

Androgen abuse is common among elite and professional athletes and in young men. Physical examination findings may include excessive muscular bulk, acne, gynecomastia, and decreased testicular volume. Low sperm counts also may be present with exogenous androgen use. Androgen abuse can result in hypogonadism and infertility, which occasionally are irreversible. This patient's normal physical examination, normal testicular volume, and absence of the vas deferens argue against this diagnosis.

Primary hypogonadism is due to testicular failure and is defined as a low testosterone level with elevated luteinizing hormone and follicle-stimulating hormone levels. Primary hypogonadism can have congenital or acquired causes. The most common congenital cause is Klinefelter syndrome (47,XXY karyotype). The extra sex chromosome results in malformation of the seminiferous tubules and typically of the Leydig cells. Physical examination is likely to reveal small, firm testes and decreased virilization. Additional manifestations include oligospermia and infertility. Klinefelter syndrome does not result in obstructive azoospermia due to absence of the vas deferens.

A clinically palpable varicocele typically affects fertility by lowering sperm motility through a local heat effect. A scrotal bulge may be noted by the clinician, and the patient may note pain that is worse with the Valsalva maneuver. Azoospermia would not be caused by varicocele alone.

Y chromosome microdeletions can be associated with oligospermia or azoospermia and small testicular volume. This chromosomal abnormality is not associated with absence of the vas deferens and is therefore not a likely cause of this patient's findings.

KEY POINT

- Congenital bilateral absence of the vas deferens is a common cause of obstructive azoospermia and is frequently associated with cystic fibrosis.

Bibliography

Stahl PJ, Schlegel PN. Genetic evaluation of the azoospermic or severely oligozoospermic male. Curr Opin Obstet Gynecol. 2012 Aug;24(4):221-8. [PMID: 22729088]

Item 82   Answer: B
Educational Objective: Manage primary adrenal failure.

Initiation of cortisol replacement therapy with a glucocorticoid (such as hydrocortisone) and mineralocorticoid (such as fludrocortisone) is the most appropriate next step in management. This patient has symptoms consistent with adrenal insufficiency (fatigue, unintentional weight loss, nausea, and vomiting); her family history of autoimmune disorders, hyperpigmentation noted on physical examination, and hyperkalemia on laboratory testing suggest primary adrenal failure. Patients with primary adrenal failure frequently have increased pigmentation over the extensor surfaces and buccal mucosa due to the excessive secretion of melanocyte-stimulating hormone, which shares a common precursor with adrenocorticotropic hormone (ACTH). Hyperkalemia occurs due to deficiency of aldosterone. The diagnosis of adrenal insufficiency is made by documenting an inappropriately low serum cortisol level. An early morning serum cortisol level that is less than 3 µg/dL (82.8 nmol/L) in the setting of signs and symptoms of cortisol deficiency is diagnostic of this disorder. Treatment should not be withheld while awaiting further diagnostic testing since adrenal insufficiency is a potentially life-threatening condition that may result in hemodynamic instability. Treatment of primary adrenal failure requires both glucocorticoid and mineralocorticoid replacement. Hydrocortisone or another long-acting agent with primarily glucocorticoid activity should be given along with a mineralocorticoid agent such as fludrocortisone.

The synthetic ACTH (cosyntropin) stimulation test is extremely sensitive for detecting either primary or secondary adrenal insufficiency. In patients with nondiagnostic basal cortisol values (4-12 µg/dL [110.4-331.2 nmol/L]), stimulation testing with synthetic ACTH is indicated. A normal response is a peak serum cortisol greater than 20 µg/dL (552 nmol/L). ACTH stimulation testing is not needed if the early morning serum cortisol level is unequivocally low, as in this patient.

Measurement of the plasma ACTH level is used to differentiate primary adrenal failure from other causes of low cortisol. In primary adrenal failure, the plasma ACTH level is typically significantly elevated (200 pg/mL [44 pmol/L]) and would confirm the diagnosis. However, withholding therapy while awaiting diagnostic confirmation would not be appropriate because of the potential life-threatening nature of primary adrenal failure.

Although prednisone is an acceptable agent for glucocorticoid replacement, it has almost pure glucocorticoid activity and would not be an appropriate single agent for treatment of primary adrenal failure in which replacement of both glucocorticoid and mineralocorticoid is required.

KEY POINT

- Cortisol replacement therapy should be initiated immediately in persons with confirmed adrenal insufficiency, which is diagnosed by an early morning serum cortisol level below 3 µg/dL (82.8 nmol/L) in the setting of signs and symptoms of cortisol deficiency.

Bibliography

Neary N, Nieman L. Adrenal insufficiency: etiology, diagnosis and treatment. Curr Opin Endocrinol Diabetes Obes. 2010 Jun;17(3):217-23. [PMID: 20375886]

Item 83   Answer: A
Educational Objective: Manage the "honeymoon" phase of type 1 diabetes mellitus.

The most appropriate management for this patient's hypoglycemia is to decrease insulin glargine and insulin aspart. The glucose toxicity present at the time of diabetic ketoacidosis has diminished with an intensive insulin regimen. Her remaining functional pancreatic beta cells have regained the ability to produce some insulin in the "honeymoon" phase, which explains the hypoglycemia on previously well-tolerated doses of insulin. The decreased need for insulin will not be long term as pancreatic beta cells continue to be destroyed over the course of type 1 diabetes. Continuing insulin, even at low doses, is recommended during the "honeymoon" phase in order to preserve beta cell function as long as possible by reducing the metabolic stress on these cells. The low-dose insulin regimen can consist of a basal and prandial insulin combination or a basal insulin regimen. She is experiencing symptomatic postprandial and fasting hypoglycemia. Decreasing the insulin aspart and insulin glargine doses would address the prandial and fasting hypoglycemia, while also still providing low-dose insulin to protect the functioning beta cells. She will require close monitoring of her blood glucose levels to determine when insulin doses should be increased as she nears the end of the "honeymoon" phase. The "honeymoon" period may persist for several weeks to months.

Meal-time insulin doses are generally reduced by 50% when pramlintide is initiated due to the risk of hypoglycemia.

The addition of pramlintide would likely exacerbate the current issue of hypoglycemia even with reduction of meal-time insulin.

The use of sliding-scale insulin without basal insulin is discouraged. When sliding-scale insulin is used without basal insulin, the likelihood of wide swings from hyperglycemia to hypoglycemia increases. Without a basal insulin regimen, she may not consistently receive daily insulin to decrease the metabolic stress on her functioning pancreatic beta cells.

Discontinuation of both insulin glargine and insulin aspart increases metabolic stress on the pancreatic beta cells and accelerates the loss of functional cells producing insulin. As pancreatic beta cell function declines toward the end of the "honeymoon" phase, the risk of diabetic ketoacidosis increases without any exogenous insulin.

KEY POINT

- Continuing insulin, even at low doses, is recommended during the "honeymoon phase" of type 1 diabetes mellitus to reduce metabolic stress on functioning beta cells and preserve any residual function for as long as possible.

Bibliography

DeWitt DE, Hirsch IB. Outpatient insulin therapy in type 1 and type 2 diabetes mellitus: scientific review. JAMA. 2003 May 7;289(17):2254-64. [PMID: 12734137]

Item 84   Answer: A

Educational Objective: Treat hypogonadism secondary to hyperprolactinemia in a male patient.

The most appropriate treatment is a dopamine agonist such as cabergoline. Hyperprolactinemia as a result of a prolactinoma is a possible cause of erectile dysfunction and decreased libido and may be successfully treated with a dopamine agonist. In addition to the sexual dysfunction associated with hyperprolactinemia, semen parameters are often abnormal; patients commonly demonstrate oligoasthenospermia (reduced sperm motility) and at times complete azoospermia. Three months of treatment are typically needed prior to return of improved semen parameters. Prolactin is secreted by the pituitary lactotroph cells under tonic inhibition by dopamine. Dopamine agonist therapy can normalize prolactin levels, reverse hypogonadism, and shrink tumors by at least 50% in almost 90% of patients. Evaluation of the infertile male with abnormal findings on semen analysis should always include investigation of the hypothalamic-pituitary-testicular (HPT) axis. Disturbances in this axis may result in failure of gonadotropin release from the anterior pituitary and insufficient testosterone production as well as absent or diminished spermatogenesis.

Clomiphene citrate is effective only when the HPT axis is intact, which does not apply for this patient. Although the indication for clomiphene citrate in the infertile male population remains controversial, some clinicians use it to increase endogenous follicle-stimulating hormone and luteinizing hormone output from the anterior pituitary to support testosterone production by Leydig cells.

Sildenafil may improve erectile dysfunction in this patient, but it will not increase endogenous testosterone levels and will not improve his hyperprolactinemic state.

Testosterone replacement therapy would be helpful to alleviate the sexual side effects of this patient's hyperprolactinemic state; however, no restoration of spermatogenesis would occur, and therefore infertility would persist. Neither testosterone replacement nor sildenafil therapy will reduce the size of the patient's prolactinoma.

KEY POINT

- Secondary hypogonadism in a male patient caused by hyperprolactinemia as a result of a prolactinoma is a possible cause of erectile dysfunction and should be treated with a dopamine agonist such as cabergoline.

Bibliography

Mann WA. Treatment for prolactinomas and hyperprolactinaemia: a lifetime approach. Eur J Clin Invest. 2011 Mar;41(3):334-42. [PMID: 20955213]

Index

Note: Page numbers followed by f and t denote figures and tables, respectively. Test questions are indicated by Q.

A

Abdominal CT scan, for androgen-producing adrenal tumor, Q52
Acarbose, for diabetes mellitus, 5t, 10t
ACE inhibitor, in diabetic nephropathy, 17
Acquired type 1 diabetes, 3
Acromegaly, 27
    causes of, 27
    clinical features and diagnosis in, 27
    transsphenoidal surgery for, Q61
    treatment of, 27–28
ACTH stimulation test, 22, 23
Adenoma
    adrenal, 32
    pituitary, 20 (see also Pituitary tumors)
    thyroid, toxic, 44
Adrenal crisis, 36
Adrenal failure, bilateral adrenal hemorrhage and, Q42
Adrenal fatigue, 38
Adrenal gland, disorders of, 29–40
    adrenal hormone excess and, 30–36
    adrenal insufficiency and, 36–39
    adrenal masses, 39–40
    related anatomy and physiology, 29, 29f
Adrenal insufficiency, 36
    during critical illness, 38–39
    primary adrenal failure, 36–38
Adrenal masses, 39–40
    imaging characteristics of, 32t
    incidentally noted, 39–40, 39f, Q50, Q60
Adrenal metastases, 39
Adrenal vein sampling (AVS), 34
Adrenocortical carcinomas (ACCs), 32, 32t, 39, 40
    surgical excision of, Q27
Adrenocorticotropic hormone (ACTH), 19, 19t
    and cortisol production, 29
    deficiency of, 22–23, 23t
Aging male, androgen deficiency in, 57–58
Aldosterone, 29
Aldosterone-producing adrenocortical adenomas, 34
Alendronate
    for osteoporosis, 69, Q78
    for Paget disease of bone, 71
Alogliptin, for diabetes mellitus, 10t
α-adrenoceptors blockers, for pheochromocytomas, 33
α-glucosidase inhibitors, for type 2 diabetes, 4, 5t, 10t
Amenorrhea, 54–55
    evaluation of, 55
    primary, 54, Q9
    secondary, 54–55
American Diabetes Association (ADA), on screening for type 2 diabetes, 1, 2t
Amiloride, in primary hyperaldosteronism, 35
Amiodarone-induced thyrotoxicosis (AIT), 46
    type 1, 46
    type 2, 46
Amitriptyline, in distal symmetric polyneuropathy, 18
Amylinomimetics, for diabetes mellitus, 10t
Anabolic steroid abuse, in men, 60
Androgen abuse, in women, 56
Androgen deficiency, in aging male, 57–58
Androgen-producing adrenal tumors, 36, Q52
Angiotensin receptor blocker (ARB), in diabetic nephropathy, 17
Anticonvulsants, in distal symmetric polyneuropathy, 18
Antidepressants, in distal symmetric polyneuropathy, 18
Antidiuretic hormone (ADH), 19
    deficiency of, 24–25
    excess of, 28

Antiresorptive therapy, in Paget disease of bone, 71, Q40
Antithyroid drugs, in Graves disease, 44
Apathetic hyperthyroidism, 42
Asherman syndrome (AS), 54, Q68
Atenolol, in thyrotoxicosis, 43
Atherosclerotic cardiovascular disease (ASCVD), 16
Autoimmune adrenalitis, and primary adrenal failure, 36
Autoimmune-mediated type 1 diabetes mellitus, 1, 3
Autonomic neuropathy, 18

B

Bariatric surgery, 8, Q49
β-adrenoceptors blockers, for pheochromocytomas, 33–34
β-blockers
    in thyroid storm treatment, 49
    in thyrotoxicosis, 43, Q10
Biguanides, for diabetes mellitus, 10t
Bilateral adrenal hemorrhage, Q42
Bisphosphonates
    in hypercalcemia, 64, 65
    in osteoporosis, 68–69
Bone mineral density (BMD), 66–67, Q12
    decline in, 67
    and fracture risk, 67
    increase in, 66
    measurement of, 67, 68t
Bromocriptine, for prolactinomas, 26

C

Cabergoline, Q84
    for Cushing disease, 28
    for prolactinomas, 26, Q19
Calcitonin, 42
    for osteoporosis, 69
Calcitriol, 62, 66
Calcium
    homeostasis and bone physiology, 61–62
    postsurgical hypoparathyroidism and supplementation intake, Q34
Calcium carbonate, in hypocalcemia, 66
Calcium citrate, in hypocalcemia, 66
Calcium-creatinine clearance ratio, 64–65
Canagliflozin, for diabetes mellitus, 10t
Capsaicin cream, 18
Cardiovascular disease (CVD), diabetes mellitus and, 16–17, 16t
Catecholamines, 29, 29f
Celiac disease, autoimmune-mediated type 1 diabetes and, 3
Central diabetes insipidus, 24–25
Central hyperthyroidism, 45
Central hypothyroidism, measurement of serum free thyroxine (T_4) level in, Q36
Chlorpropamide, for diabetes mellitus, 10t
Clomiphene citrate, 57, Q64
Continuous glucose monitoring (CGM), 7, Q53
Continuous subcutaneous insulin infusion (CSII) therapy, 7–9
Corticotrophin-releasing hormone (CRH), 19, 28
Cortisol, 29
Critical illness, adrenal function during, 38–39
Cushing disease, 28–29
Cushing syndrome (CS), 28, 30–32
    causes of, 30, 30t
    clinical manifestations of, 30, 30f, 31t
    CT of adrenal glands in, Q5
    diagnosis of, 30–32, 31f, Q5, Q48
    endogenous, 30
    iatrogenic, 30, Q23
    imaging studies in, 32, 32t
    and pseudo-Cushing syndrome, 30
    treatment of, 32
Cystic fibrosis, and infertility, Q81

D

Dapagliflozin, for diabetes mellitus, 10t
Denosumab
    in hypercalcemia, 65
    in osteoporosis, 69
Desmopressin, in central diabetes insipidus, 25
Destructive thyroiditis, 44
Dexamethasone
    in primary adrenal failure, 38t
    in secondary cortisol deficiency, 23
1-mg dexamethasone suppression test, Q48
DHEA, in primary adrenal failure, 37, 38t
Diabetes mellitus, 1
    and chronic kidney disease, Q51
    classification of, 1, 3t
        insulin deficiency, 1, 3, 3t
        insulin resistance, 3–5, 3t
        uncommon types, 3t, 5
    complications of
        acute, 14, 15f, 15t
        chronic, 16–18, 16t
    diagnostic criteria for, 1, 2t
    elevated plasma glucose levels in, 1
    insulin therapy in
        basal and prandial insulin, in hospitalized patient, Q47
        timing issues with, Q38
    management of, 5–6, 6t
        blood glucose monitoring, 7, 7t
        nonpharmacologic approaches, 7–8
        patient education, 6–7
        pharmacologic therapy, 8–11, 10t
    screening for, 1, 2t
    type 1, 1, 3, 3t (see also Type 1 diabetes)
    type 2, 4, 5t (see also Type 2 diabetes mellitus)
Diabetes self-management education (DSME), 6–7
Diabetes self-management support (DSMS), 6–7
Diabetic amyotrophy, 18
Diabetic complications, and glycemic targets, Q14
Diabetic foot ulcers, 18
Diabetic ketoacidosis (DKA), 3, 14, 15f, 15t, Q24
Diabetic nephropathy, 16t, 17
Diabetic neuropathy, 16t, 17–18, Q66
Diabetic retinopathy, 17
Diet and exercise, for prevention/delay of type 2 diabetes, 4, 5t
Dipeptidyl peptidase-4 (DPP-4) inhibitors, for diabetes mellitus, 9, 10t
Distal symmetric polyneuropathy (DPN), 18
Dopamine agonists (DA), for prolactinomas, 26
Drug-induced thyroid dysfunction, 46, 47t
Dual-energy x-ray absorptiometry (DEXA) scan, 64, 67, Q12, Q43
Duloxetine
    in diabetic polyneuropathy, Q66
    in distal symmetric polyneuropathy, 18

E

Epinephrine, 29
Eplerenone, in primary hyperaldosteronism, 35
Estrogen agonists and antagonists, for osteoporosis, 69
Estrogen replacement, in hypergonadotropic hypogonadism, 54–55
Euthyroid sick syndrome (ESS), 48, Q13
Exenatide, for diabetes mellitus, 10t
Exercise
    for diabetes management, 8
    and hypoglycemia, 12, Q35

F

Familial hyperparathyroidism, and hypercalcemia, 65
Familial hypocalciuric hypercalcemia (FHH), 64–65
    urine calcium and creatinine levels in, measurement of, Q37
Fasting hyperglycemia, Q4
Fasting hypoglycemia, 13
Fasting plasma glucose (FPG), 1, 2t, Q57
Female reproductive disorders
    amenorrhea, 54–55
    female infertility, 56–57
    female reproduction, physiology of, 53, 53f
    hyperandrogenism syndromes, 55–56
Fine-needle aspiration (FNA), 42
    of thyroid nodules, 51, 51t, Q8
Fludrocortisone, in primary adrenal failure, 38t, Q44, Q82
Fluid resuscitation, in hypercalcemia, 65
Follicle-stimulating hormone (FSH), 19, 19t, 53

Foot care, in diabetic patient, 18
Foot ulcers, in diabetic patient, 18
Fracture Risk Assessment Tool (FRAX) calculator, 67–68
Fractures
    osteoporosis and, 67
    prediction of risk of, 67–68
Framingham Risk Score, 4

G

Gabapentin, in distal symmetric polyneuropathy, 18
Gestational diabetes mellitus, 5
    complications related to, 5
    screening for, 5
    therapy for, 5
Gigantism, 27
Gliclazide, for diabetes mellitus, 10t
Glimepiride, for diabetes mellitus, 10t
Glipizide, for diabetes mellitus, 10t
Glucagon-like peptide 1 (GLP-1) mimetics, for diabetes mellitus, 9, 10t
Glucocorticoids
    in hypercalcemia, 65
    in lymphocytic hypophysitis, 20
    in primary adrenal failure, 37–38, 38t, Q82
    in thyroid storm treatment, 49
Glucose metabolism, disorders of. See also specific disorder
    diabetes mellitus, 1–11
    hyperglycemia, 11–12
    hypoglycemia, 12–14
Glutamic acid decarboxylase (GAD65), 1
Glyburide, for diabetes mellitus, 10t
Glycemic targets, and diabetic complications, Q14
Goiter, 41
    multinodular, 51–52
    simple, 52
Gonadotropin-producing pituitary adenomas, 28
Gonadotropin-releasing hormone (GnRH), 19, 53
Graves disease, 43–44
Graves ophthalmopathy, 44, Q70
Growth hormone (GH), 19
    deficiency of, 24
    excess of, 27 (see also Acromegaly)
Gynecomastia, 60–61
    causes of, 60–61
    examination in, 61

H

Hashimoto thyroiditis, and hypothyroidism, 45
Hemochromatosis, diagnosis of, Q30
Hemodialysis, in hypercalcemia, 65, Q75
Hemoglobin A_{1c} testing, 1, 2t, 7, 7t
    disadvantages of, 1
    in patient with diabetes mellitus and chronic kidney disease, Q51
Hirsutism, 55–56
Honeymoon phase, insulin therapy in, 3
Human chorionic gonadotropin (HCG) testing, 55
Hydrocortisone
    after adrenalectomy in patient with Cushing syndrome, Q39
    in primary adrenal failure, 38t, Q82
    in secondary cortisol deficiency, 23
25-Hydroxyvitamin D, 61, 62
Hyperandrogenism syndromes, 55–56
Hypercalcemia, 62–66
    causes of, 62, 63t
    clinical features of, 62
    diagnosis of, 62, 63f
    non-parathyroid hormone–mediated, 65, Q22
    parathyroid hormone–mediated, 62–65
    treatment of, 65–66
Hyperglycemia, management of, 11
    hospitalized patients with diabetes mellitus, 11–12
    hospitalized patients without diabetes mellitus, 12
Hyperglycemic hyperosmolar syndrome (HHS), 14, 15f, 15t
Hypergonadotropic hypogonadism, Klinefelter syndrome and, Q58
Hyperprolactinemia, 25–27, 25t, Q80, Q84
    antipsychotics and, Q11
    causes of, 25–26, 25t
    clinical features and diagnosis, 26
    and secondary amenorrhea, 54
    therapy for, 26

Hyperthyroidism
  during pregnancy, Q1
  subclinical, 45
  triiodothyronine (T$_3$) level, measurement of, Q21
Hypocalcemia
  clinical features of, 66
  diagnosis and causes of, 66
  hypoparathyroidism and, 66
  low magnesium level and, Q28
  treatment of, 66
Hypoglycemia
  and altered mental status, Q20
  definition of, 12
  exercise-induced, Q35
  in patients with diabetes mellitus, 12–13
  in patients without diabetes mellitus, 13
    differential diagnosis of, 13t
    fasting hypoglycemia, 13
    postprandial hypoglycemia, 13
  in patient without diabetes mellitus, Q67
Hypoglycemic unawareness, 18
  treatment of, Q76
Hypogonadism, 57–59
  androgen deficiency in aging male, 57–58
  desire for fertility and therapy for, Q32
  evaluation of, 58, 59f
  primary, 57
  secondary, 57
  testosterone replacement therapy for, 58–59, 60t
Hypogonadotropic hypogonadism, 54
  GnRH deficiency and, 24
  hemochromatosis and, Q30
Hypoparathyroidism
  and hypocalcemia, 66
  postsurgical, Q34
Hypopituitarism, 21–22
  adrenocorticotropic hormone deficiency, 22–23, 23t
  causes of, 21, 22t
  central diabetes insipidus, 24–25
  gonadotropin deficiency, 24
  growth hormone deficiency, 24
  panhypopituitarism, 25
  Sheehan syndrome and, 22
  thyroid-stimulating hormone deficiency, 23–24
Hypothalamic amenorrhea, and GnRH deficiency, 24
Hypothalamic-pituitary-ovarian axis, 53
Hypothermia, in myxedema coma, 49
Hypothyroid, 44
Hypothyroidism
  causes of, 45
  central, Q36
  evaluation of, 45
  management of, 45–46
  medication induced, 45
  in pregnancy, Q41
Hysterosalpingogram (HSG), for tubal patency, Q73

I
Ibandronate, for osteoporosis, 69
Idiopathic type 1 diabetes, 3
Incidentally noted adrenal mass, 39–40, 39f, Q50, Q60
Infertility
  female, 56–57
  male, 60
Insulin resistance, 3
  gestational diabetes, 5
  metabolic syndrome, 3–4, 4t
  obesity and, 3
  type 2 diabetes mellitus, 4, 5t
Insulin therapy, for type 1 diabetes, 8–9, 8t, Q63, Q83. *See also* Diabetes mellitus
Intrapetrosal sinus sampling (IPSS), 28
Iodine deficiency, 41
Iodine drops, in thyroid storm treatment, 49
Ionized calcium level, testing for, Q31

J
Jod-Basedow phenomenon, 44

K
Kallmann syndrome, and GnRH deficiency, 24
Karyotype testing, Q58

Ketoacidosis, diabetic, 3, 14, 15f, 15t, Q24
Ketoconazole, in Cushing disease, 28
Klinefelter syndrome, Q58
  and primary hypogonadism, 57

L
Lactic acidosis, 9
Laparoscopic adrenalectomy, 35
Laser photocoagulation, in diabetic retinopathy, 17
Late autoimmune diabetes in adults (LADA), 3
Late-night (LN) salivary cortisol, 30–32
Letrozole, 57
Levothyroxine
  for hypothyroidism, 45, Q16
  hypothyroidism from pituitary dysfunction and dosage of, Q56
  for hypothyroidism in pregnancy, Q41
Lifestyle modifications, in diabetes management, 4, 5
Linagliptin, for diabetes mellitus, 10t
Lipase inhibitors, for prevention/delay of type 2 diabetes, 4, 5t
Liraglutide, for diabetes mellitus, 10t
Lithium, and hypercalcemia, 65
Loop diuretics, in hypercalcemia, 65
Low-dose dexamethasone suppression test (LDST), 30–31, 40
Low triiodothyronine (T3) syndrome, 48
Luteinizing hormone (LH), 19, 19t, 53, Q77
Lymphocytic hypophysitis, 20
Lymphocytic thyroiditis, 40

M
Male reproductive disorders
  anabolic steroid abuse, 60
  gynecomastia, 60–61
  hypogonadism, 57–59
  male infertility, 60
  male reproduction, physiology of, 57, 57f
Malignancy-associated hypercalcemia, 65
Maturity-onset diabetes of young (MODY), 5
Medical nutrition therapy, for diabetes management, 7–8
Medullary thyroid cancer (MTC), 53
  plasma fractionated metanephrine levels in, Q74
Meglitinides, for diabetes mellitus, 10t
Menstrual cycle, 53
Mental status changes
  hypoglycemia and, Q20
  in myxedema coma, 49
Metabolic bone disease, 66
Metabolic syndrome, 3
  and cardiovascular disease (CVD), 3
  definition of, 3, 4t
  Endocrine Society on screening for, 4
  and type 2 diabetes mellitus, 3
  10-year CVD risk, calculation of, 4
Metformin, for type 2 diabetes, 4, 5t, 9, 10t, Q29
Methimazole
  in Graves ophthalmopathy, Q70
  in thyrotoxicosis, 43
Metoprolol, in subacute thyroiditis, Q10
Metyrapone, in Cushing disease, 28
Microprolactinomas, in asymptomatic patients, Q65
Miglitol, for diabetes mellitus, 10t
Mineralocorticoid antagonist, in primary hyperaldosteronism, 35
Mineralocorticoids, in primary adrenal failure, 37, 38t
Mitotane, 40
Mixed meal tolerance test, 13
Multinodular goiter, 44, 51–52
Multiple daily injection (MDI) insulin therapy, 7, 8
Multiple endocrine neoplasia syndrome (MEN), 65
Multiple endocrine neoplasia syndrome type 2 (MEN2), Q2
Myxedema coma, 49

N
Nateglinide, for diabetes mellitus, 10t
National Osteoporosis Foundation, on osteoporosis evaluation, 67
Nerve compression syndromes, 18
Nonthyroidal illness syndrome, 48
Norepinephrine, 29
Normocalcemic primary hyperparathyroidism, 64

O
Oral glucose tolerance test (OGTT), 1, 2t
Orlistat, for prevention/delay of type 2 diabetes, 5t

Osteonecrosis of jaw, 68
Osteopenia, 66–68. *See also* Osteoporosis
Osteoporosis
    annual reassessment in, 69
    BMD testing and DEXA scan, 67–68, Q12, Q43
    bone mineral density loss and, 67, Q25
    defined, 67
    diagnosis of, 67–68
    hypercortisolism and risk of, Q43
    National Osteoporosis Foundation and Endocrine Society
        recommendations, 70
    physiology related to, 66–67
    risk assessment and screening guidelines, 67, 67t, 68t
    secondary causes of, 68, Q25
    treatment of, 68–69
    vertebral imaging, 68
    vitamin D and, 69–70
Overnight blood glucose monitoring, Q4

P
Paget disease of bone, 70–71, Q40
    clinical manifestation, 70, 71f
    diagnosis of, 71
    treatment for, 71
Pamidronate, for Paget disease of bone, 71
Panhypopituitarism, 25
    hormone replacement therapy in, Q56
Paragangliomas, 32–34
Parathyroid carcinoma, 64
Parathyroidectomy, for primary hyperparathyroidism, 63,
        Q17
Parathyroid hormone (PTH), 61, 62. *See also* Hypercalcemia
Paroxetine, in distal symmetric polyneuropathy, 18
Pasireotide, in Cushing disease, 28
Patient education, for diabetes management, 6–7
Pegvisomant, 27
Phenoxybenzamine, for pheochromocytomas, 33, Q55
Pheochromocytomas, 32–34, 32t, 34t, Q55, Q74
    diagnosis of, 33
    multiple endocrine neoplasia (MEN) syndromes and, 33, 33t
    radiographic localization of, 33
    treatment of, 33–34
Physiologic insulin therapy, for type 1 diabetes, 8–9, 8t
Pioglitazone, for diabetes mellitus, 5t, 10t
Pituitary adenoma, 20. *See also* Pituitary tumors
Pituitary apoplexy, 21–22, Q7
Pituitary gland disorders
    anatomy and physiology related to, 18–20, 19f, 19t
    hypopituitarism, 21–25
    pituitary hormone deficiency and excess, testing for, 19t
    pituitary hormone excess, 25–29
    pituitary tumors, 20–21, 20f
Pituitary tumors, 20
    empty sella, 21
    functional, 25
    incidentally noted, 20–21
    macroadenoma, 20, 20f
    mass effects of, 21
    microadenoma, 20
    nonfunctioning, 21
    sellar mass, approach to, 20
Plasma aldosterone concentration (PAC), 34, 35t
Plasma aldosterone-plasma renin activity ratio, Q71
Plasma free metanephrines, measurement of, Q50
Plasma renin activity (PRA), 34, 35t
Polycystic ovary syndrome (PCOS), 54, 55–56, Q64
    elevated resting luteinizing hormone levels in, Q77
    estrogen-progestin oral contraceptive pills in, Q26, Q54
Polyuria, hypercalcemia and, 65
Pooled Cohort Equation, 4, 16
Postmenopausal women
    fracture risk in, 67
    osteoporosis treatment in, 68–69
Postpartum thyroiditis, 44
Postprandial hyperglycemia, Q69
    in pregnancy, 5
Postprandial hypoglycemia, 13
Potassium chloride, in diabetic ketoacidosis, Q24
Pramlintide, for diabetes mellitus, 10t
Prediabetes, 1
Prednisolone, in primary adrenal failure, 38t

Prednisone
    in primary adrenal failure, 38t, Q44
    in secondary cortisol deficiency, 23
Pregabalin, in distal symmetric polyneuropathy, 18
Pregnancy
    diabetes in, 5
    thyroid function and disease during, 46, Q1
    hypothyroidism in, Q41
    prolactinoma in, 26–27
    and secondary amenorrhea, 54
    thionamides use during, 48
    thyroid function in, 46–48, 48f
    visual field testing during, Q3
Premature ovarian insufficiency (POI), 54
Pretibial myxedema, 43
Primary adrenal failure, 36–38, Q82
    causes and clinical features, 36, 37t
    diagnosis of, 36–37
    prednisone and fludrocortisone in, Q44
    treatment of, 37–38, 38t
Primary amenorrhea, 54, Q9
Primary hyperaldosteronism (PA), 34–36, 35t
Primary hyperparathyroidism, 62–64, 64t, Q2
    parathyroidectomy for, 63, Q17
    and vitamin D deficiency, Q46
Primary hypogonadism, 57
Primary hypothyroidism, and hyperprolactinemia, 26
Primary thyroid lymphoma, 52, Q45
Progesterone challenge test, 55
Prolactin, 19
Prolactinoma, 25
    in pregnancy, 26–27, Q3
    therapy for, 26
Propranolol, in thyrotoxicosis, 43
Propylthiouracil (PTU)
    for hyperthyroidism during pregnancy, Q1
    for thyrotoxicosis, 43
Pseudo-Cushing syndrome, 30
Pseudogynecomastia, 61
Pseudohypercalcemia, 61, Q31
Pseudohypocalcemia, 61

R
Radioactive iodine ablation
    for thyrotoxicosis, 43
    for toxic nodules, 44
Radioactive iodine uptake (RAIU), 42, Q18
Raloxifine, for osteoporosis, 69
Receptor activator of nuclear factor κB (RANK) ligand inhibitors, for
        osteoporosis, 69
Repaglinide, for diabetes mellitus, 10t
Resistant hypertension, Q71
Risedronate
    for osteoporosis, 69
    for Paget disease of bone, 71
Risperidone, and hyperprolactinemia, Q11
Rosiglitazone
    for diabetes mellitus, 10t
    for prevention/delay of type 2 diabetes, 5t

S
Sarcoidosis, hypercalcemia in, Q22
Saxagliptin, for diabetes mellitus, 10t
Secondary amenorrhea, 54–55
Secondary hypogonadism, 57
Secondary hypothyroidism, 23–24
Self-monitoring of blood glucose (SMBG), 7
Serum ferritin level and transferrin saturation, measurement of, Q30
Sheehan syndrome, hypopituitarism and, 22
Sitagliptin, for diabetes mellitus, 10t
Smoking cessation, for prevention/delay of type 2 diabetes, 5t
Sodium-glucose transporter-2 (SGLT2) inhibitors, for diabetes mellitus, 9, 10t
Somatostatin analogues, in acromegaly, 27
Spironolactone, in primary hyperaldosteronism, 35, Q79
Stereotactic radiosurgery, in acromegaly, 27
Subclinical hyperthyroidism, 45
Subclinical hypothyroidism, 46, Q16
Sulfonylureas
    for diabetes mellitus, 10t
    and hypoglycemia, Q20
Syndrome of inappropriate ADH secretion (SIADH), 28

T

Teriparatide, for osteoporosis, 69
Tertiary hyperparathyroidism, 64
Testicular failure. *See* Primary hypogonadism
Testosterone replacement therapy, 58–59, 60t
Thiazide diuretics, and hypercalcemia, 65
Thiazolidinediones
    for diabetes mellitus, 10t
    for prevention/delay of type 2 diabetes, 4, 5t
Thionamides
    in thyroid storm treatment, 49
    in thyrotoxicosis, 43
Thyroglobulin (TgAb), 42
Thyroid autoantibody measurement, 41
Thyroid cancer, 52–53
    and adjuvant radioactive iodine therapy, Q62
    incidence of, 52
    medullary, 53
    staging and prognosis of, 52
    treatment of, 52–53
    types of, frequency of, 52, 52t
Thyroidectomy, for substernal goiter, Q72
Thyroid emergencies, 48–49
Thyroid function, in pregnancy, 46–48, 48f
Thyroid function test, in elderly patient, Q59
Thyroid gland
    anatomy and physiology, 40–41
    disorders of
        euthyroid sick syndrome, 48
        functional, 42–46
        in pregnancy, 46–48, 48f
        structural, 50–52
        thyroid cancers, 52–53, 52f
        thyroid emergencies, 48–49
    function of, evaluation of, 41–42
    hormones of, 41
Thyroid hormone replacement therapy, 45
Thyroid hormone therapy, in myxedema coma, 49
Thyroiditis, 44
    autoimmune-mediated type 1 diabetes and, 3
    destructive, 44
    Hashimoto, 45
    painful, 44
    painless, 44
    postpartum, 44
    subacute, Q10
Thyroid nodules, 50–51
    evaluation of, 50–51, 50f, Q18
    fine-needle aspiration of, 51, 51t, Q8
    history and physical examination, 50
    incidentally discovered, 50
    types of, 50t
Thyroid peroxidase (TPO), 41
Thyroid-stimulating hormone (TSH), 19, 19t, 41
    deficiency of, 23–24
    in elderly patient, Q59
Thyroid-stimulating hormone–secreting tumors, 28
Thyroid-stimulating immunoglobulins (TSI) autoantibodies, 42
Thyroid storm, 48–49, Q33
    diagnosis of, 49
    treatment of, 49
Thyrotoxicosis, 42
    evaluation of, 42–43
    management of, 43
    symptoms of, 42–43
Thyrotropin receptor (TRAb), 41
Thyroxine (T$_4$), 41

Tissue transglutaminase antibody testing, Q15
Tolbutamide, for diabetes mellitus, 10t
Toxic adenoma, 44
Transsphenoidal pituitary decompression, Q7
Transsphenoidal tumor resection
    in acromegaly, 27
    in Cushing disease, 28
Transvaginal ultrasound, for Asherman syndrome, Q68
Triiodothyronine (T$_3$), 41, Q21
Troglitazone, for prevention/delay of type 2 diabetes, 5t
T-score, 67
Turner syndrome, 54
Type 1 diabetes, 1, 3t, Q14. *See also* Diabetes mellitus
    acquired, 3
    autoimmune-mediated, 1, 3
    idiopathic, 3
    insulin deficiency and, 1
    therapy for, 8–9, 8t, Q83
Type 2 diabetes mellitus, 4, Q29. *See also* Diabetes mellitus
    diagnosis of, Q57
    epidemiology of, 4
    etiology of, 4
    ketosis-prone patients with, 4, Q6
    metabolic syndrome and, 3
    obesity and, 4
    prevention/delay of, strategies for, 4, 5t
    therapy for, 9–11, 10t

U

Ulcers, foot, in diabetic patient, 18
Urine albumin excretion, elevated, 16t, 17
24-hour urine free cortisol (UFC), 30, 31
U.S. Preventive Services Task Force (USPSTF)
    BMD testing and vertebral imaging, recommendations for, 68t
    on screening for type 2 diabetes, 1, 2t

V

Valproate, in distal symmetric polyneuropathy, 18
Venlafaxine, in distal symmetric polyneuropathy, 18
Vertebral fractures, osteoporosis and, 67–69
Vildagliptin, for diabetes mellitus, 10t
Viral infections, and type 1 diabetes mellitus, 1
Visual field testing, 21
    during pregnancy, Q3
Vitamin D, 61–62
    hypercalcemia, 62–66
    hypocalcemia, 66
    production of, 62f
    sources of, 61t
Vitamin D$_2$ (ergocalciferol), 61
Vitamin D$_3$ (cholecalciferol), 61, Q46
Vitamin D deficiency, 69–70, Q15
Voglibose, for diabetes mellitus, 5t, 10t
Volume repletion, for hypercalcemia, 65

W

Weight loss, for prevention of type 2 diabetes, 4
Whipple triad, 13
Wolff-Chaikoff effect, 46

Z

Zoledronic acid
    for hypercalcemia, 65
    for osteoporosis, 69
    for Paget disease of bone, 71
Z-score, 67

A — NAME AND ADDRESS (Please complete.)

Last Name _____ First Name _____ Middle Initial _____

Address _____

Address cont. _____

City _____ State _____ ZIP Code _____

Country _____

Email address _____

ACP®
American College of Physicians
Leading Internal Medicine, Improving Lives

Medical Knowledge Self-Assessment Program® 17

TO EARN *AMA PRA CATEGORY 1 CREDITS™* YOU MUST:

1. Answer all questions.
2. Score a minimum of 50% correct.

===

TO EARN *FREE* INSTANTANEOUS *AMA PRA CATEGORY 1 CREDITS™* ONLINE:

1. Answer all of your questions.
2. Go to **mksap.acponline.org** and enter your ACP Online username and password to access an online answer sheet.
3. Enter your answers.
4. You can also enter your answers directly at **mksap.acponline.org** without first using this answer sheet.

To Submit Your Answer Sheet by Mail or FAX for a $15 Administrative Fee per Answer Sheet:

1. Answer all of your questions and calculate your score.
2. Complete boxes A–F.
3. Complete payment information.
4. Send the answer sheet and payment information to ACP, using the FAX number/address listed below.

B — Order Number

(Use the Order Number on your MKSAP materials packing slip.)

C — ACP ID Number

(Refer to packing slip in your MKSAP materials for your ACP ID Number.)

COMPLETE FORM BELOW ONLY IF YOU SUBMIT BY MAIL OR FAX

Last Name _____ First Name _____ MI

Payment Information. Must remit in US funds, drawn on a US bank.

The processing fee for each paper answer sheet is $15.

☐ Check, made payable to ACP, enclosed

Charge to ☐ **VISA** ☐ MasterCard ☐ AMERICAN EXPRESS ☐ **DISCOVER**

Card Number _____

Expiration Date _____ / _____   Security code (3 or 4 digit #s) _____
　　　　　　　　　MM　　　　YY

Signature _____

Fax to: 215-351-2799

Mail to:
Member and Customer Service
American College of Physicians
190 N. Independence Mall West
Philadelphia, PA 19106–1572

D

TEST TYPE	Maximum Number of CME Credits
○ Cardiovascular Medicine	21
○ Dermatology	12
○ Gastroenterology and Hepatology	16
○ Hematology and Oncology	22
○ Neurology	16
○ Rheumatology	16
○ Endocrinology and Metabolism	14
○ General Internal Medicine	26
○ Infectious Disease	19
○ Nephrology	19
○ Pulmonary and Critical Care Medicine	19

E

CREDITS CLAIMED ON SECTION
(1 hour = 1 credit)

Enter the number of credits earned on the test to the nearest quarter hour. Physicians should claim only the credit commensurate with the extent of their participation in the activity.

F

Enter your score here.

Instructions for calculating your own score are found in front of the self-assessment test in each book.

You must receive a minimum score of 50% correct.

_____ %

Credit Submission Date: _____

1 Ⓐ Ⓑ Ⓒ Ⓓ Ⓔ   46 Ⓐ Ⓑ Ⓒ Ⓓ Ⓔ   91 Ⓐ Ⓑ Ⓒ Ⓓ Ⓔ   136 Ⓐ Ⓑ Ⓒ Ⓓ Ⓔ
2 Ⓐ Ⓑ Ⓒ Ⓓ Ⓔ   47 Ⓐ Ⓑ Ⓒ Ⓓ Ⓔ   92 Ⓐ Ⓑ Ⓒ Ⓓ Ⓔ   137 Ⓐ Ⓑ Ⓒ Ⓓ Ⓔ
3 Ⓐ Ⓑ Ⓒ Ⓓ Ⓔ   48 Ⓐ Ⓑ Ⓒ Ⓓ Ⓔ   93 Ⓐ Ⓑ Ⓒ Ⓓ Ⓔ   138 Ⓐ Ⓑ Ⓒ Ⓓ Ⓔ
4 Ⓐ Ⓑ Ⓒ Ⓓ Ⓔ   49 Ⓐ Ⓑ Ⓒ Ⓓ Ⓔ   94 Ⓐ Ⓑ Ⓒ Ⓓ Ⓔ   139 Ⓐ Ⓑ Ⓒ Ⓓ Ⓔ
5 Ⓐ Ⓑ Ⓒ Ⓓ Ⓔ   50 Ⓐ Ⓑ Ⓒ Ⓓ Ⓔ   95 Ⓐ Ⓑ Ⓒ Ⓓ Ⓔ   140 Ⓐ Ⓑ Ⓒ Ⓓ Ⓔ

6 Ⓐ Ⓑ Ⓒ Ⓓ Ⓔ   51 Ⓐ Ⓑ Ⓒ Ⓓ Ⓔ   96 Ⓐ Ⓑ Ⓒ Ⓓ Ⓔ   141 Ⓐ Ⓑ Ⓒ Ⓓ Ⓔ
7 Ⓐ Ⓑ Ⓒ Ⓓ Ⓔ   52 Ⓐ Ⓑ Ⓒ Ⓓ Ⓔ   97 Ⓐ Ⓑ Ⓒ Ⓓ Ⓔ   142 Ⓐ Ⓑ Ⓒ Ⓓ Ⓔ
8 Ⓐ Ⓑ Ⓒ Ⓓ Ⓔ   53 Ⓐ Ⓑ Ⓒ Ⓓ Ⓔ   98 Ⓐ Ⓑ Ⓒ Ⓓ Ⓔ   143 Ⓐ Ⓑ Ⓒ Ⓓ Ⓔ
9 Ⓐ Ⓑ Ⓒ Ⓓ Ⓔ   54 Ⓐ Ⓑ Ⓒ Ⓓ Ⓔ   99 Ⓐ Ⓑ Ⓒ Ⓓ Ⓔ   144 Ⓐ Ⓑ Ⓒ Ⓓ Ⓔ
10 Ⓐ Ⓑ Ⓒ Ⓓ Ⓔ   55 Ⓐ Ⓑ Ⓒ Ⓓ Ⓔ   100 Ⓐ Ⓑ Ⓒ Ⓓ Ⓔ   145 Ⓐ Ⓑ Ⓒ Ⓓ Ⓔ

11 Ⓐ Ⓑ Ⓒ Ⓓ Ⓔ   56 Ⓐ Ⓑ Ⓒ Ⓓ Ⓔ   101 Ⓐ Ⓑ Ⓒ Ⓓ Ⓔ   146 Ⓐ Ⓑ Ⓒ Ⓓ Ⓔ
12 Ⓐ Ⓑ Ⓒ Ⓓ Ⓔ   57 Ⓐ Ⓑ Ⓒ Ⓓ Ⓔ   102 Ⓐ Ⓑ Ⓒ Ⓓ Ⓔ   147 Ⓐ Ⓑ Ⓒ Ⓓ Ⓔ
13 Ⓐ Ⓑ Ⓒ Ⓓ Ⓔ   58 Ⓐ Ⓑ Ⓒ Ⓓ Ⓔ   103 Ⓐ Ⓑ Ⓒ Ⓓ Ⓔ   148 Ⓐ Ⓑ Ⓒ Ⓓ Ⓔ
14 Ⓐ Ⓑ Ⓒ Ⓓ Ⓔ   59 Ⓐ Ⓑ Ⓒ Ⓓ Ⓔ   104 Ⓐ Ⓑ Ⓒ Ⓓ Ⓔ   149 Ⓐ Ⓑ Ⓒ Ⓓ Ⓔ
15 Ⓐ Ⓑ Ⓒ Ⓓ Ⓔ   60 Ⓐ Ⓑ Ⓒ Ⓓ Ⓔ   105 Ⓐ Ⓑ Ⓒ Ⓓ Ⓔ   150 Ⓐ Ⓑ Ⓒ Ⓓ Ⓔ

16 Ⓐ Ⓑ Ⓒ Ⓓ Ⓔ   61 Ⓐ Ⓑ Ⓒ Ⓓ Ⓔ   106 Ⓐ Ⓑ Ⓒ Ⓓ Ⓔ   151 Ⓐ Ⓑ Ⓒ Ⓓ Ⓔ
17 Ⓐ Ⓑ Ⓒ Ⓓ Ⓔ   62 Ⓐ Ⓑ Ⓒ Ⓓ Ⓔ   107 Ⓐ Ⓑ Ⓒ Ⓓ Ⓔ   152 Ⓐ Ⓑ Ⓒ Ⓓ Ⓔ
18 Ⓐ Ⓑ Ⓒ Ⓓ Ⓔ   63 Ⓐ Ⓑ Ⓒ Ⓓ Ⓔ   108 Ⓐ Ⓑ Ⓒ Ⓓ Ⓔ   153 Ⓐ Ⓑ Ⓒ Ⓓ Ⓔ
19 Ⓐ Ⓑ Ⓒ Ⓓ Ⓔ   64 Ⓐ Ⓑ Ⓒ Ⓓ Ⓔ   109 Ⓐ Ⓑ Ⓒ Ⓓ Ⓔ   154 Ⓐ Ⓑ Ⓒ Ⓓ Ⓔ
20 Ⓐ Ⓑ Ⓒ Ⓓ Ⓔ   65 Ⓐ Ⓑ Ⓒ Ⓓ Ⓔ   110 Ⓐ Ⓑ Ⓒ Ⓓ Ⓔ   155 Ⓐ Ⓑ Ⓒ Ⓓ Ⓔ

21 Ⓐ Ⓑ Ⓒ Ⓓ Ⓔ   66 Ⓐ Ⓑ Ⓒ Ⓓ Ⓔ   111 Ⓐ Ⓑ Ⓒ Ⓓ Ⓔ   156 Ⓐ Ⓑ Ⓒ Ⓓ Ⓔ
22 Ⓐ Ⓑ Ⓒ Ⓓ Ⓔ   67 Ⓐ Ⓑ Ⓒ Ⓓ Ⓔ   112 Ⓐ Ⓑ Ⓒ Ⓓ Ⓔ   157 Ⓐ Ⓑ Ⓒ Ⓓ Ⓔ
23 Ⓐ Ⓑ Ⓒ Ⓓ Ⓔ   68 Ⓐ Ⓑ Ⓒ Ⓓ Ⓔ   113 Ⓐ Ⓑ Ⓒ Ⓓ Ⓔ   158 Ⓐ Ⓑ Ⓒ Ⓓ Ⓔ
24 Ⓐ Ⓑ Ⓒ Ⓓ Ⓔ   69 Ⓐ Ⓑ Ⓒ Ⓓ Ⓔ   114 Ⓐ Ⓑ Ⓒ Ⓓ Ⓔ   159 Ⓐ Ⓑ Ⓒ Ⓓ Ⓔ
25 Ⓐ Ⓑ Ⓒ Ⓓ Ⓔ   70 Ⓐ Ⓑ Ⓒ Ⓓ Ⓔ   115 Ⓐ Ⓑ Ⓒ Ⓓ Ⓔ   160 Ⓐ Ⓑ Ⓒ Ⓓ Ⓔ

26 Ⓐ Ⓑ Ⓒ Ⓓ Ⓔ   71 Ⓐ Ⓑ Ⓒ Ⓓ Ⓔ   116 Ⓐ Ⓑ Ⓒ Ⓓ Ⓔ   161 Ⓐ Ⓑ Ⓒ Ⓓ Ⓔ
27 Ⓐ Ⓑ Ⓒ Ⓓ Ⓔ   72 Ⓐ Ⓑ Ⓒ Ⓓ Ⓔ   117 Ⓐ Ⓑ Ⓒ Ⓓ Ⓔ   162 Ⓐ Ⓑ Ⓒ Ⓓ Ⓔ
28 Ⓐ Ⓑ Ⓒ Ⓓ Ⓔ   73 Ⓐ Ⓑ Ⓒ Ⓓ Ⓔ   118 Ⓐ Ⓑ Ⓒ Ⓓ Ⓔ   163 Ⓐ Ⓑ Ⓒ Ⓓ Ⓔ
29 Ⓐ Ⓑ Ⓒ Ⓓ Ⓔ   74 Ⓐ Ⓑ Ⓒ Ⓓ Ⓔ   119 Ⓐ Ⓑ Ⓒ Ⓓ Ⓔ   164 Ⓐ Ⓑ Ⓒ Ⓓ Ⓔ
30 Ⓐ Ⓑ Ⓒ Ⓓ Ⓔ   75 Ⓐ Ⓑ Ⓒ Ⓓ Ⓔ   120 Ⓐ Ⓑ Ⓒ Ⓓ Ⓔ   165 Ⓐ Ⓑ Ⓒ Ⓓ Ⓔ

31 Ⓐ Ⓑ Ⓒ Ⓓ Ⓔ   76 Ⓐ Ⓑ Ⓒ Ⓓ Ⓔ   121 Ⓐ Ⓑ Ⓒ Ⓓ Ⓔ   166 Ⓐ Ⓑ Ⓒ Ⓓ Ⓔ
32 Ⓐ Ⓑ Ⓒ Ⓓ Ⓔ   77 Ⓐ Ⓑ Ⓒ Ⓓ Ⓔ   122 Ⓐ Ⓑ Ⓒ Ⓓ Ⓔ   167 Ⓐ Ⓑ Ⓒ Ⓓ Ⓔ
33 Ⓐ Ⓑ Ⓒ Ⓓ Ⓔ   78 Ⓐ Ⓑ Ⓒ Ⓓ Ⓔ   123 Ⓐ Ⓑ Ⓒ Ⓓ Ⓔ   168 Ⓐ Ⓑ Ⓒ Ⓓ Ⓔ
34 Ⓐ Ⓑ Ⓒ Ⓓ Ⓔ   79 Ⓐ Ⓑ Ⓒ Ⓓ Ⓔ   124 Ⓐ Ⓑ Ⓒ Ⓓ Ⓔ   169 Ⓐ Ⓑ Ⓒ Ⓓ Ⓔ
35 Ⓐ Ⓑ Ⓒ Ⓓ Ⓔ   80 Ⓐ Ⓑ Ⓒ Ⓓ Ⓔ   125 Ⓐ Ⓑ Ⓒ Ⓓ Ⓔ   170 Ⓐ Ⓑ Ⓒ Ⓓ Ⓔ

36 Ⓐ Ⓑ Ⓒ Ⓓ Ⓔ   81 Ⓐ Ⓑ Ⓒ Ⓓ Ⓔ   126 Ⓐ Ⓑ Ⓒ Ⓓ Ⓔ   171 Ⓐ Ⓑ Ⓒ Ⓓ Ⓔ
37 Ⓐ Ⓑ Ⓒ Ⓓ Ⓔ   82 Ⓐ Ⓑ Ⓒ Ⓓ Ⓔ   127 Ⓐ Ⓑ Ⓒ Ⓓ Ⓔ   172 Ⓐ Ⓑ Ⓒ Ⓓ Ⓔ
38 Ⓐ Ⓑ Ⓒ Ⓓ Ⓔ   83 Ⓐ Ⓑ Ⓒ Ⓓ Ⓔ   128 Ⓐ Ⓑ Ⓒ Ⓓ Ⓔ   173 Ⓐ Ⓑ Ⓒ Ⓓ Ⓔ
39 Ⓐ Ⓑ Ⓒ Ⓓ Ⓔ   84 Ⓐ Ⓑ Ⓒ Ⓓ Ⓔ   129 Ⓐ Ⓑ Ⓒ Ⓓ Ⓔ   174 Ⓐ Ⓑ Ⓒ Ⓓ Ⓔ
40 Ⓐ Ⓑ Ⓒ Ⓓ Ⓔ   85 Ⓐ Ⓑ Ⓒ Ⓓ Ⓔ   130 Ⓐ Ⓑ Ⓒ Ⓓ Ⓔ   175 Ⓐ Ⓑ Ⓒ Ⓓ Ⓔ

41 Ⓐ Ⓑ Ⓒ Ⓓ Ⓔ   86 Ⓐ Ⓑ Ⓒ Ⓓ Ⓔ   131 Ⓐ Ⓑ Ⓒ Ⓓ Ⓔ   176 Ⓐ Ⓑ Ⓒ Ⓓ Ⓔ
42 Ⓐ Ⓑ Ⓒ Ⓓ Ⓔ   87 Ⓐ Ⓑ Ⓒ Ⓓ Ⓔ   132 Ⓐ Ⓑ Ⓒ Ⓓ Ⓔ   177 Ⓐ Ⓑ Ⓒ Ⓓ Ⓔ
43 Ⓐ Ⓑ Ⓒ Ⓓ Ⓔ   88 Ⓐ Ⓑ Ⓒ Ⓓ Ⓔ   133 Ⓐ Ⓑ Ⓒ Ⓓ Ⓔ   178 Ⓐ Ⓑ Ⓒ Ⓓ Ⓔ
44 Ⓐ Ⓑ Ⓒ Ⓓ Ⓔ   89 Ⓐ Ⓑ Ⓒ Ⓓ Ⓔ   134 Ⓐ Ⓑ Ⓒ Ⓓ Ⓔ   179 Ⓐ Ⓑ Ⓒ Ⓓ Ⓔ
45 Ⓐ Ⓑ Ⓒ Ⓓ Ⓔ   90 Ⓐ Ⓑ Ⓒ Ⓓ Ⓔ   135 Ⓐ Ⓑ Ⓒ Ⓓ Ⓔ   180 Ⓐ Ⓑ Ⓒ Ⓓ Ⓔ